GET READY WITH MEREDITH

First published in the United States of America in 2026 by
Rizzoli International Publications, Inc.
49 West 27th Street
New York, NY 10001
www.rizzoliusa.com

Publisher: Charles Miers
Associate Publisher: Anthony Petrillose
Editors: Gisela Aguilar and Julie Schumacher
Design and Art Direction: Graphic Services
Production Manager: Colin Hough Trapp
Editorial Coordination: Hannah Satzke
Managing Editor: Lynn Scrabis
Design Coordinator: Tim Biddick
Agent: Sydney Shiffman, CAA

ISBN: 978-0-8478-7687-7
Library of Congress Control Number: 2026937156

Printed in China
2026 2027 2028 2029 / 10 9 8 7 6 5 4 3 2 1

The authorized representative in the EU for product safety and compliance is Mondadori Libri S.p.A., via Gian Battista Vico 42, Milan, Italy, 20123, www.mondadori.it

Visit us online:
Instagram: @RizzoliBooks
Facebook.com/RizzoliNewYork
Youtube.com/user/RizzoliNY

MIX
Paper | Supporting responsible forestry
FSC™ C005748
FSC www.fsc.org

GET READY WITH MEREDITH

SKIN, GLAM, FASHION, GET UNREADY WITH ME

MEREDITH DUXBURY

RIZZOLI
NEW YORK

New York Paris London Milan

FOREWORD
by Charlotte Tilbury

In the world of beauty, trends move fast—techniques evolve, and the definition of creativity is constantly being rewritten by new voices and fresh perspectives. Every so often, though, someone emerges who does more than just follow the moment—they shape it. That is exactly what Meredith has achieved.

She has become the face of the digital era of beauty; she celebrates experimentation and unapologetic self-expression. Meredith's work exists at the intersection of artistry, confidence, and the internet's extraordinary ability to amplify creativity. Her self-expression through beauty inspires millions—there is such an unmistakable sense of fun in her approach—a willingness to play with products, experiment, and break conventions in a way that reminds us why so many people fall in love with makeup in the first place.

For millions of people scrolling through their phones late at night or between moments in their day, Meredith's videos offered something magnetic. Perhaps it was the audacity of her technique—foundation applied boldly and excessively. Perhaps it was the fluid transformation from bare skin to luminous glamour. Or perhaps it was simply the sense that beauty could be playful again.

In an industry built on rules, Meredith, like me, dared to question them. Traditional makeup artistry often teaches precision above all else: the right brush, the right amount of product, the right sequence of steps. Meredith arrived on the scene with a different message. She reminded people that makeup is not prescriptive—it is tactile, it is emotional, it is personal.

Her approach sparked conversation across the beauty community, and that conversation became part of the magic. Beauty has always thrived on dialogue: between artists and audiences, between tradition and innovation. Meredith's voice added a new chapter to that dialogue—one defined by boldness and experimentation.

But beyond the viral moments and headline-grabbing techniques, what truly defines Meredith's work is her instinct for transformation and artistry.

Makeup, at its best, is storytelling. A smoky eye can evoke drama. A bold lip can capture confidence. Skin illuminated with layers of foundation and highlighter can become a statement of presence. Meredith understands this instinctively. Each look she creates is not merely a tutorial—it is a performance of color, texture, and light.

The pages ahead punctuate her journey in experimentation and artistry as she continues to evolve through the worlds of beauty, fashion, culture, and beyond.

The digital age has transformed how beauty is shared. Meredith was part of the first generation of creators to occupy this new landscape. As you move through these pages, you will see echoes of the long history of beauty that came before: the luminous skin of Hollywood glamour, the fearless color of editorial fashion, the sculptural precision of classic makeup artistry. Meredith's work sits within that lineage even as it pushes at its boundaries.

Her style is bold, yes—but it is also joyful. This book captures that energy, celebrating the joy of transformation. Because at the heart of Meredith Duxbury's work lies a simple truth: Beauty is not about perfection. It is about possibility.

CHARLOTTE TILBURY
MBE - President, Chairman, Chief Creative Officer, and Founder of Charlotte Tilbury Beauty

AN INTRODUCTION
by Meredith Duxbury

This book offers a glimpse into my personal life, the ways the beauty, fashion, and modeling industries have shaped me, and the different roles they have played in my journey to get to where I am today. It's a reflection of everything I've lived and learned and a guide to my favorite beauty tips, rituals, and creative practices that I genuinely love and return to again and again.

I was never a conventional learner. I've always learned best through experience by being hands-on, curious, and willing to explore things for myself. Creating this book has taught me so much about who I am and who I'm becoming. It reminded me that it's okay not to live life by a playbook—that it's okay to rewrite the rules, to take detours, and to trust your own instincts.

Life can feel like a roller coaster at times. There were moments when I found myself wondering, *How did I get here?* And every time, the answer was the same: I followed my passion. I followed my love for art, beauty, and creation. I let the world around me inspire my work, and then I use that work to inspire new versions of myself. Along the way, I learned how easy it is to look outward for validation and reassurance, but also how powerful it is to realize that everything you need is already within you. Sometimes, you just have to slow down, dig a little deeper, and truly get to know yourself.

This book is for those who love to color outside the lines. For the ones who challenge expectations, push boundaries, and refuse to give up on their vision. It's for the creatives who explore new forms of expression, even when it means standing apart from the norm. It's for anyone searching for a safe space to feel seen, understood, and inspired.

My hope is that as you move through each chapter, you'll learn to love yourself a little more. That you'll give yourself permission to grow, to evolve, and to show yourself grace. And that you'll walk away feeling empowered to create a life that feels true to you.

I want to thank my supporters for being on this journey with me and for being there through each and every era. I am inspired by you all and love this community we have created together.

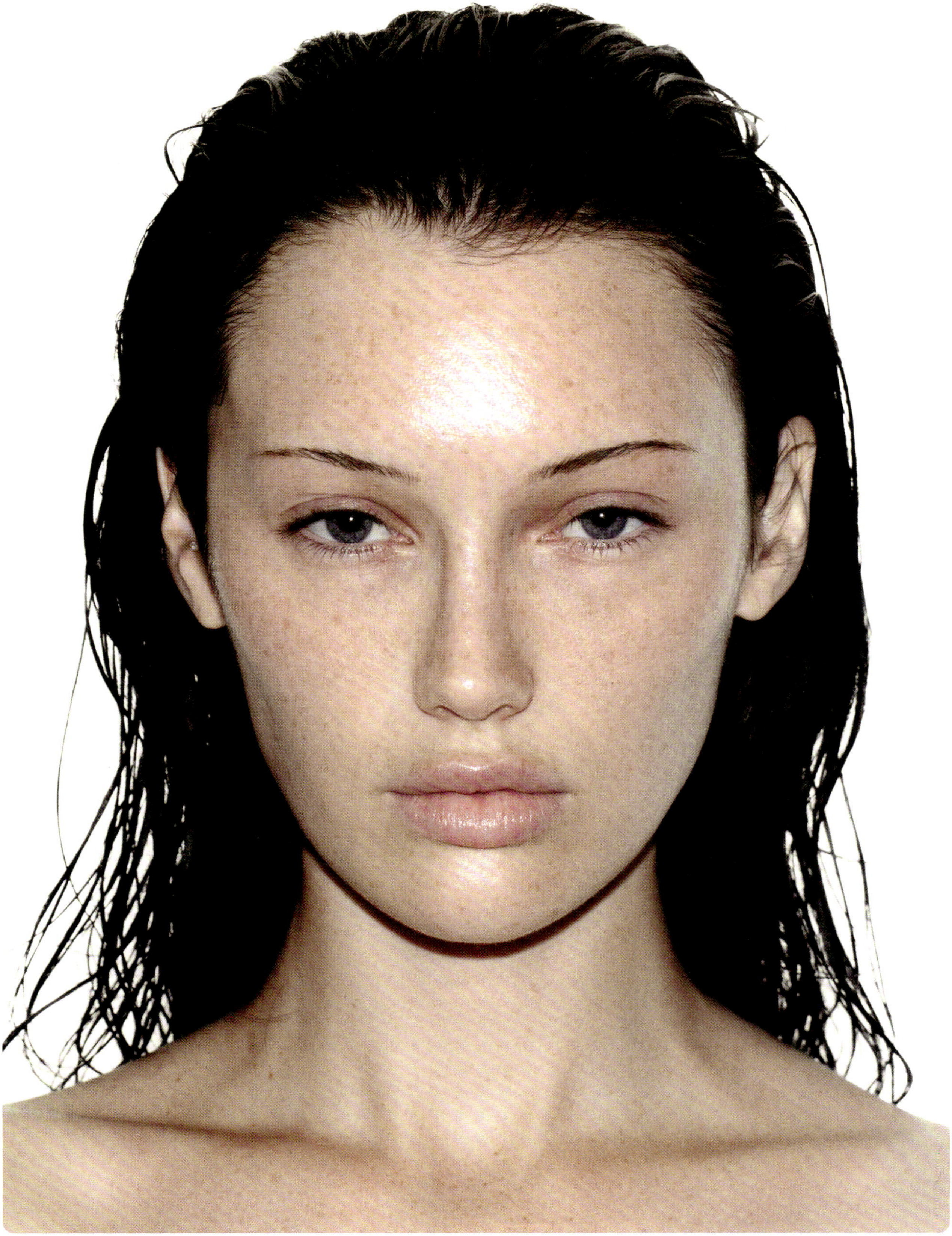

SKIN

GLAM

FASHION

SKIN

1

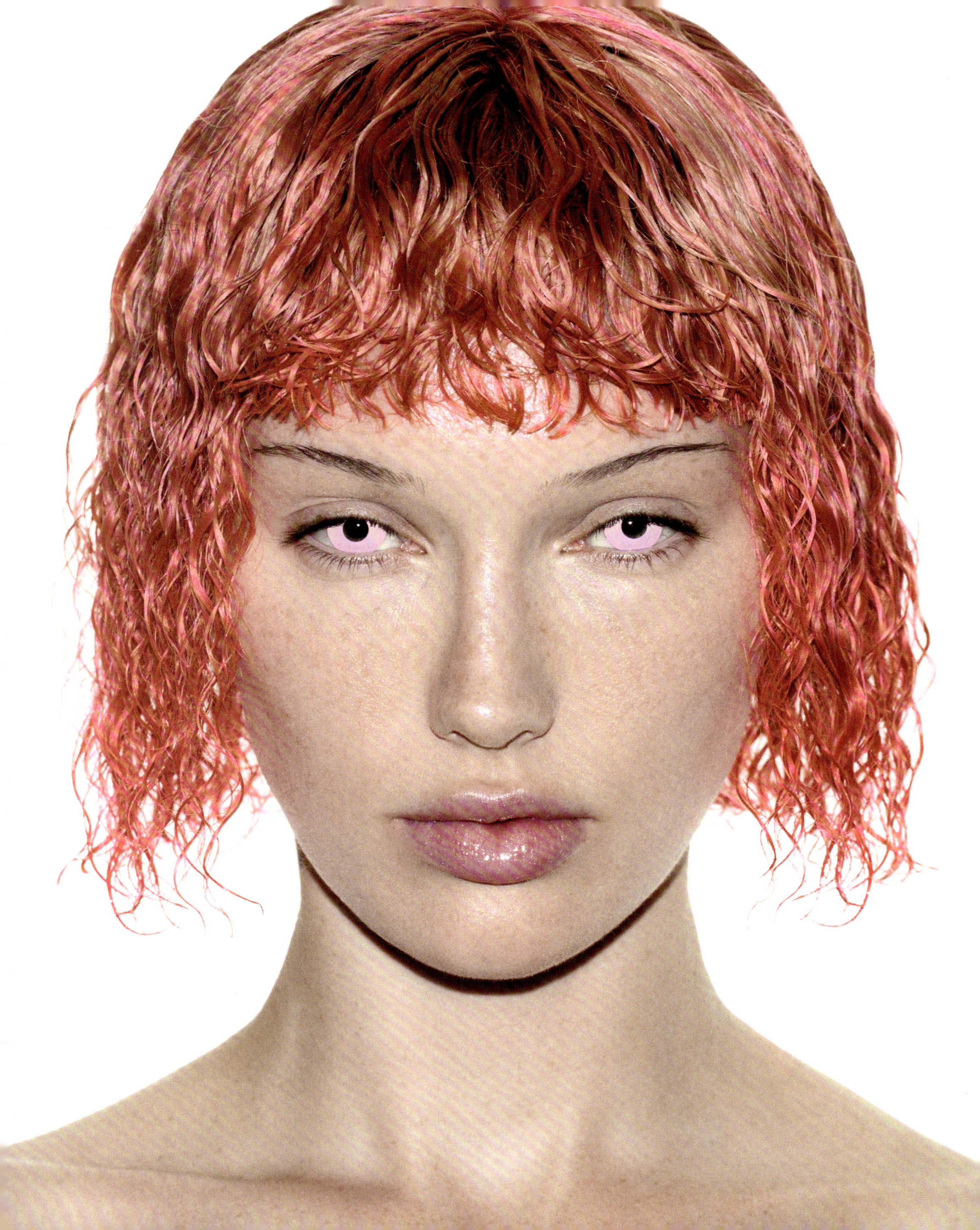

Skin has been, and will always be, my first canvas. Skin is where it all begins, and here is where I'll tell you about how I got to where I am today. I get inspired looking at my bare face in the mirror, envisioning all the different ways I can transform myself into another character for the day through glam. For me, skin holds emotions, memories, and some of the most intimate moments we share with ourselves. Sometimes we tend to treat our skin like a report card…like it's proof of how good we are at taking care of ourselves. We use it to judge ourselves in the worst ways without even realizing it, when in reality, our skin is our biggest ally. It's never going to be perfect, at times it will be messy, complicated, and confusing; but that is life…

I've had days where I loved my freckles like they were little sun-kisses, and days where I wanted to cover every single one of them up. Learning to love your differences and things that make you unique will make you feel so much more freedom in loving yourself. Reality is, we've taught ourselves that confidence and skin are tied together in ways I wish they weren't. Reframe your thinking. Learning to treat my skin like a friend instead of an enemy has helped me accept the reality of it all, that if you don't work through it rather than against it, you're going to feel so defeated time and time again. Workshop, listen, and nurture. Come back to the basics.

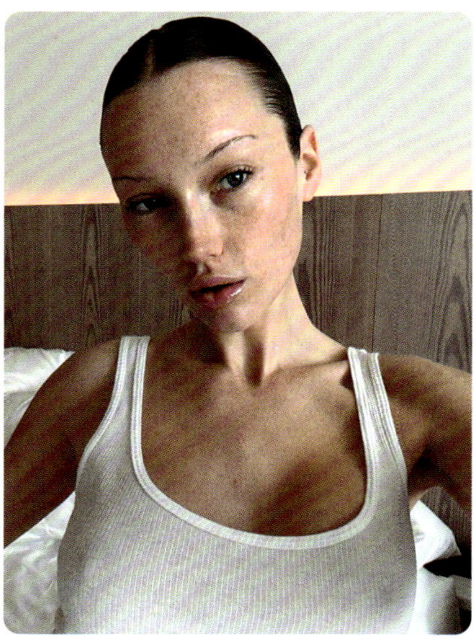

Skincare is such an important part of my morning and nighttime routine. Taking time to nurture my skin helps me feel better overall and gives me a moment to care for myself.

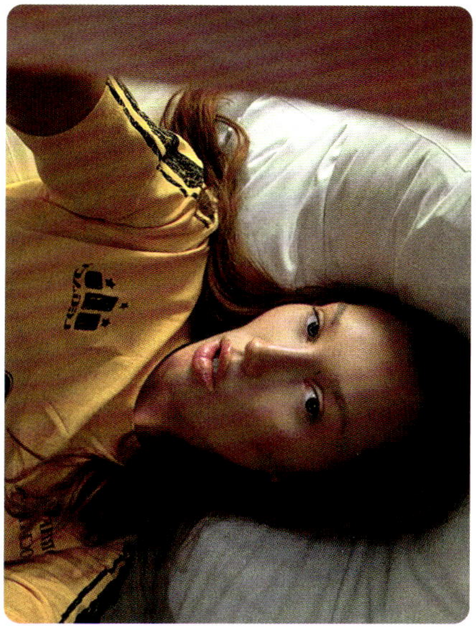

I love taking time when I'm feeling my best to lean into that moment, whether it's snapping a quick selfie or just allowing myself to soak in that confidence, whatever it is!

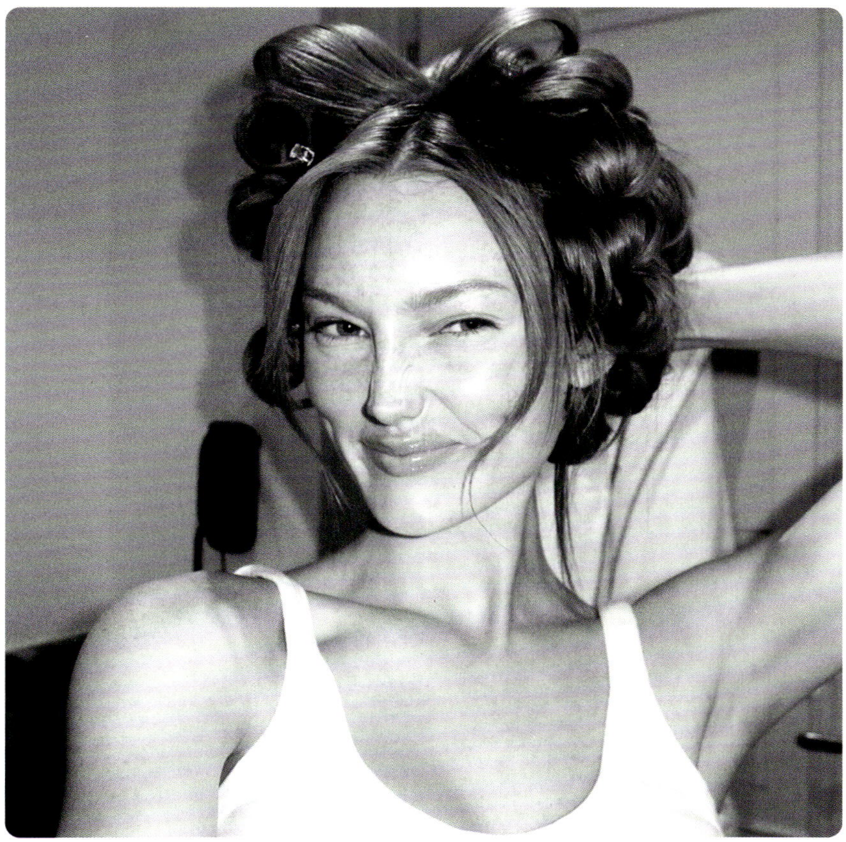

I think we can all agree that getting ready and putting on a good playlist is one of the best parts of the night! I never skip my skincare before getting into glam because it's a part of my process that I really enjoy and makes me feel like I'm treating myself.

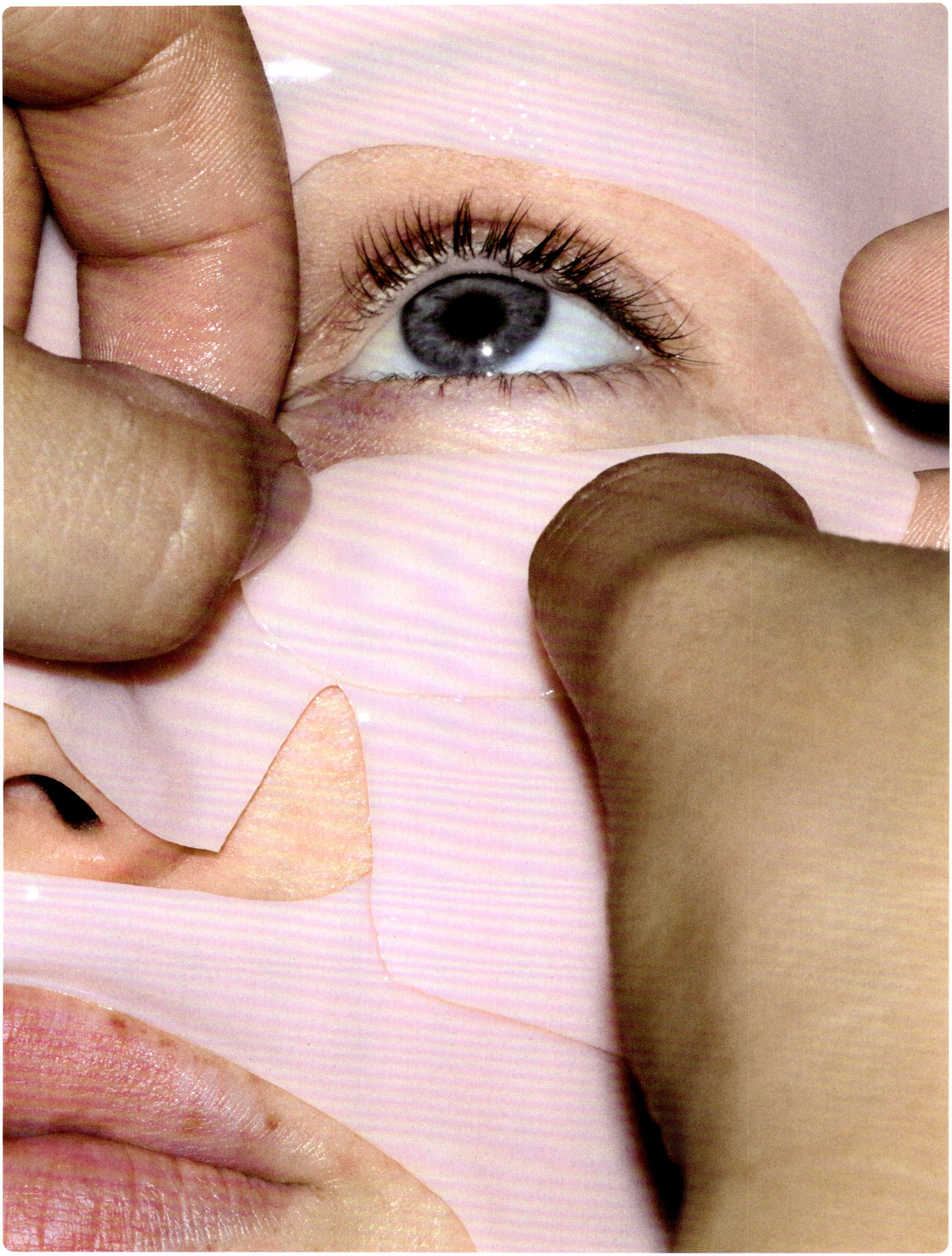

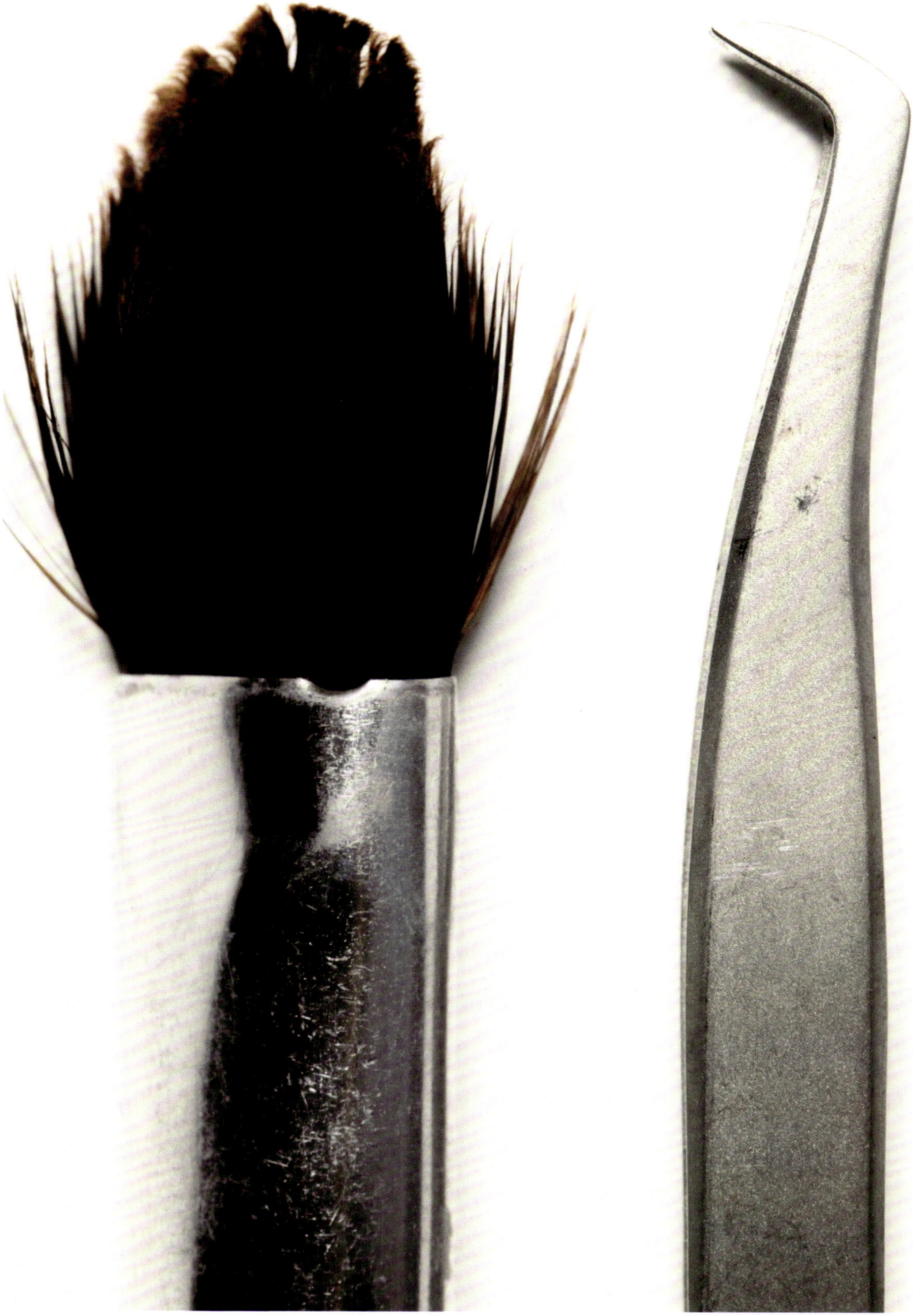

Q Has being an online person changed your relationship with beauty?*

*DAISE BEDOLLA is a creative producer, social media strategist, and writer
She is a Beauty Editor and Producer at Glossier.

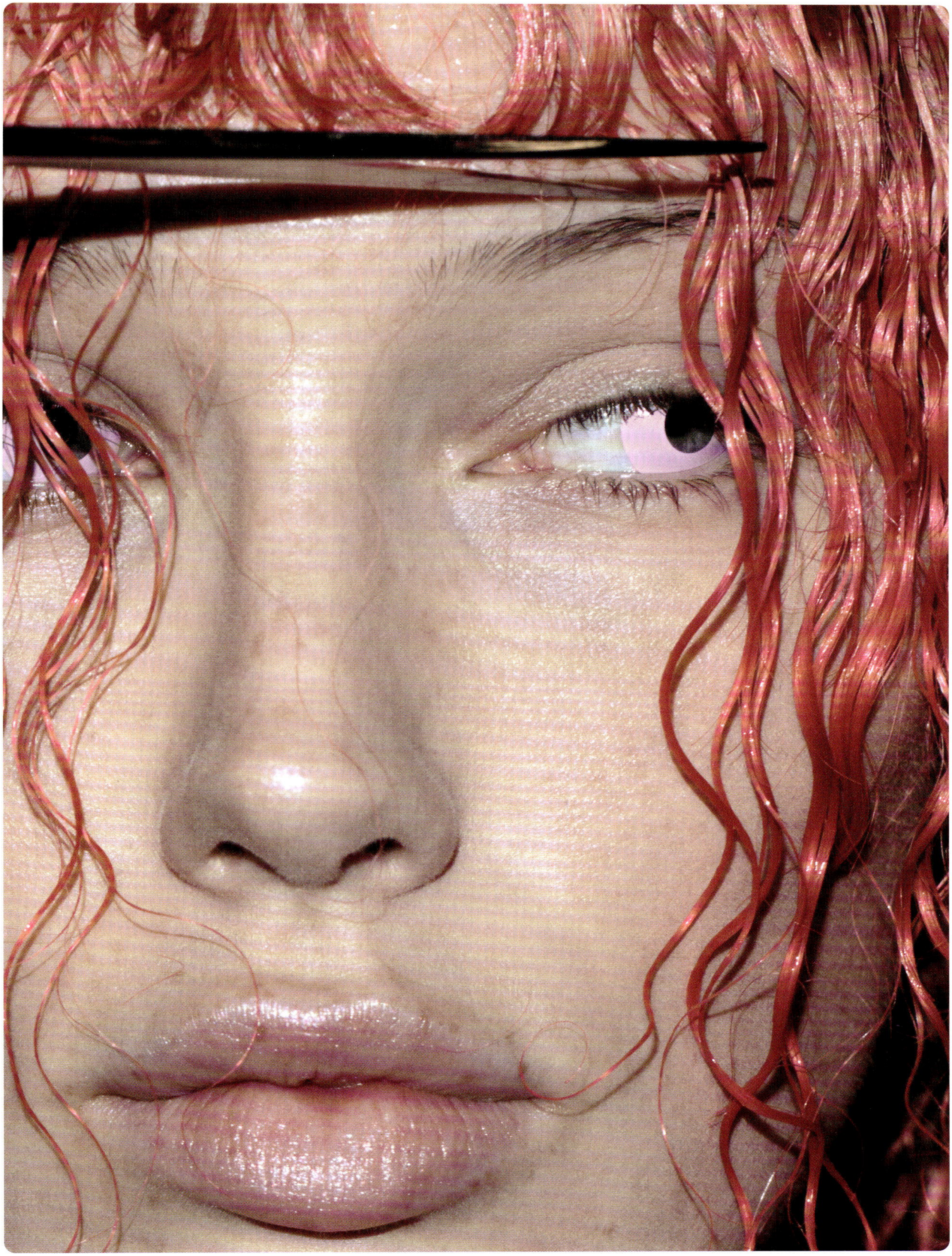

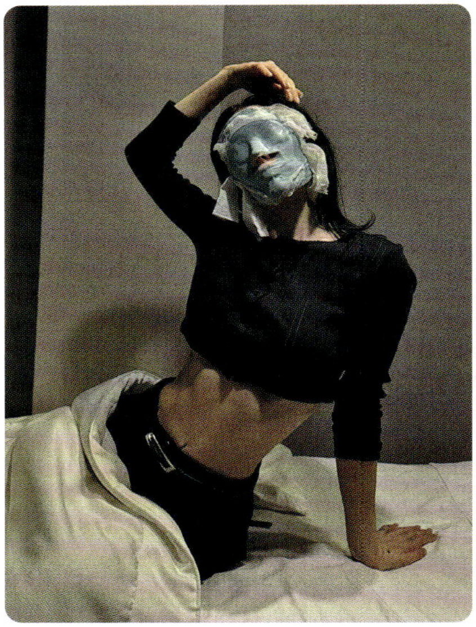

Facial I got at the BLS Clinic in Seoul, Korea. They do the best facials and are experts in everything skincare. This was specifically a hydro facial, which helped to exfoliate, extract, and hydrate my skin all in one treatment.

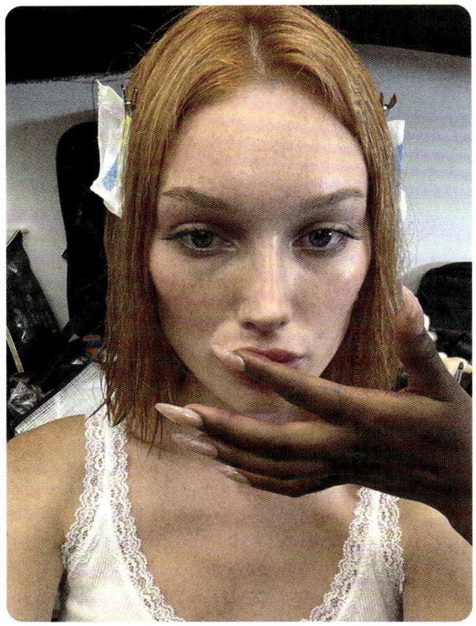

Me backstage in hair and makeup at GCDS, my first runway show ever!!! I loved this look. It was so angelic, the fluttery corner lashes and pink lip. I remember, Giuliano Calza, the creative director, told me he just wanted me to feel my best and most comfortable, which was so sweet to hear coming into an industry that was very intimidating to me.

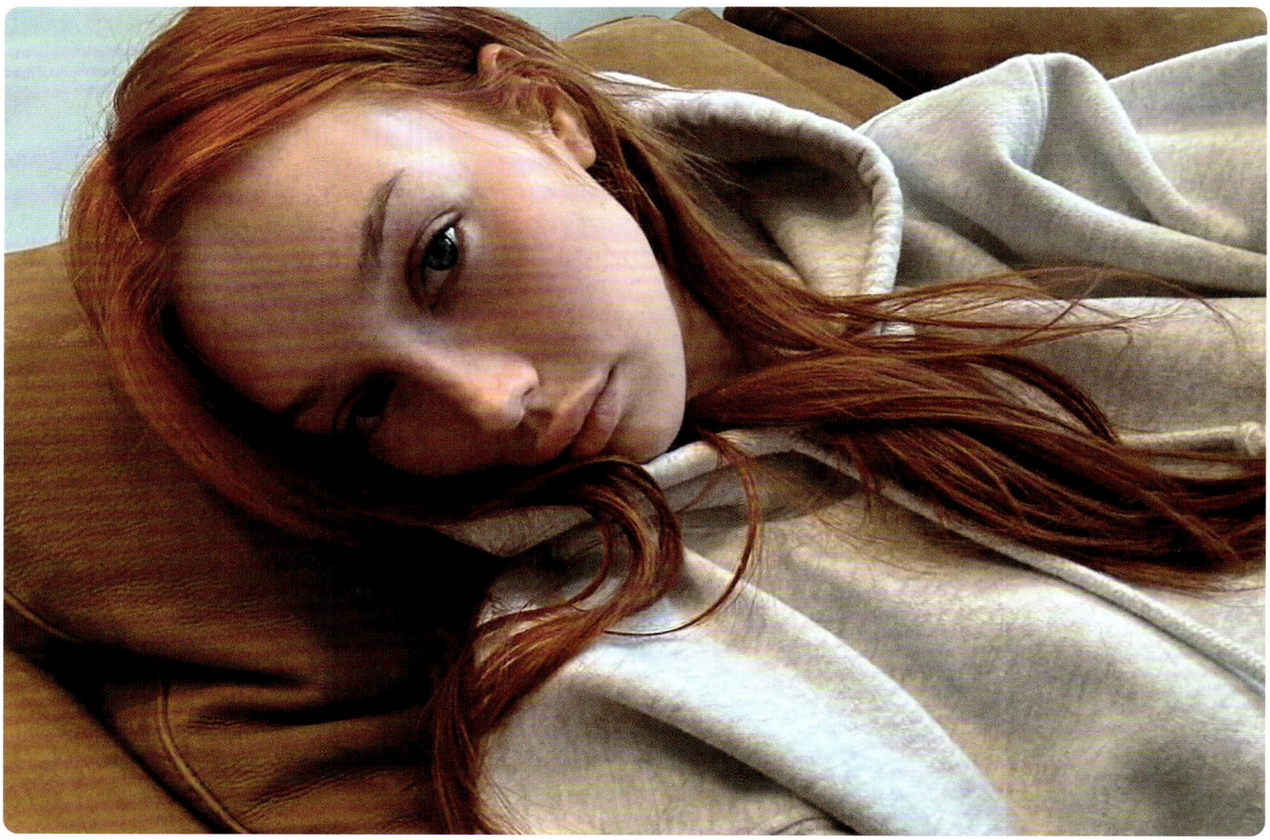

My red hair era!!! I love how different hair colors can bring out different tones in my skin. This definitely brought out more of my pink undertones and complemented my freckles nicely.

A People praised me when I showed my freckles and my skin. They asked me to show the "natural look" more. They tried to turn my love for makeup into a negative thing. They didn't understand that I was using makeup because I like being creative and making art on my face, so creating a natural look just didn't scratch that itch for me. I got online to show fun looks and have fun with makeup.

I know that a lot of people really enjoy seeing the different looks. So as much as I have come to love showing my freckles, it was hard to hear people say I should stop covering them up, because for me, makeup isn't covering up—it's creating.

Q Tell us. How did we get here? Where does this story *really* begin…?

A Since day one, I have always felt some sort of creative spark inside me. I was rebellious, I pushed limits, and I didn't like to follow the rules. I felt a lot of my creativeness was misunderstood. I always wanted to do things differently and make my own rules, outside of the ones that society accepted. Passion is the leading drive of my story. I wouldn't be where I am today without my love for art, creativity, and expression. I thrived off of coloring outside the lines—it was a thrill I got from trying something that hadn't been explored yet. This is where my foundation technique came into play.

Q What sparked your need to share?

A I liked the idea of having a community of people who all enjoy the same things and share the same passions. I didn't feel like I got that through my community at school, so I wanted to look outward to see if I could build it myself. Social media was a way for me to express my creativity in my own way and not have anyone controlling it. My videos were truly up to me to make. I could post when I wanted. There was no one telling me how, what, or when to post. It was a fully free outlet for me.

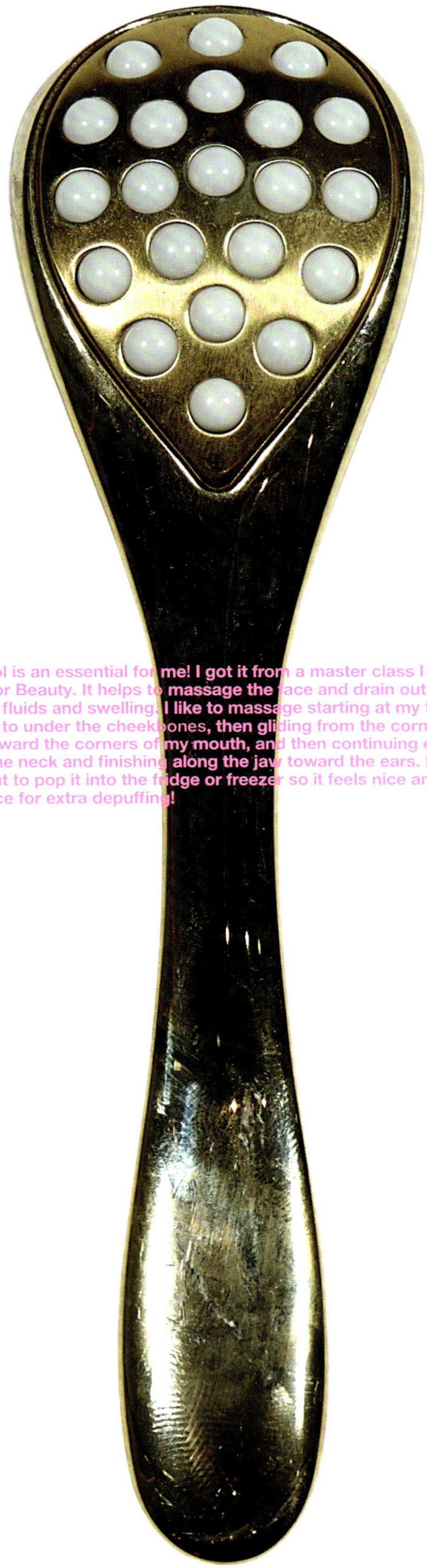

This tool is an essential for me! I got it from a master class I took with Dior Beauty. It helps to massage the face and drain out any unwanted fluids and swelling. I like to massage starting at my temples, moving to under the cheekbones, then gliding from the corners of my nose toward the corners of my mouth, and then continuing everything down the neck and finishing along the jaw toward the ears. PRO TIP: It's great to pop it into the fridge or freezer so it feels nice and icy on your face for extra depuffing!

Q Do you remember the first video you ever made?

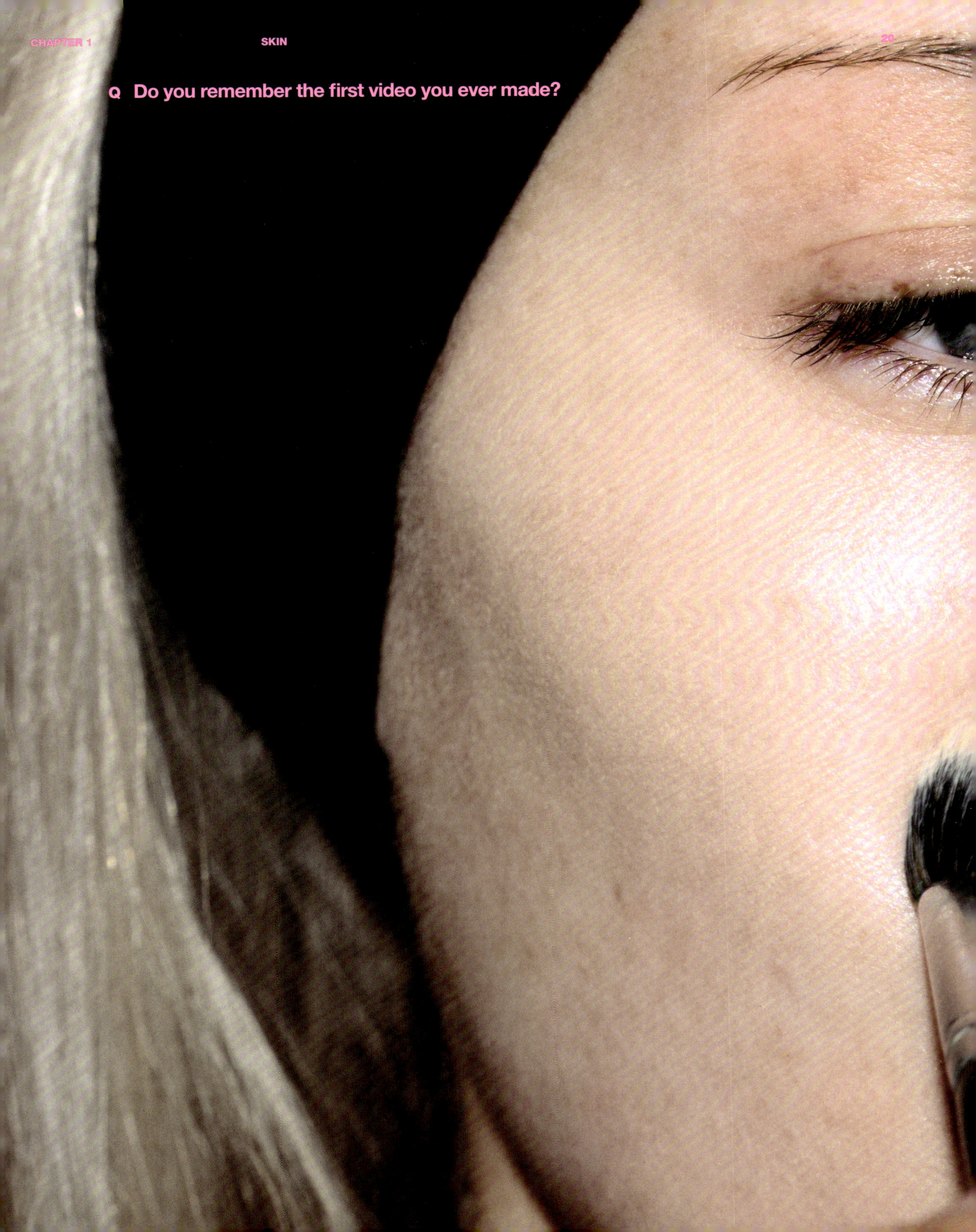

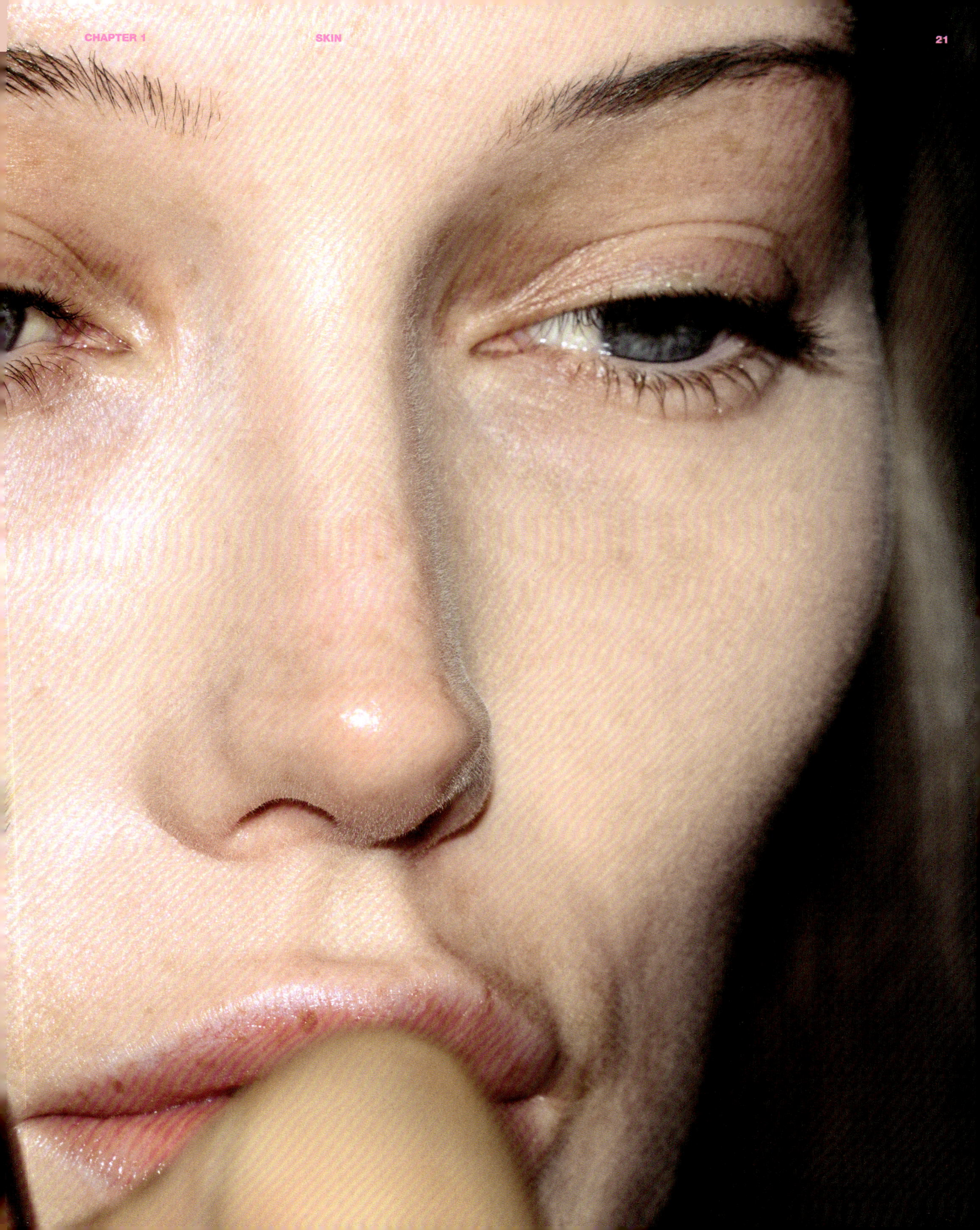

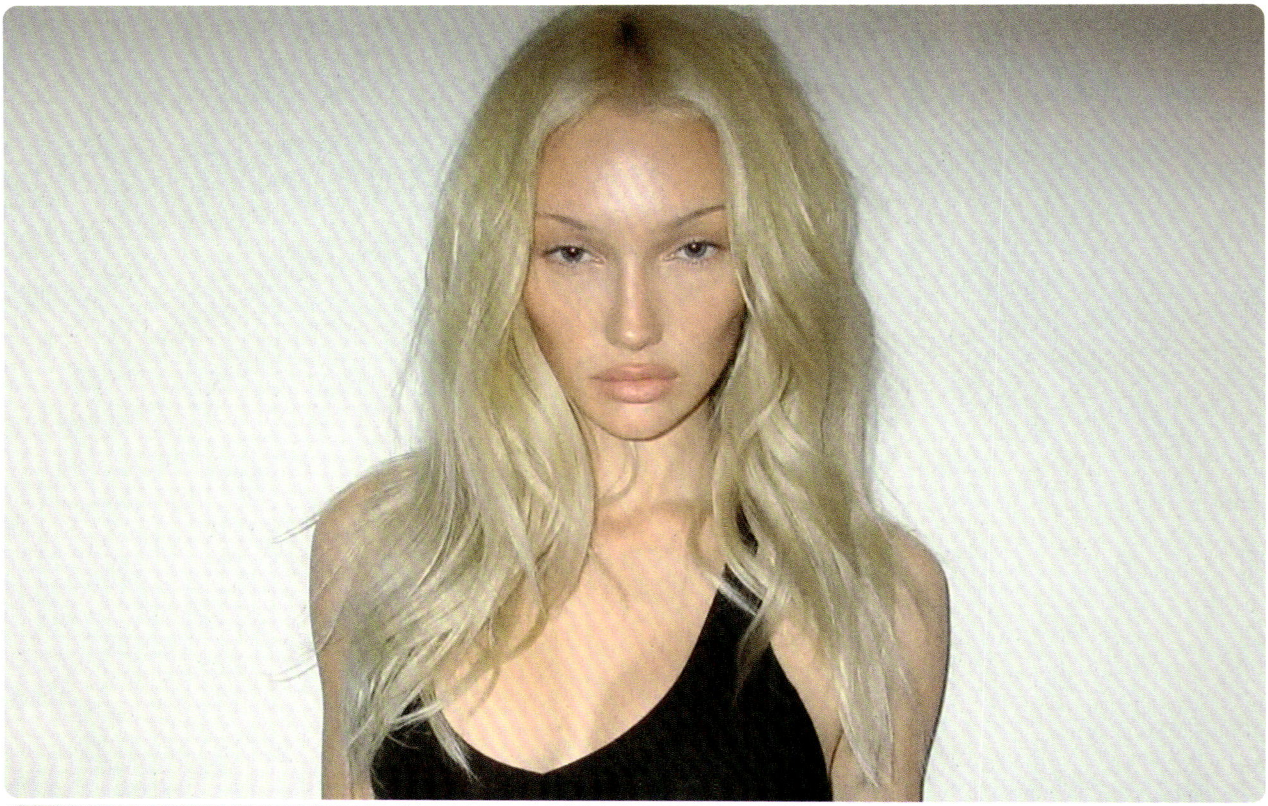

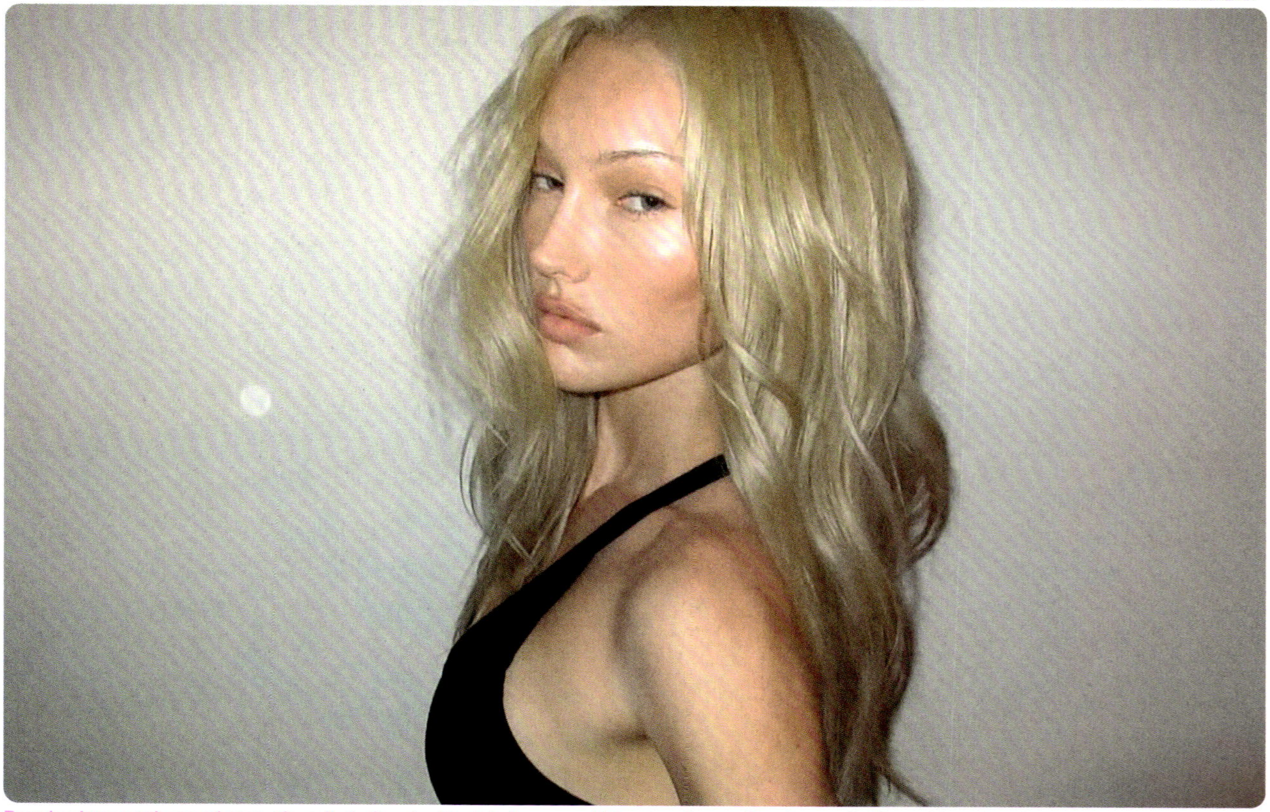

People always ask me what my favorite hair color I've tried was, and it's a tough question for me. I will say I love how blonde hair brought out my softer features with my eyes and skin. During this era, I really leaned into softer glam, focusing on glowy skin. My favorite product combo during this time was the Charlotte Tilbury Flawless Filter and the Beauty Light Wand.

TOP: Beachy skin is always my favorite. There's nothing like a long day at the beach, leaving feeling sun-kissed and golden. CENTER: Another favorite facial massaging tool! I love the dual-ended sides to get into those smaller crevices. This one is from RoC Skincare—I love a metal tool because they're super sturdy and last a long time. BELOW : Change and growth are a major part of coming into yourself and getting older, but never lose sight of the little kid in you. It's going to keep you grounded and is a reminder to be kind to yourself!

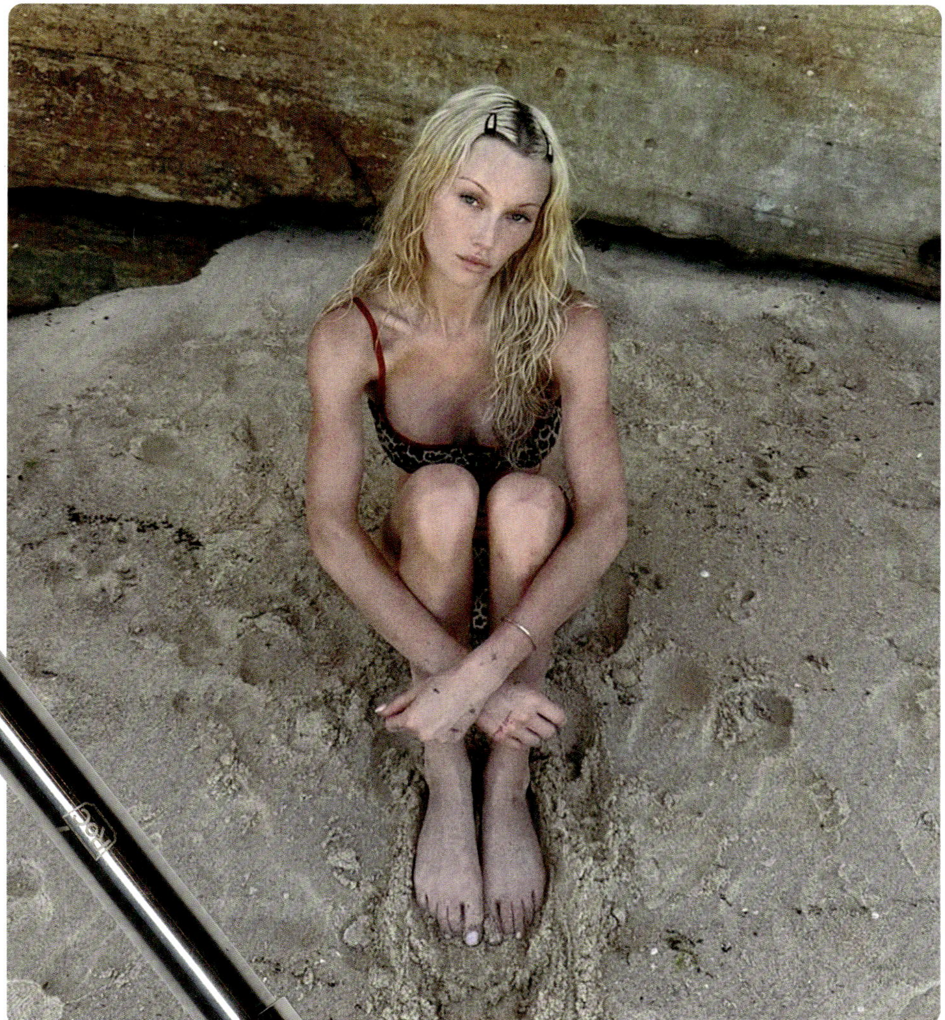

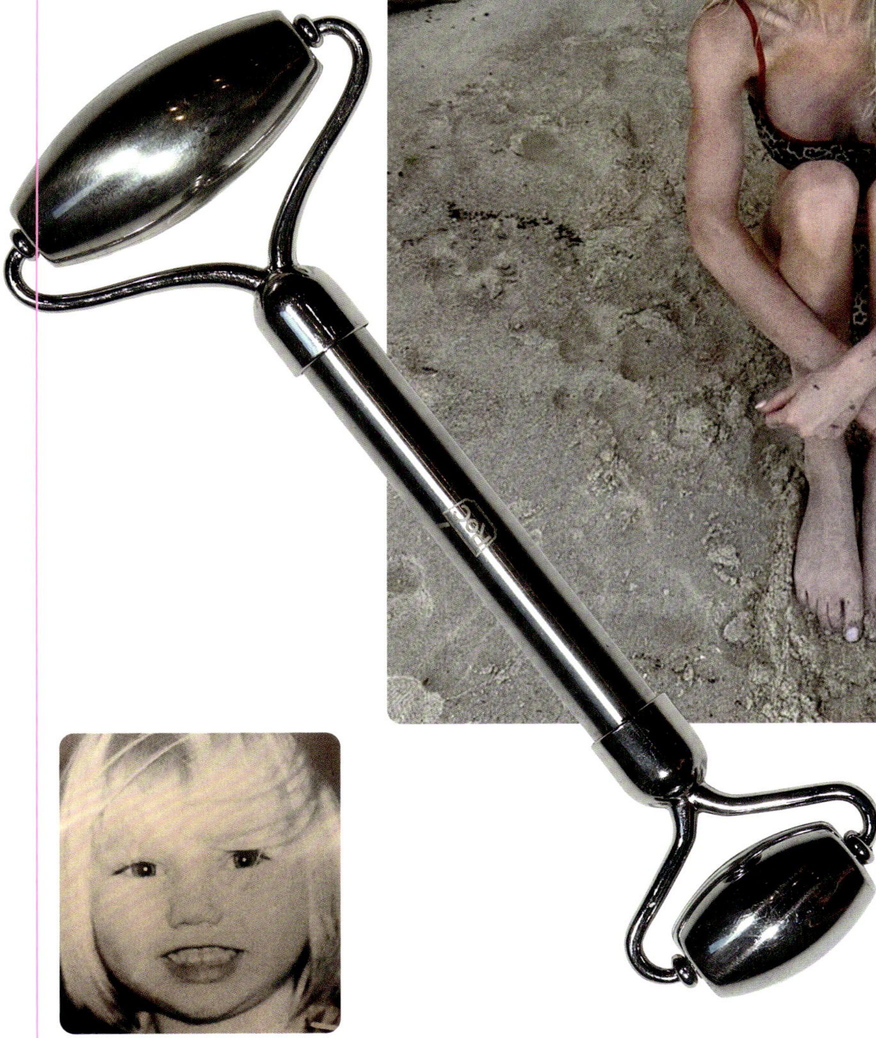

A The first one that I remember posting and being really proud of was a YouTube video where I made a DIY Scrabble ring. I know that sounds so random, but that's how YouTube was at the time…all the girls on there that I followed and looked up to were always doing these DIY projects. I've always had a passion for DIY and making art, so this was a really fun era for me.

And I think the second video I made was a "what's in my bag" video, which was another trend on YouTube at the time. I remember pulling out the Maybelline Colossal Mascara and the Baby Lips (iconic, iykyk). I remember saving up from doing chores around the house to be able to buy these it-girl beauty products.

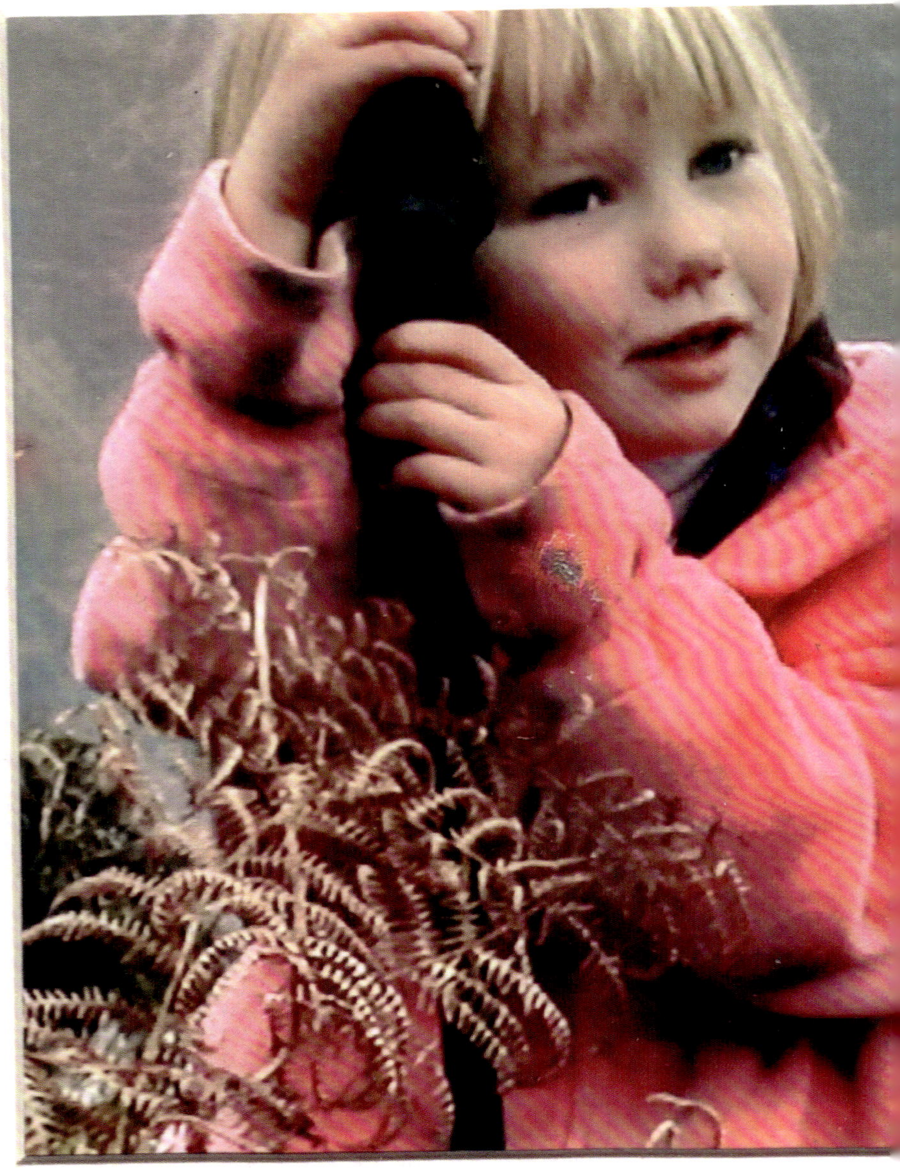

Moments like this are so special to me because they remind me of the other side of me that many people don't see online. I didn't grow up in glitz and glam. A lot of my childhood was hiking, camping, and fishing with my dad!

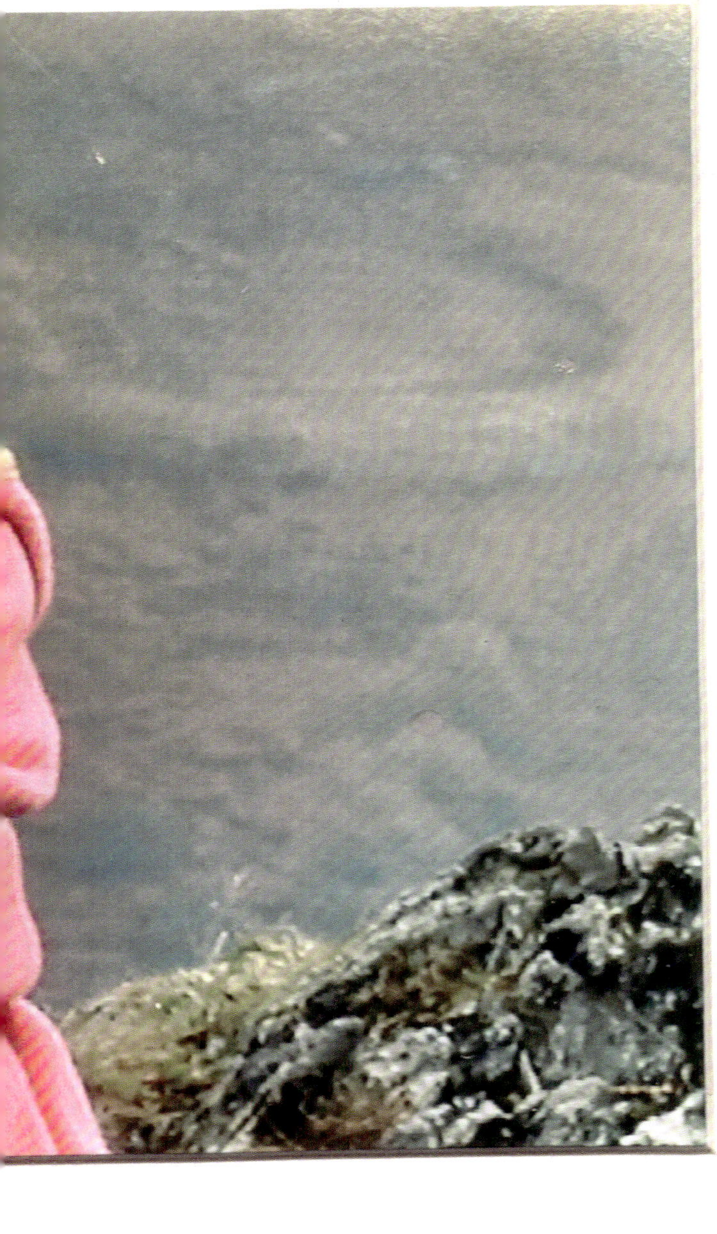

Q How old were you?

A I was twelve or thirteen years old. I had always been playing with makeup before that. YouTube was really my outlet for my creativity at the time. It was a platform where I was able to create these fun videos as well as play around with editing, and that was a fun part of the creative process for me. Personally, I found it difficult to grow my audience on YouTube, so when TikTok arrived, it felt like a second chance to do what I always loved doing while sharing my passion with a different audience.

When I started posting on TikTok, I was like, "Oh! This really works for me…." I liked how the app worked and appreciated the short, quick videos. I have ADHD, so it was very easy for my brain to work at that pace. Even when I watch YouTube, I play it on 2x speed. I think TikTok just happened to be the perfect app for me. I told myself, "Okay, you can't care what people think. Just do you and post it."

Q I'm curious about your parents' reactions.

A Growing up, I was a little bit of a rebel. I got in trouble with my parents a few times, and I remember hating it when they would take my social media away because it was really a creative place for me to turn to. But they always loved that I was super-creative and made these videos—they always supported my creative ideas.

I asked my mom to put me into art classes, and she was super supportive of it!! I also remember asking my dad for help. We had a tool shed in the backyard, and I asked him if I could turn it into a little filming studio—I spent hours filming videos there.

So my parents were very supportive. But I don't think they knew the extent to which it would become a career for me. And, of course, I didn't know that at that time either.

Q How would little Meredith feel if she saw you now?

A She would be in shock at her success but deep down knowing she was going to make it happen because she's been manifesting since day one!

When Covid hit, I was in college with only one semester to go before graduating. I didn't know if I was going to be able to move to New York City and if I was going to be able to get a job there because of how expensive and competitive it is. I had no money saved to move to New York, so I couldn't go there without a job. If I didn't come up with a plan, I was going to have to stay at my parents' home and work there until I saved up. I told myself, "I'm going to make this TikTok thing happen and blow up by June, or the end of my college semester." I told myself, "This is your plan. There is no other option."

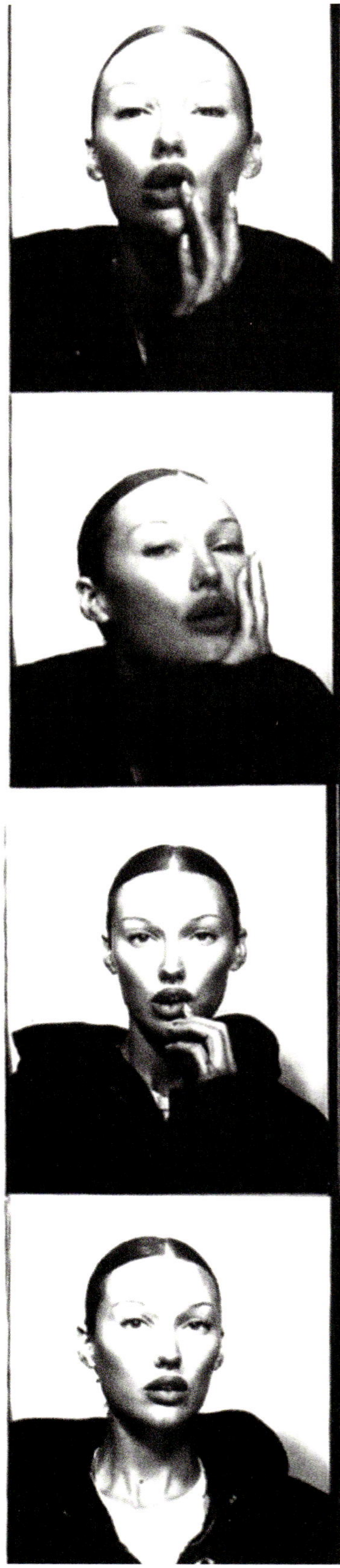

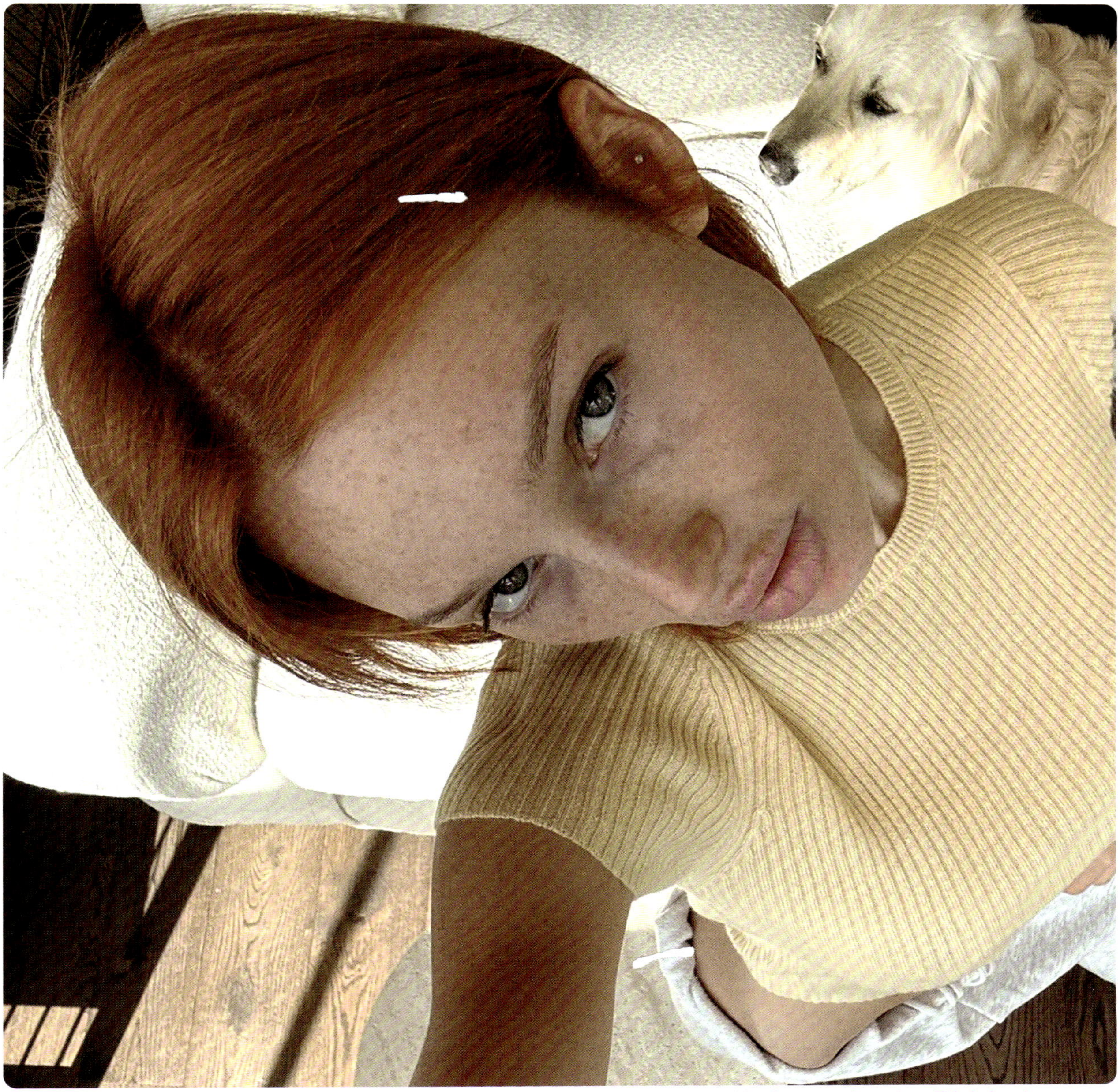

This was taken right after I dyed my hair from blonde to red! I love being a chameleon and morphing into new characters. This hair color was so fun and brought out a new side to me. I also took a risk and chopped my hair into a bob. Very invigorating!

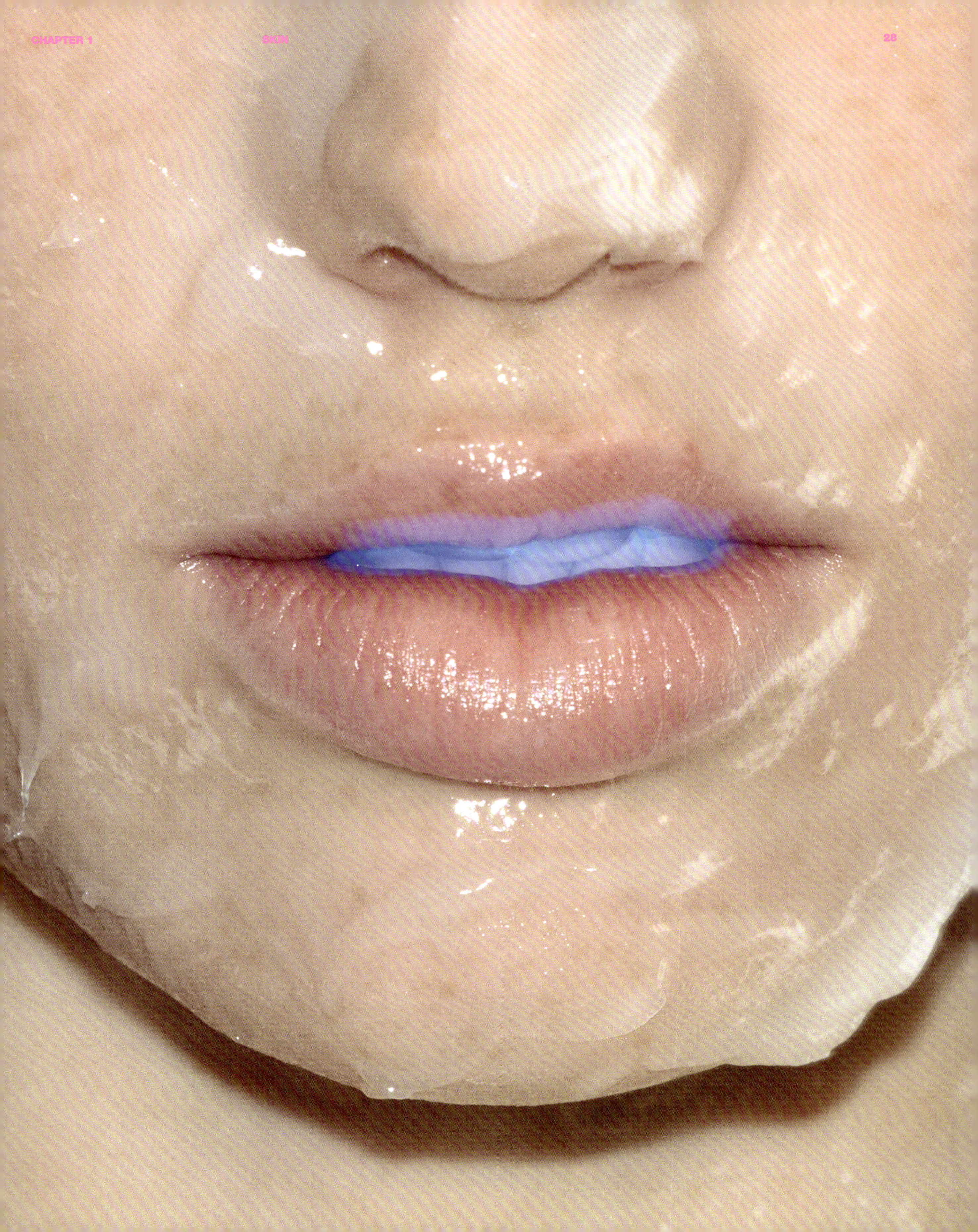

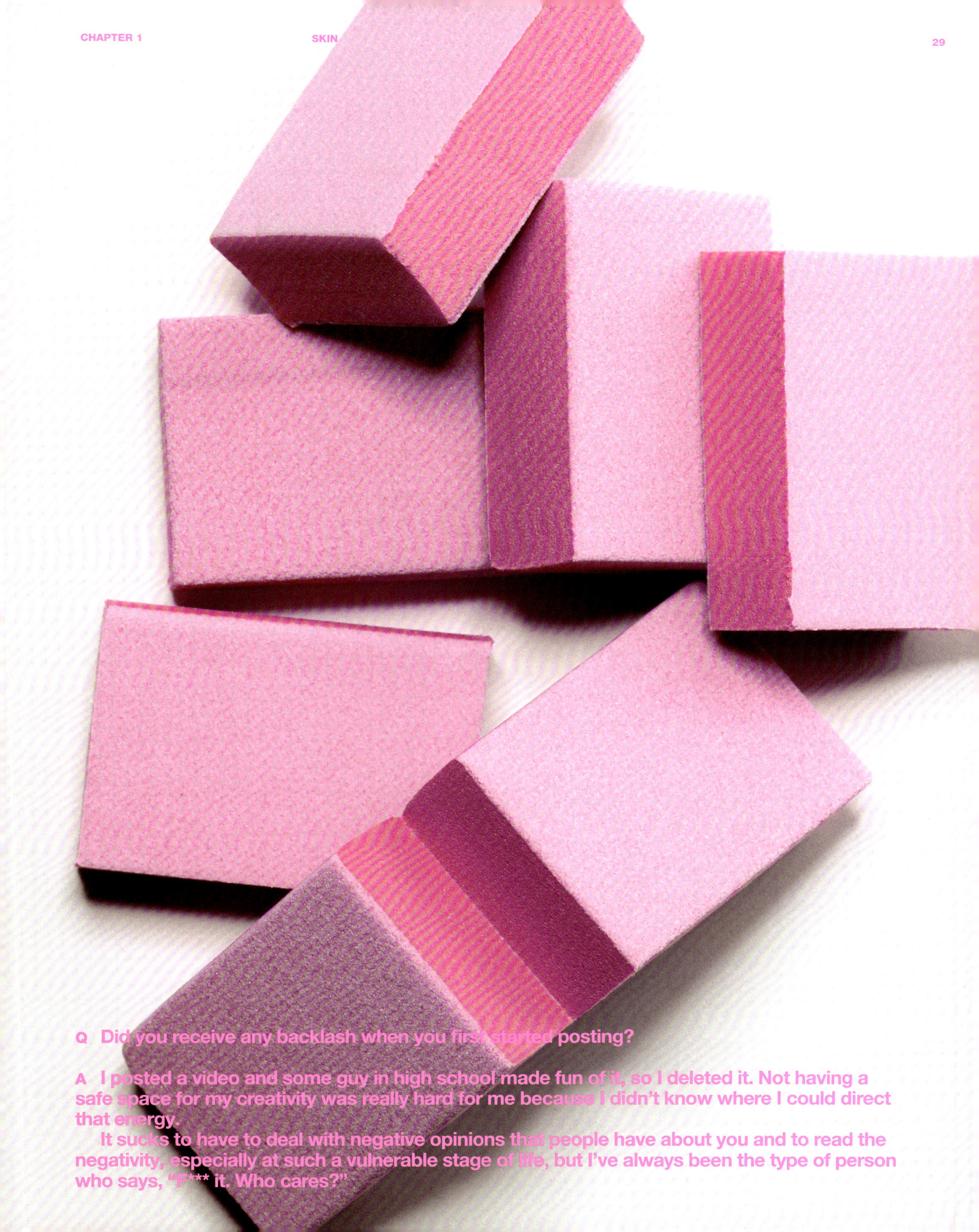

Q Did you receive any backlash when you first started posting?

A I posted a video and some guy in high school made fun of it, so I deleted it. Not having a safe space for my creativity was really hard for me because I didn't know where I could direct that energy.

It sucks to have to deal with negative opinions that people have about you and to read the negativity, especially at such a vulnerable stage of life, but I've always been the type of person who says, "F*** it. Who cares?"

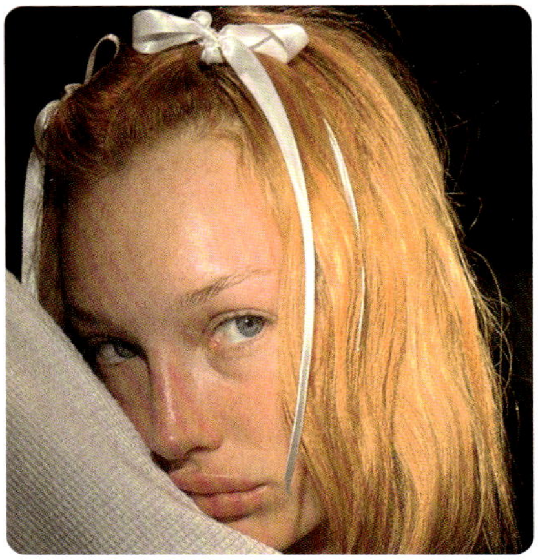

This was taken during Paris Fashion Week in 2023.

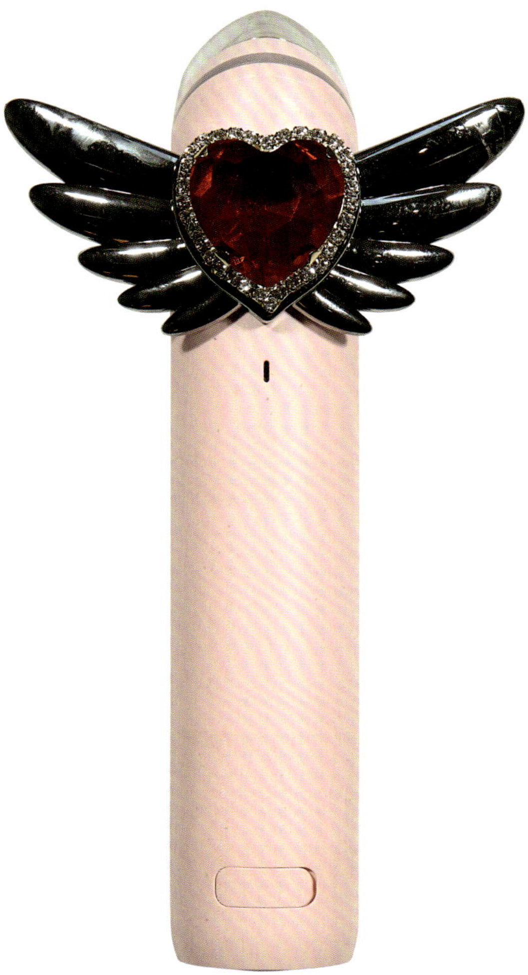

The most helpful tool ever! This is the Medicube Age-R Booster Pro Angel Edition. It helps to boost product absorption, tighten pores, improve elasticity, and increase skin radiance. It has six different functions and uses electroporation and microcurrent features.

Q Where does that confidence come from?

A I've always hated people telling me what to do. I like to take control of my own life and own my decisions, so I think it came from just growing up with that mindset.

Q When did you realize that you were becoming successful?

A It clicked to me when I reviewed my TikTok analytics. I was like, "Oh, my God! There are 60 million people per week watching me, and it just keeps growing and growing." The numbers were insane. In one month, I grew from one million followers to seven million, and from there, a million per week for a few more weeks, until I unfortunately got hacked and was locked out of my account for a month. This was really hard for me because TikTok became a place of community and support for me. I was able to share my passion with people who also loved what I was doing.

During Covid, I felt as if I was living in a little bubble in my apartment. Seeing the numbers was hard to grasp. And then, when lockdown was over, and I started going out again, people would recognize me on the streets or in the grocery store.

Q When did you realize that your work had made you so public-facing?

A For me, it was moments with my supporters and audience. It's funny because at first it feels like you're being approached by a stranger on the street, but then they share with you how you've impacted their life and inspired them, and it ends up becoming a really intimate, special moment.

Q Are there consequences to sharing information about yourself in your videos?

A When you invite people online into your life, and you reveal a lot of information, you are opening yourself up to scrutiny by some people who believe that they are entitled to know every single specific detail about you. It gets to be a little slippery because you want to share and you want to involve them, but, at the same time, you have to protect your own mental health, peace, and privacy.

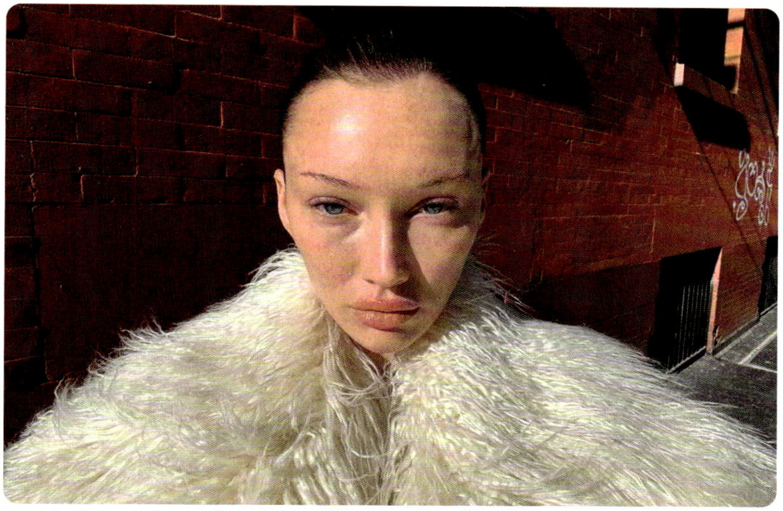

TOP: Let's normalize under-eye bags! I've always had them. Honestly, I've just started to play into the aesthetic of them instead of trying to hide them. CENTER: You guys know me and my 90s brows. This is my favorite tool to maintain that sharp, skinny brow. I just lightly shave right above my brow every week or so, and it keeps them nice and crisp. I also use this tool to dermaplane my skin from time to time. Dermaplaning is basically using a razor to exfoliate the skin by removing the top layer of dead skin cells and peach fuzz, leaving smoother skin.

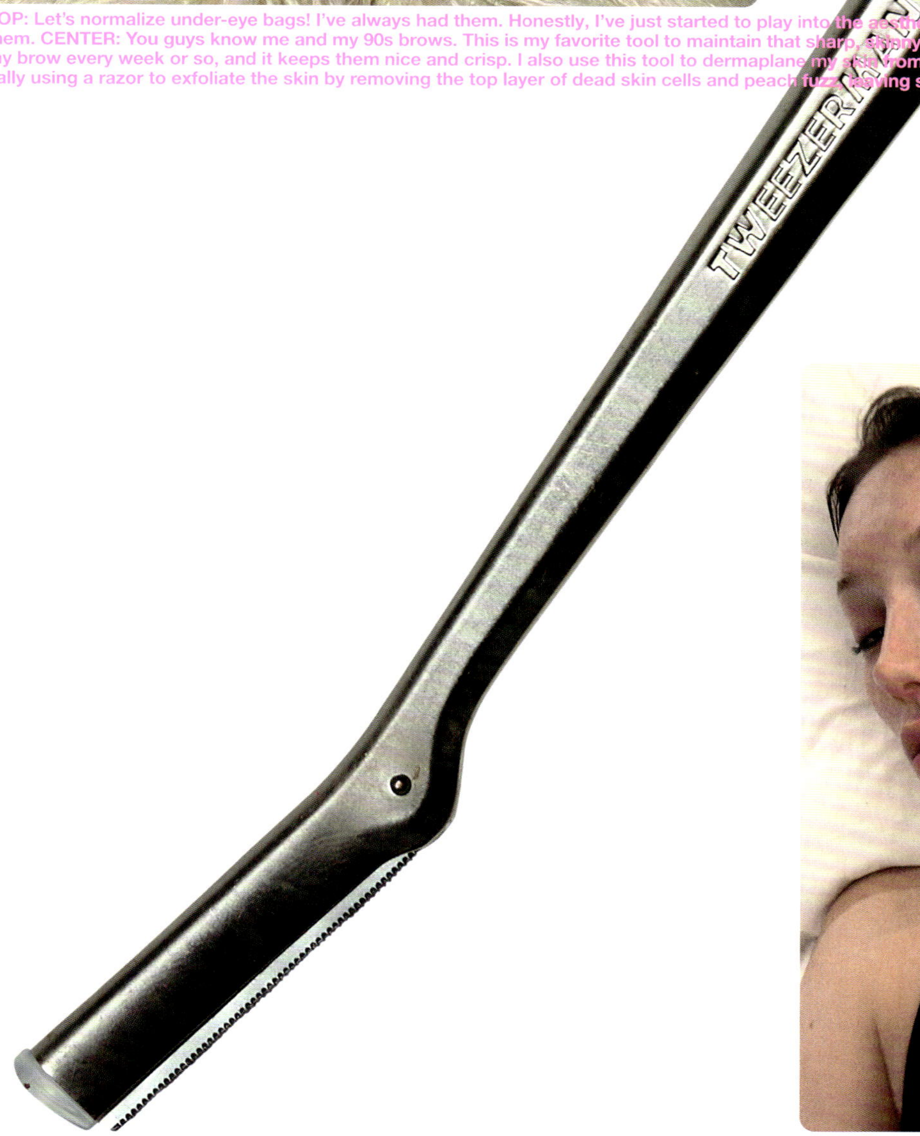

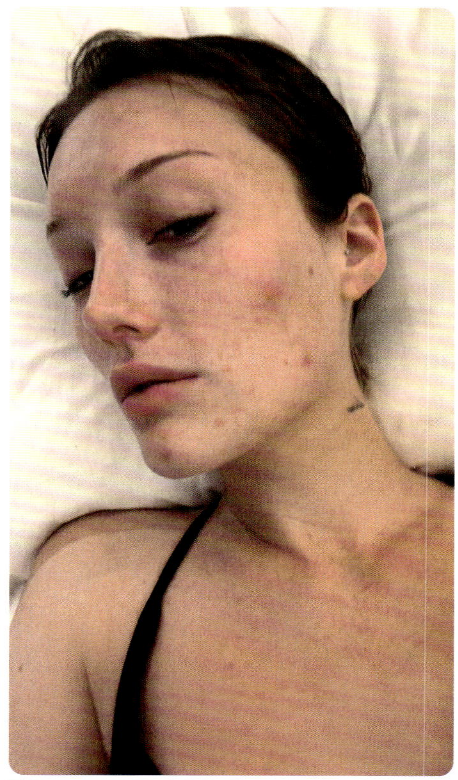

This was my skin right before a runway show during the middle of Milan Fashion Week.

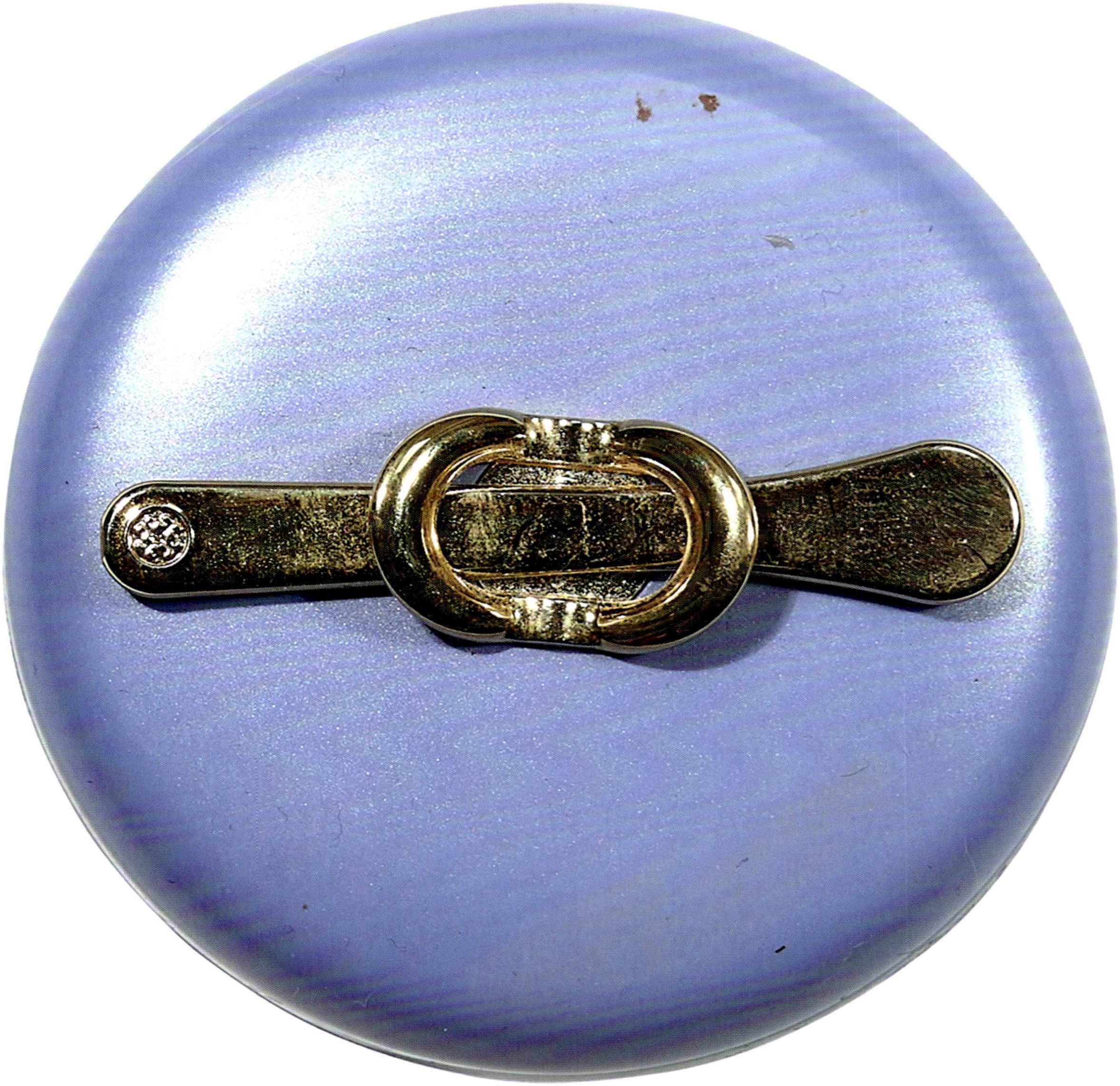

TATCHA DEWY SKIN CREAM
I'm very particular about what moisturizers I use because I have such sensitive skin. This TATCHA one has been a staple for me for years. It also acts as a great base before applying makeup. It's on the richer, thicker side, so dry-skin girlies, you'll love this!

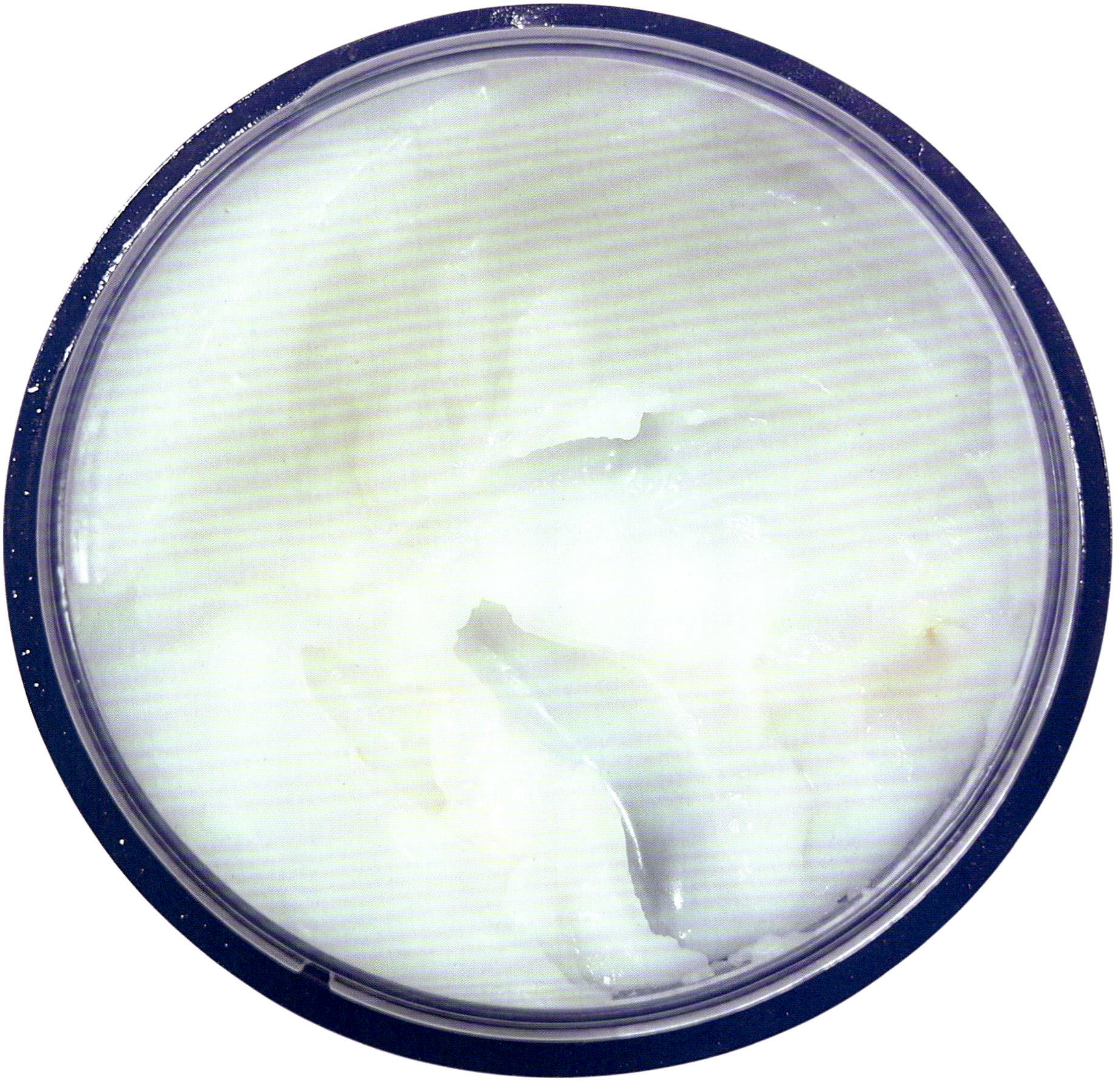

CLINIQUE TAKE THE DAY OFF CLEANSING BALM
This is one of the most underrated products. It's a melting balm that is a game-changer for removing stubborn makeup. The buttery balm melts into an oil-like consistency. It's great to use before going in with your cleanser.

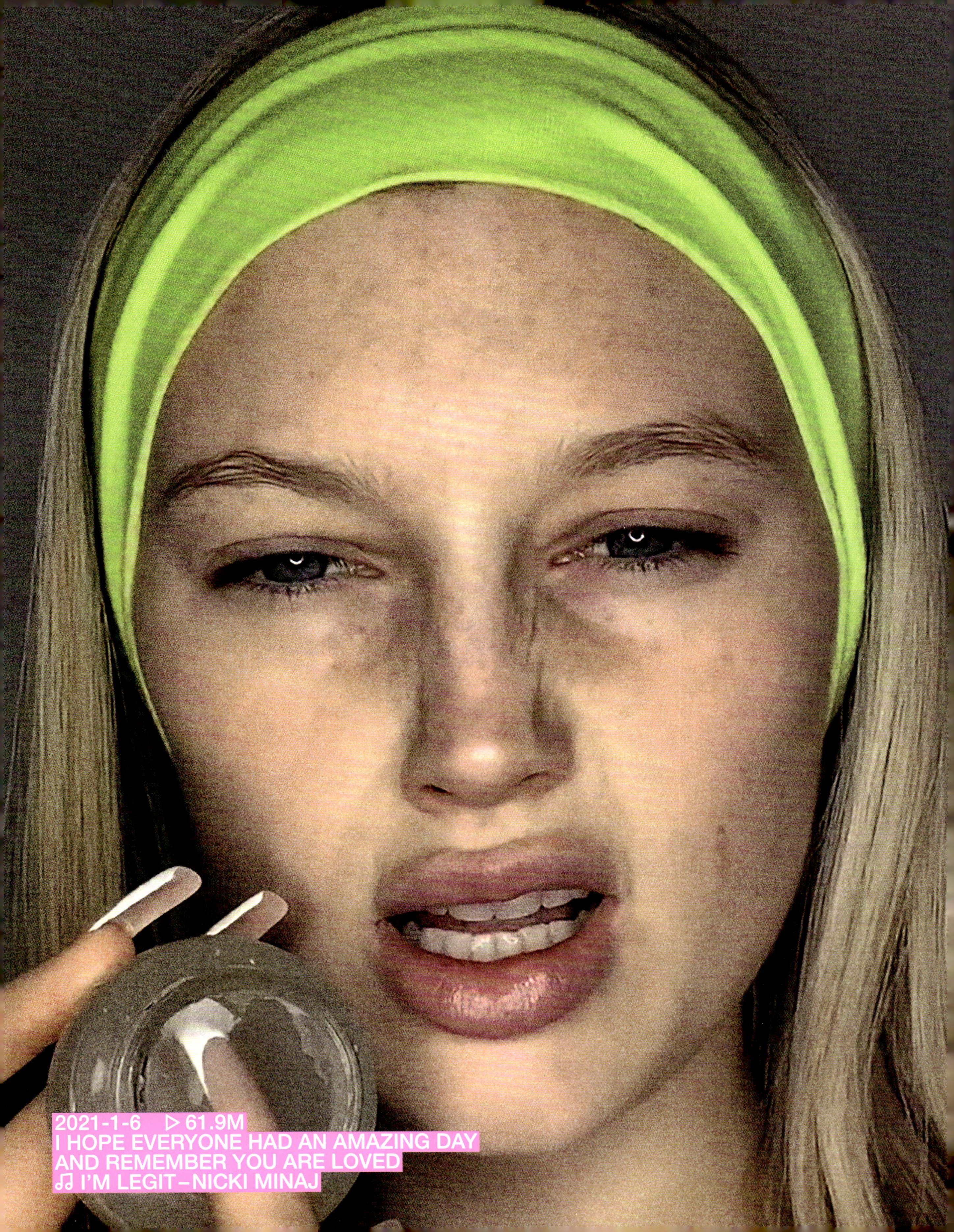
2021-1-6 ▷ 61.9M
I HOPE EVERYONE HAD AN AMAZING DAY
AND REMEMBER YOU ARE LOVED
♫ I'M LEGIT–NICKI MINAJ

"YOUR PERSONALITY IS GOING TO LEAVE A LONGER IMPRESSION THAN YOUR SKIN EVER WILL"

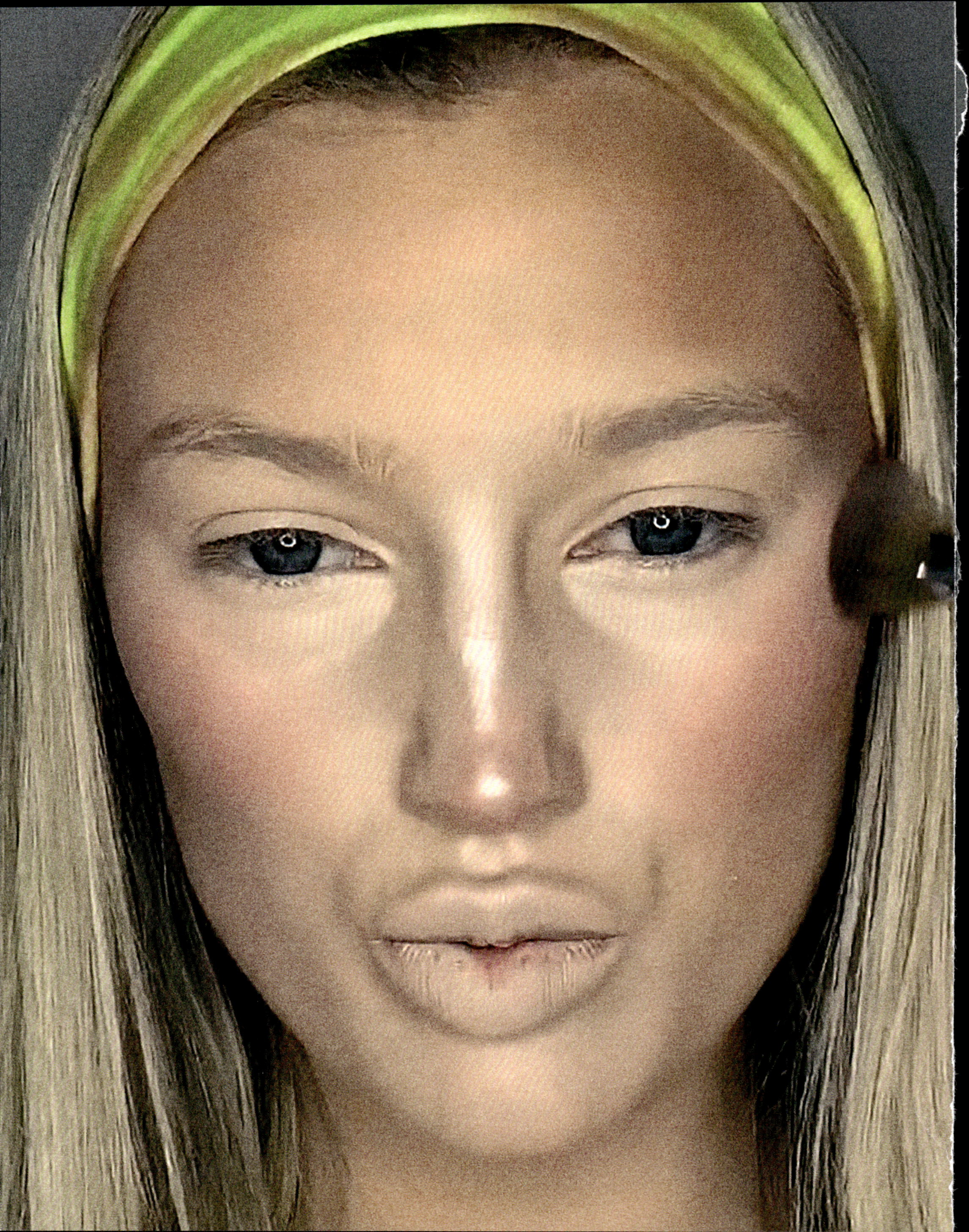

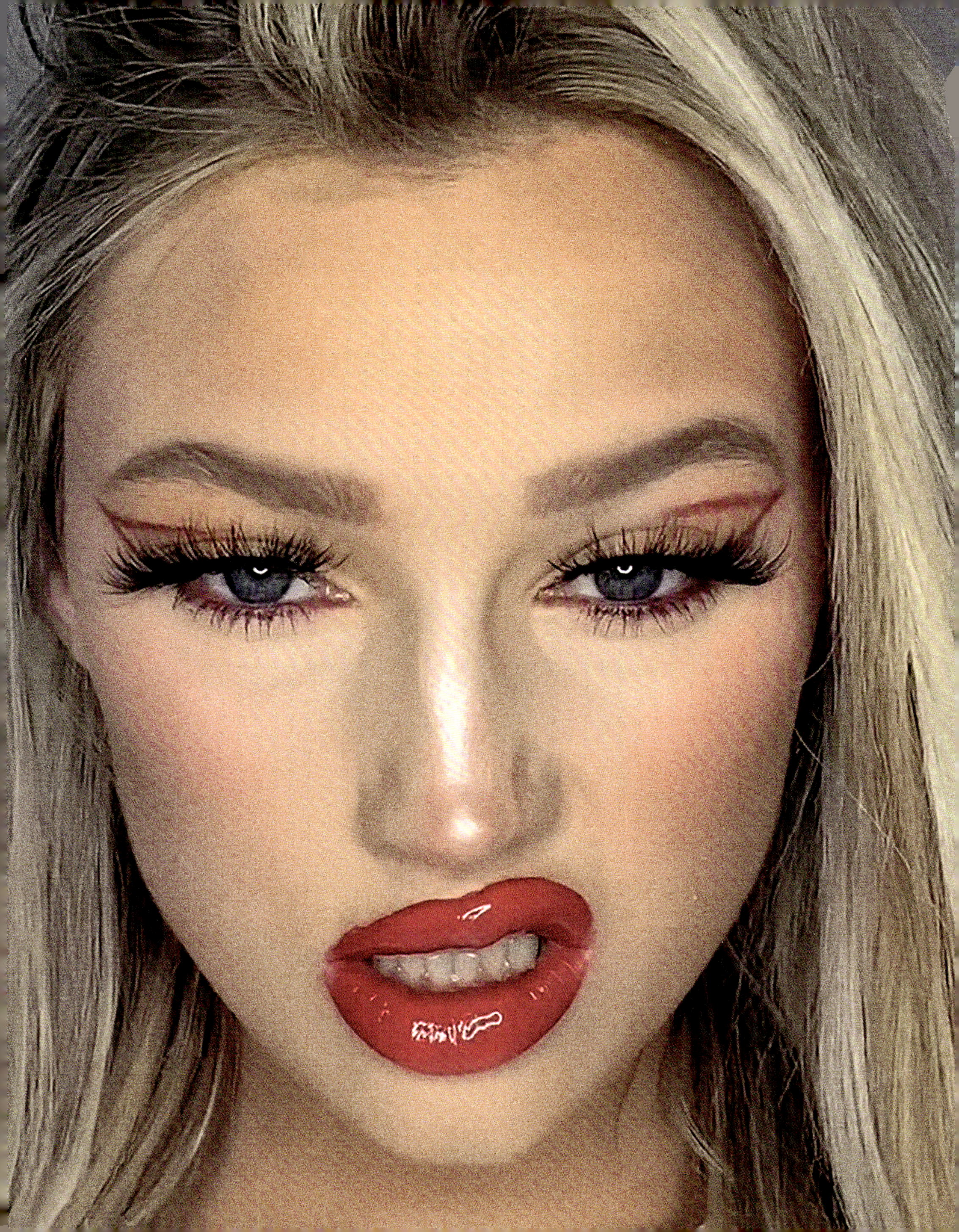

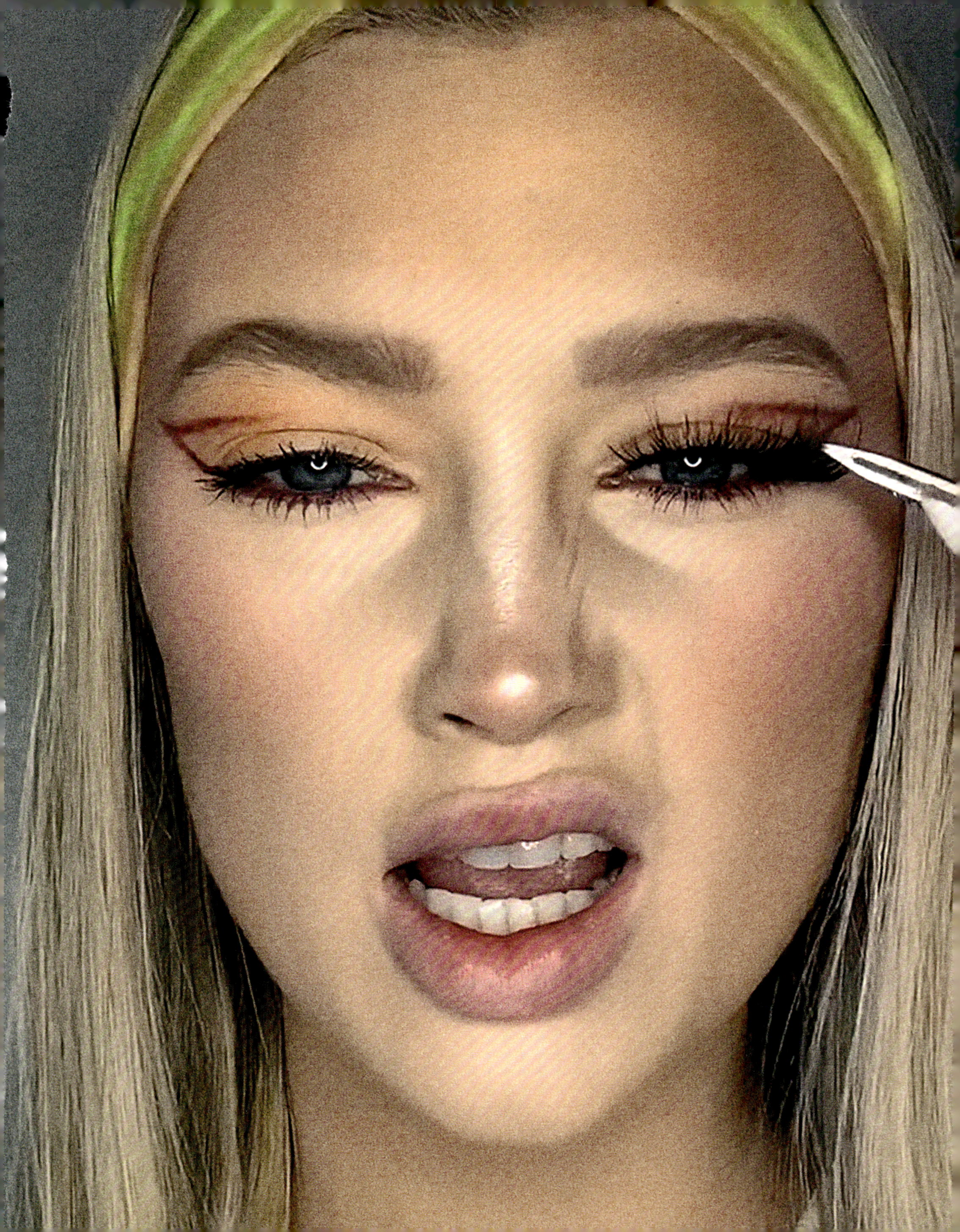

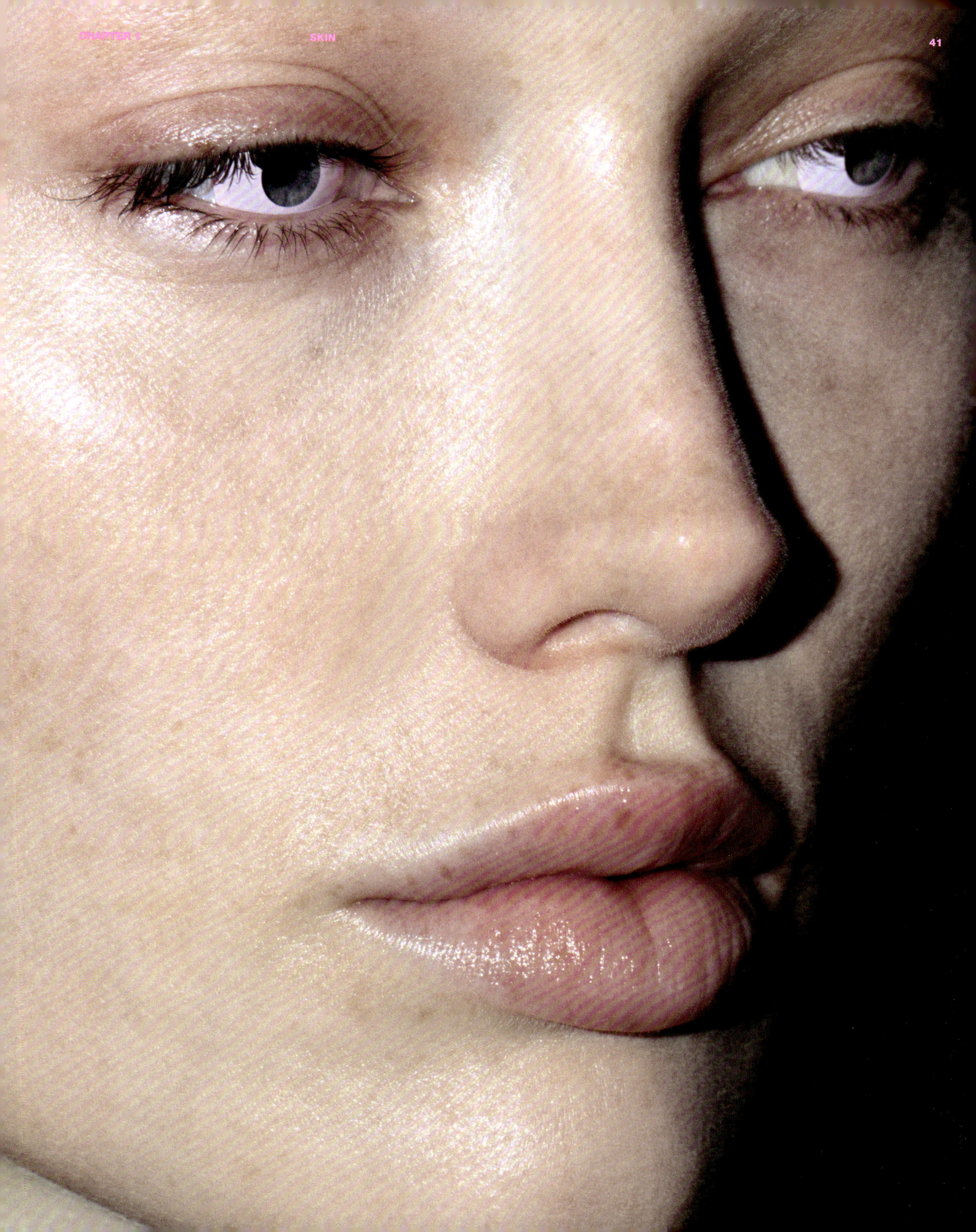

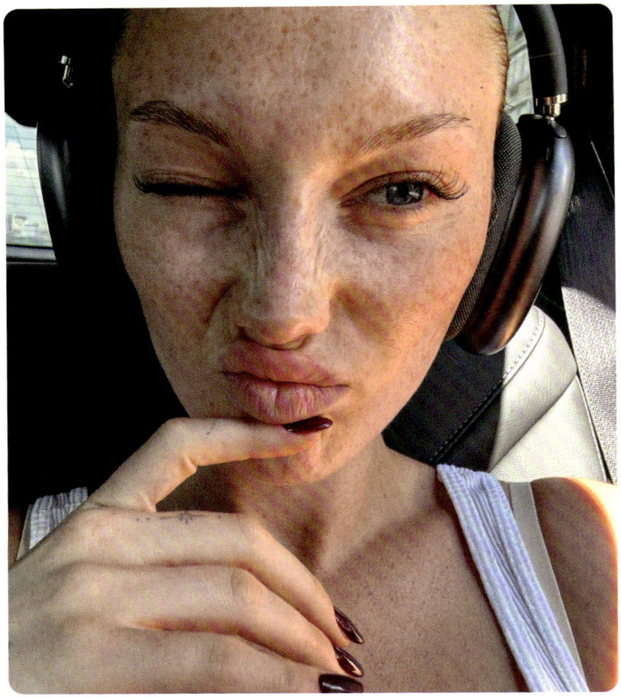
Kisses to the camera! My freckles were really popping here.

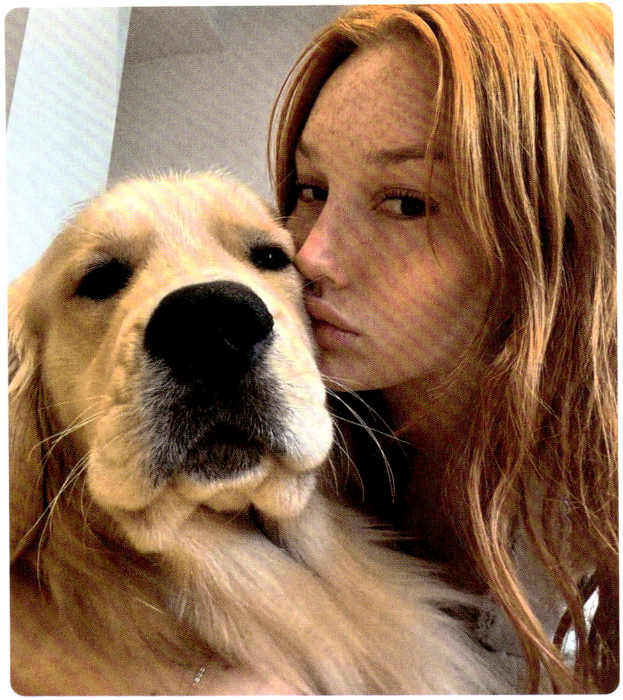
Through all the glam and fun moments, experimenting with different looks, it's always nice to come back to yourself and appreciate your natural self. My favorite thing to do is hang barefaced with the pups!

Q You've sort of grown up online...

A It's insane because I have such a large digital footprint of my twenties. I've gone through so many eras, each era documented online, which is crazy and also scary because I'm not the same person I was five years ago.

We're always changing, and we make mistakes. Maybe we don't resonate with the style we once had. But, of course, at the core, we're still the same person.

Q Is it really tough not to feel like you have space to mess up when millions of people are watching.

A Yeah. I've always tried not to be a controversial makeup person. I believe makeup should be fun, and I just want to inspire people. Of course, I want to be honest if I don't like a product. I try to speak the truth and say it in a respectful way.

This happened to me with a product from Jones Road that I reviewed on TikTok. I applied the product using my foundation technique, and I personally didn't have the best experience with it. It simply wasn't meant for my technique. Some people took my review and ran with it, twisting it into a scandal when it really was never meant to be that serious. It ended up selling great for the brand, though. It just goes to show how the internet loves drama.

After that experience, I told myself, "Okay, I'm not going to do negative reviews anymore. I'm still going to be honest, but I'm not going to create negative reviews because it only creates negative attention and gossip." For some people, that may get them further along in their career, but that's not for me. I always want to have a positive reputation.

Q What goes through your head when you read something negative?

A I would never, ever, ever feel comfortable getting online and posting a negative comment on someone else's page. I find it so uncomfortable. I honestly get secondhand embarrassment when I read negative comments because these people have gone out of their way to be mean.

When I see negative comments or hate on my page, I just remind myself how much fun I'm having with my content and that it's made me be able to live the life I have always wished for.

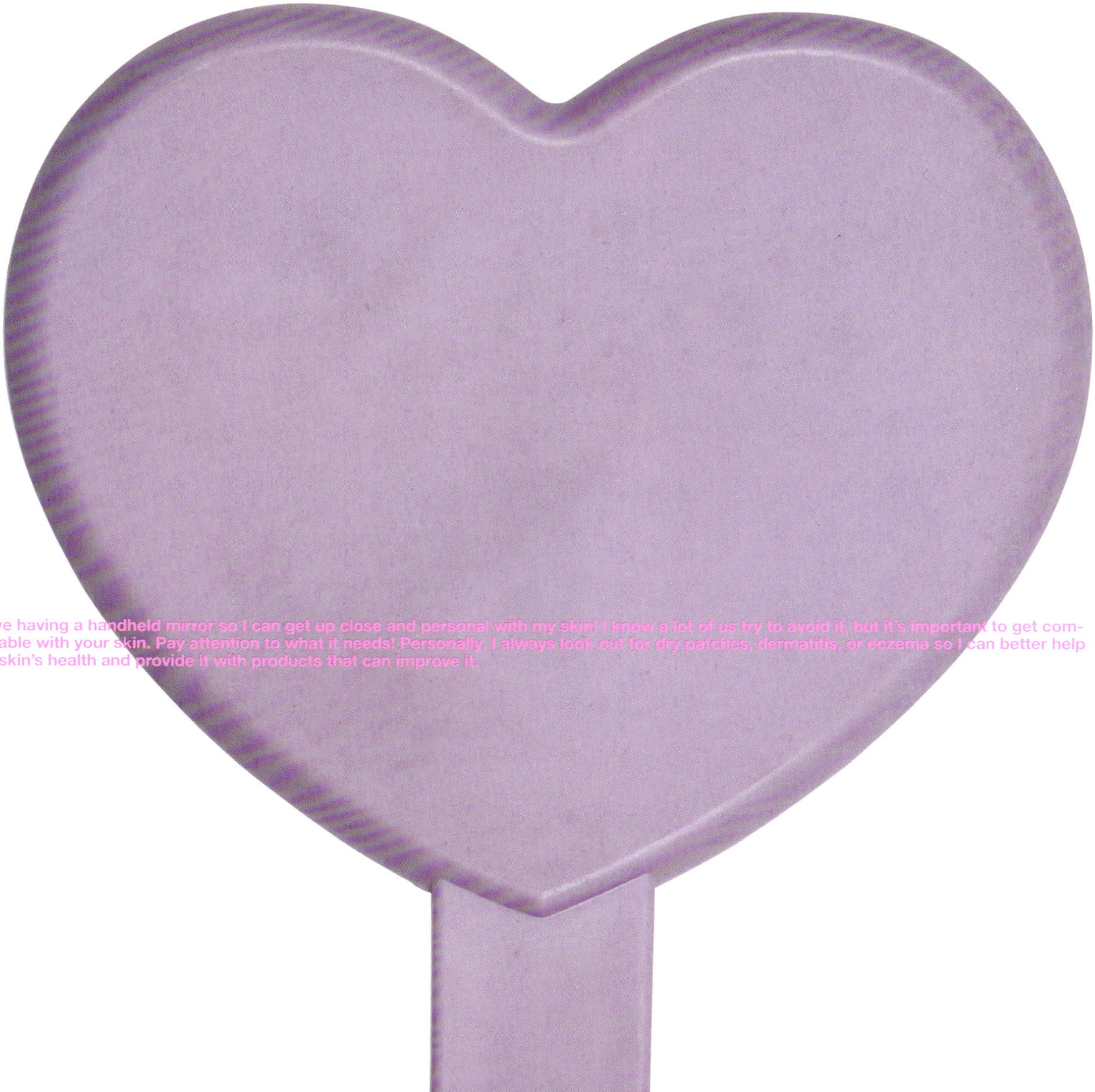

I love having a handheld mirror so I can get up close and personal with my skin! I know a lot of us try to avoid it, but it's important to get comfortable with your skin. Pay attention to what it needs! Personally, I always look out for dry patches, dermatitis, or eczema so I can better help my skin's health and provide it with products that can improve it.

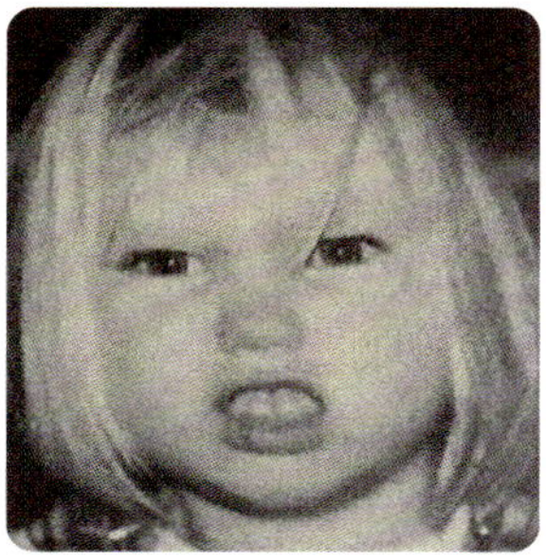

Next time you are talking down to yourself, think of little you, ask if you would say those things to your younger self? Your younger self would be so proud of how far you've come and would hate to see you speak to yourself negatively.

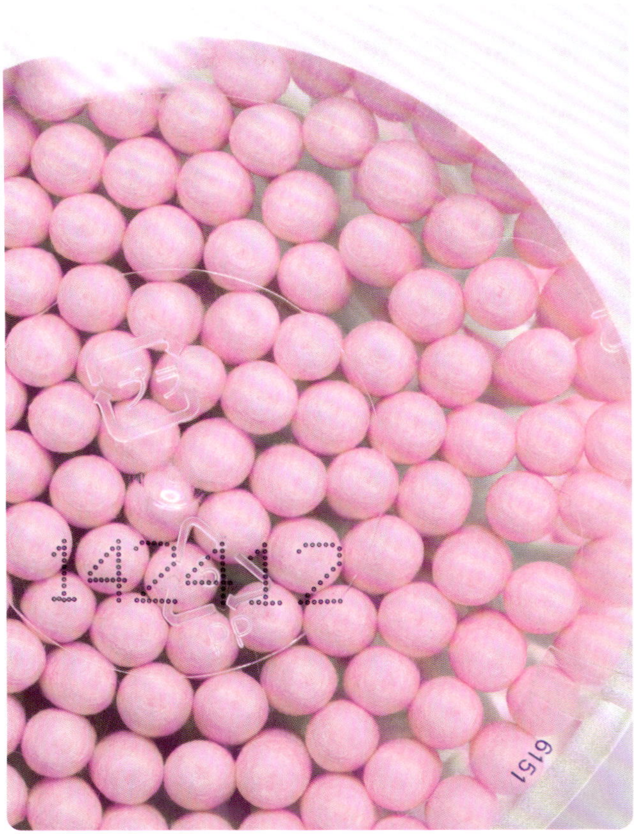

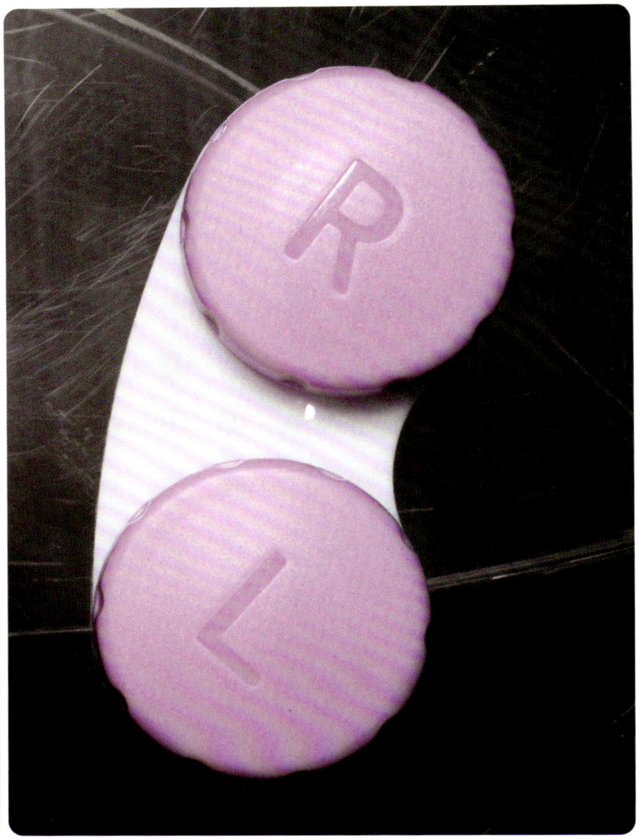
R
L

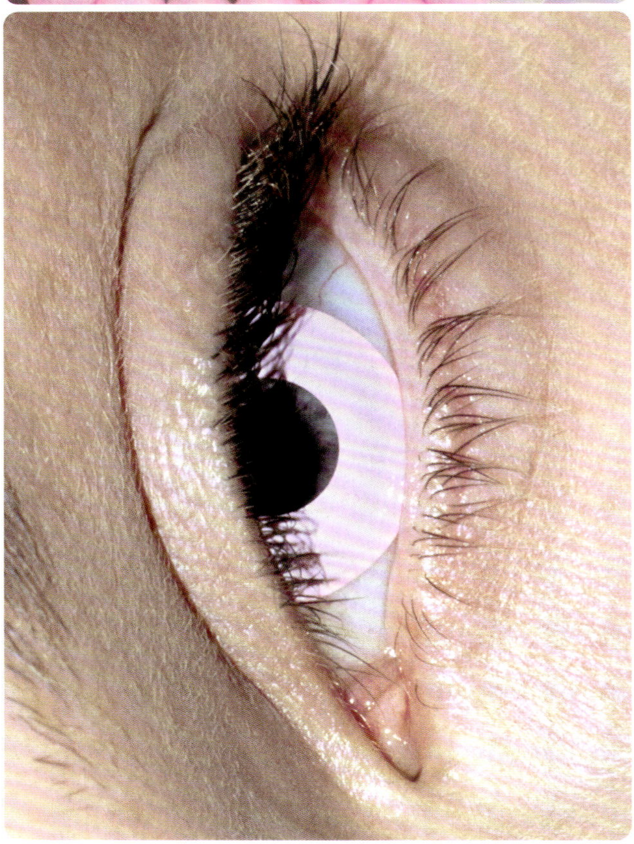

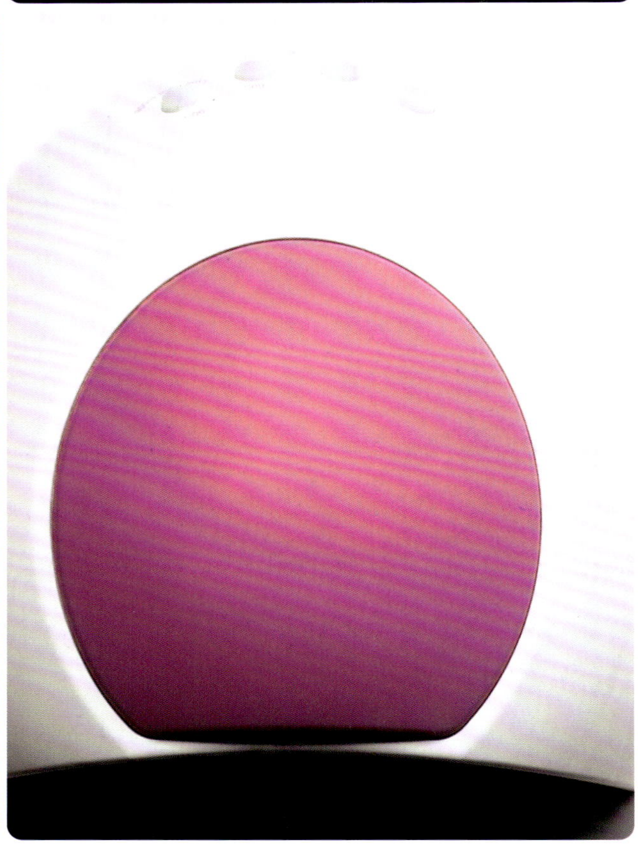

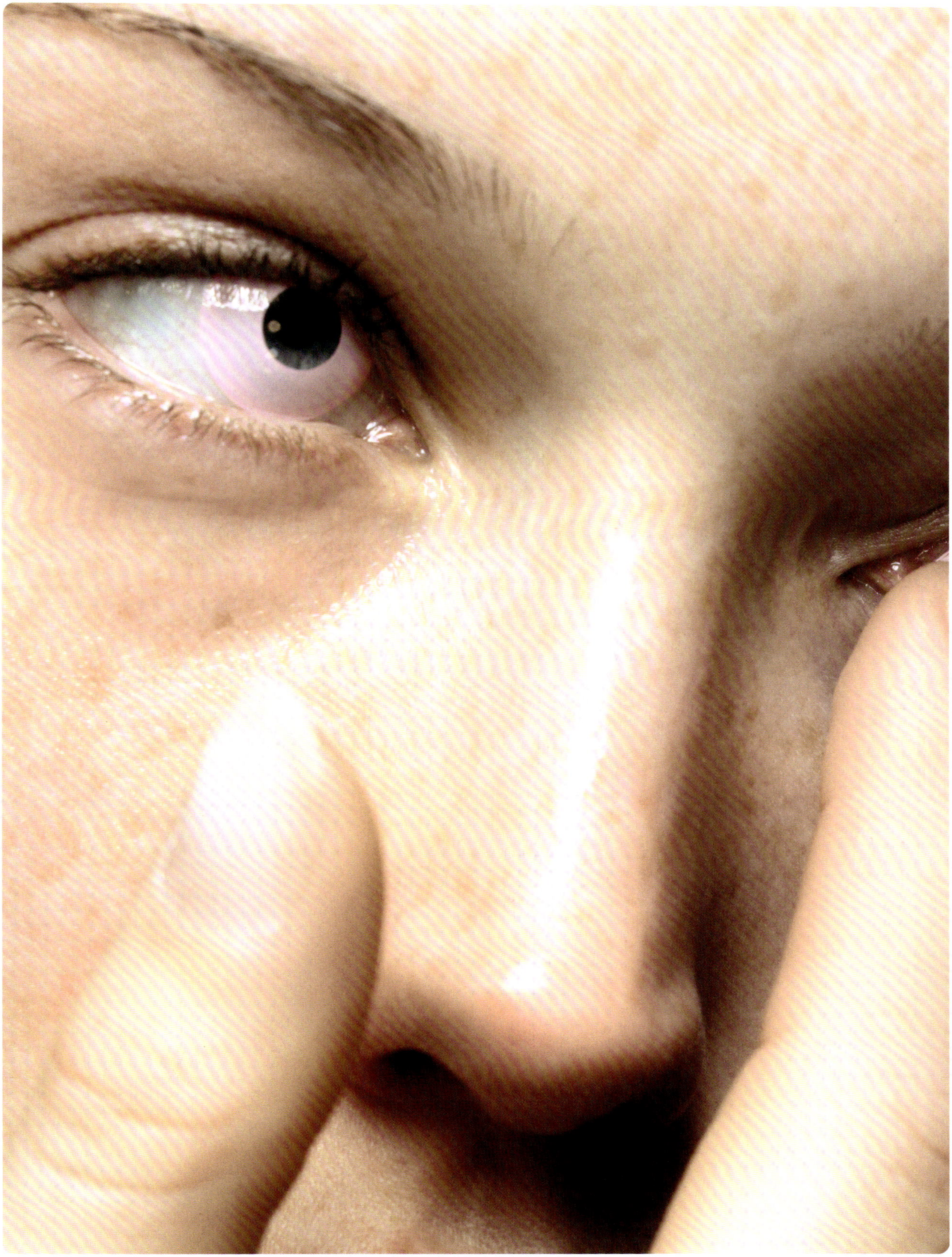

Q What comes to mind when you look at your earlier content?

A I'm proud of every piece of content I've made. Of course, when I look back, I might think, "Oh, my God. That's a hard watch." It's kind of like when you record and listen to your own voice. You think you sound weird. Looking at earlier content makes me so happy because I see how much fun I was having. I did not give a f***. And I was confident, that's all that matters.

I love going back and looking at the old videos just to see how far I've come. And I also like going back and still seeing those comments from my community. There are people I recognize who've commented for four years in a row, and I'm like, "This is crazy."

Q Is there a look that you ask yourself, "What was I thinking, and why did nobody stop me?"

A Yes, one of the looks was like pink threw up on me, but again, it's all about creativity!

Q Do you remember what inspired some of these specific looks?

A I'm very sporadic with my ideas, and my inspiration comes from all over the place. I get really inspired through color, so my favorite way to get inspired sometimes is just by picking up an eyeshadow palette!

Q Did you ever go outside in these glam looks?

A I would do full glam for a night out or event for sure. But I was also pumping out so much content back-to-back that I would just wipe it right off and go on to creating the next look! A lot of the time, I would have crazy costume jewelry on and a fun top so people would think I was attending some fancy event, but in reality, I had pj's on the bottom…

Q How tied is your confidence to your skin?

A It's definitely tied pretty closely, and I think a lot of us feel that way. For me, feeling good about myself is what makes me confident. If you have acne or blemishes, you don't always feel yourself, but that's okay! It's just about working through it and finding how to take care of your skin and use products that make you feel most confident in those moments.

I've struggled with perioral dermatitis, and it definitely plays into how I feel about my appearance. You start to ask yourself, "What am I doing wrong?" It makes you feel like you've failed your skin. In reality, a lot of this stuff is out of our control, or it's products we've been told are good for us, but in reality aren't. This is why education about product ingredients and paying attention to what your skin *actually* needs is so crucial.

With the dermatitis, I tried everything to get rid of it. I switched my toothpaste because I heard it could have been the fluoride causing it. I was on doxycycline for a month. I even switched my entire skincare routine. It's all trial and error.

If I have a breakout it's more hormone-related, but everyone is different, and that's why it's important not to judge someone for their skin—you don't know their health and what causes these issues for them.

Q Have you spoken about your eczema and dermatitis with your followers?

A I've spoken about my dermatitis, and it's actually really nice because I feel like people get very involved and want to help find a solution. They also want to find a solution for themselves. People will go through all the comments, workshopping solutions together.

Whenever I have an issue, I go to TikTok for a solution because I know people will come up with some crazy ones that I'm not finding elsewhere on the internet.

Q Some people in your comments say you should embrace your freckles more, and you should stop wearing foundation. What has actually helped you to embrace your freckles?

A I would say learning how to do editorial-style makeup and doing more in the fashion industry helped me embrace my freckles. In fashion and modeling, they really do embrace the "raw" you. Working in editorial-style makeup forced me to get comfortable with my skin.

I would go to castings without any makeup on. When I did shoots, I felt like the editorial makeup actually complemented my freckles. Before that, I could never find a style of makeup that I liked to see my freckles with.

Q What is the difference between editorial makeup and the style of makeup that you were doing?

A With editorial makeup, it's very, very natural on the skin, but then it focuses more on a fun lip, an eye, or a cool lash. There's a little bit of concealer use, but it really is just accentuating other areas of your face. The style of makeup that I was doing at the time and was most comfortable with was full glam, so freckles and all were covered.

Q Do you ever talk to your skin like a friend or an enemy? What do you say to it?

A I try my best to talk to my skin like a friend, and I workshop with her. It's easy to look in the mirror and think, "Are you kidding me? Why is my skin doing this today?" I'll mostly try and look at other factors, and I'll be like, "My skin is my bestie, she needs me right now lol."

Q Tell me some affirmations, rituals, mantras, or tiny habits that bring you back to yourself when you're not feeling your best.

A I remind myself that the feeling is temporary. There are always solutions that you can use to come back to yourself and your good skin. Your skin doesn't define you or your overall appearance. There are so many things that go into how someone looks. It's not just about your skin. Your personality, humor, and kindness are part of your appearance. It sounds so cliché, but it's true. A lot of people, when they meet you, are thinking more about your personality and the conversation they're having with you than the pimple on your face.

It's so hard because you look in the mirror and think omg, this is my worst nightmare. But when you meet someone, they don't think that. They're not going to remember you as the girl who had the pimple. They're going to remember you as the girl who is nice, funny, supportive, or whatever type of energy you're giving off.

Q If you had a message written on your mirror to look at every day, what would it say?

A "Hot a** b*tch," or something like that hahaha. Honestly, I'd love to read that every morning and be like, "Hell, yeah, I am."

Q And what color lipstick is it written in?

A Nude…duh! My go-to.

Q When you're not in the mood to get fully ready, and you need to fake-out to everyone that you have your life together, what's the number one thing you are going to do?

A Moisturized lip, and my hair needs to look good. I think that combo can really trick people into thinking you've got it all together.

I heard this quote from Austin Butler. He said, "Embarrassment is an underexplored emotion. Go out there and make a fool of yourself." Whenever I'm embarrassed, or I send a text to a guy, and I'm flirting, and I'm like, "Ooooops! Maybe I shouldn't have said that…" I'm like, "No, it's not that serious. Who cares?"

I find confidence in that quote because it's true: Embarrassment is just a short-lived feeling. You live only once, and you can't be scared about sending a text or saying something a little unhinged.

Q We've talked about the pressure of being judged for doing anything with your skin or appearance. You have been really open about your experience using filler. How has your perspective on fillers evolved over time?

A I think that there's a lot of pressure growing up to fit certain beauty standards, and I think that's where my negative feelings about filler and Botox come into play, because I never want someone to feel like they have to do it to feel pretty. But my other point of view on it is that you should be able to do these things to make yourself feel better if you want to, and you shouldn't be scrutinized for it.

When I was growing up, I always wanted plumper lips, but I think the beauty standard took it too far with the amount of filler I got in my lips. I think if there wasn't so much pressure, I would have just done a smaller amount of filler and kept it looking more natural.

1

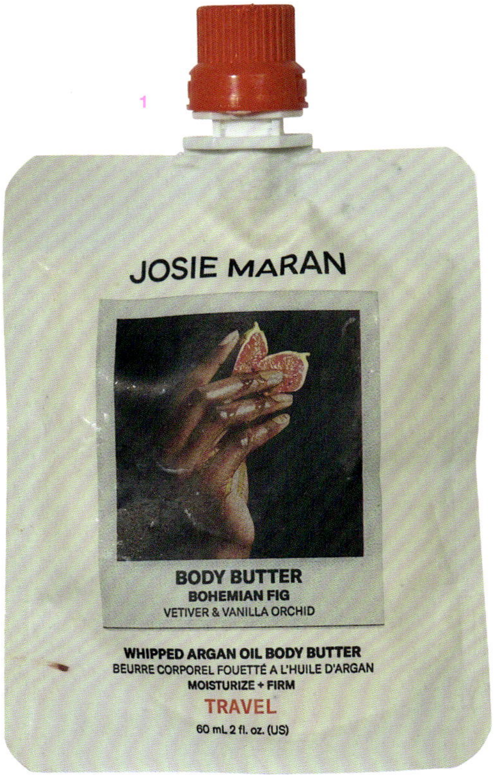

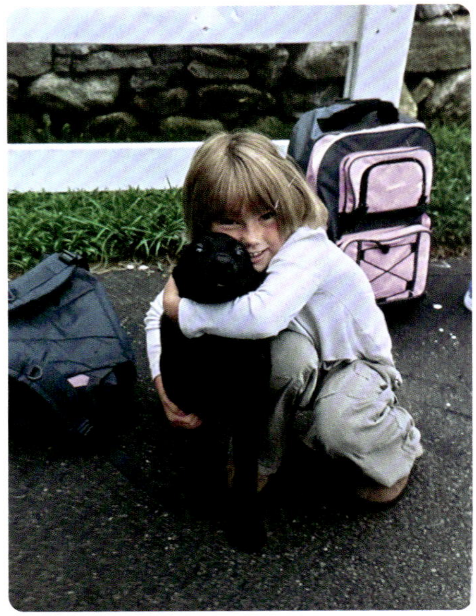

This is me before getting on the bus to elementary school, giving my dog, Oxford, one last hug before the day began. At that age, we never stood in the mirror picking ourselves apart or listing everything we wanted to change. We just were. It's important to return to that version of yourself sometimes and carry a piece of her with you. Please be gentle with yourself.

PRODUCT HIGHLIGHTS:
1. The key to a glowy, smooth body is to keep up with moisturizing, especially in the winter. This is one from Josie Maran, which is one of my favorites. I love these little to-go packs! It also smells absolutely delicious. 2. I love a nice sharp pair to trim my brows and make them snatched! You know me and my 90s skinny brows, hehe. 3. Tweezers are a crucial tool in my makeup bag. I use them for everything—from tweezing my brows, to placing my false lashes on, to sticking gems on my face. I have about twenty pairs, lol. 4. The Laneige Water Bank Blue Hyaluronic Intensive Moisturizer is another amazing moisturizer that helped heal my skin barrier and calm my perioral dermatitis.

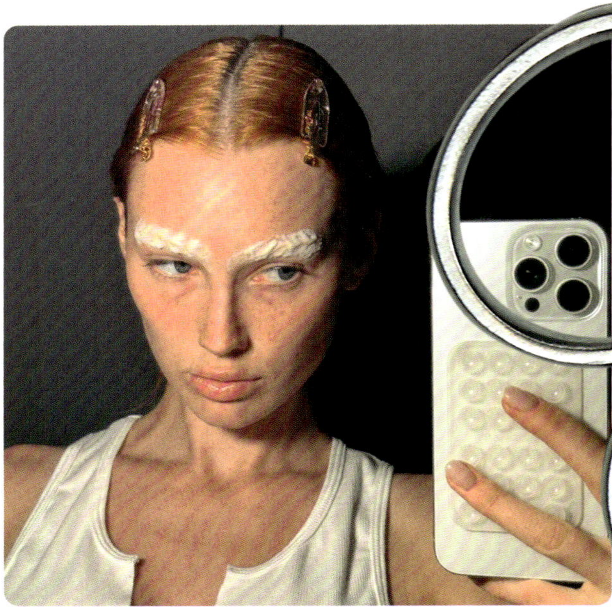

2

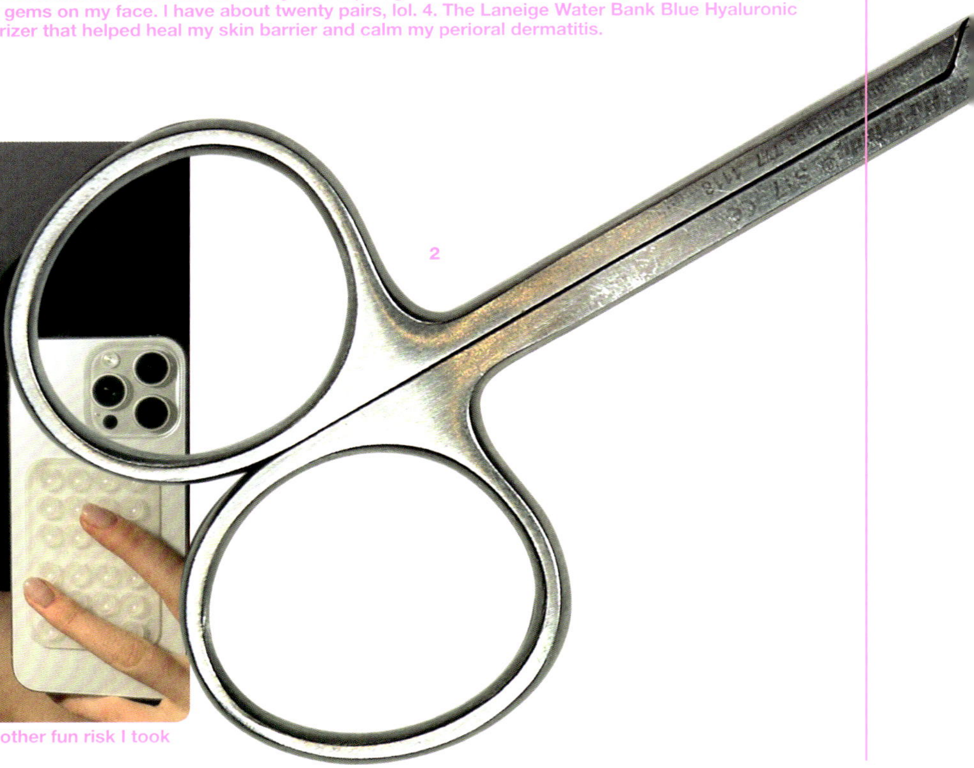

Who doesn't love a bleached brow? This was another fun risk I took during New York Fashion Week.

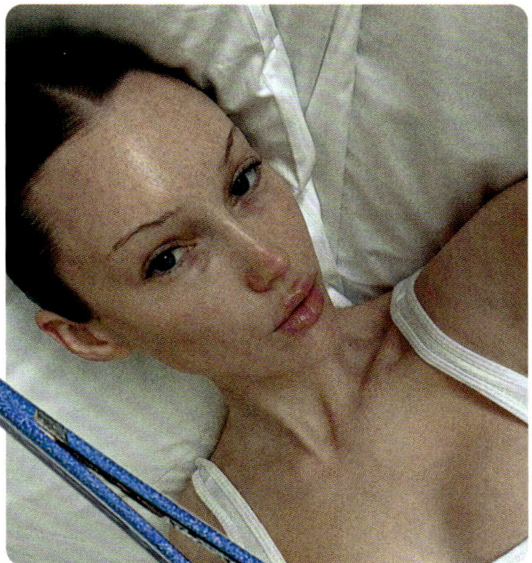

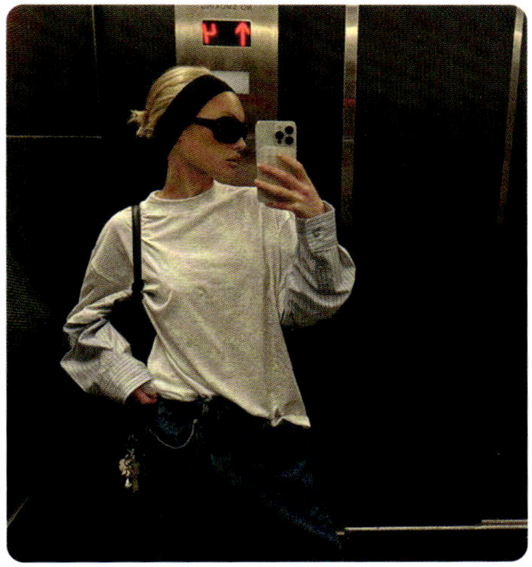

Let your skin breathe from time to time! If that means stepping out the door with a big pair of sunnies on to make you feel more put together, then so be it!

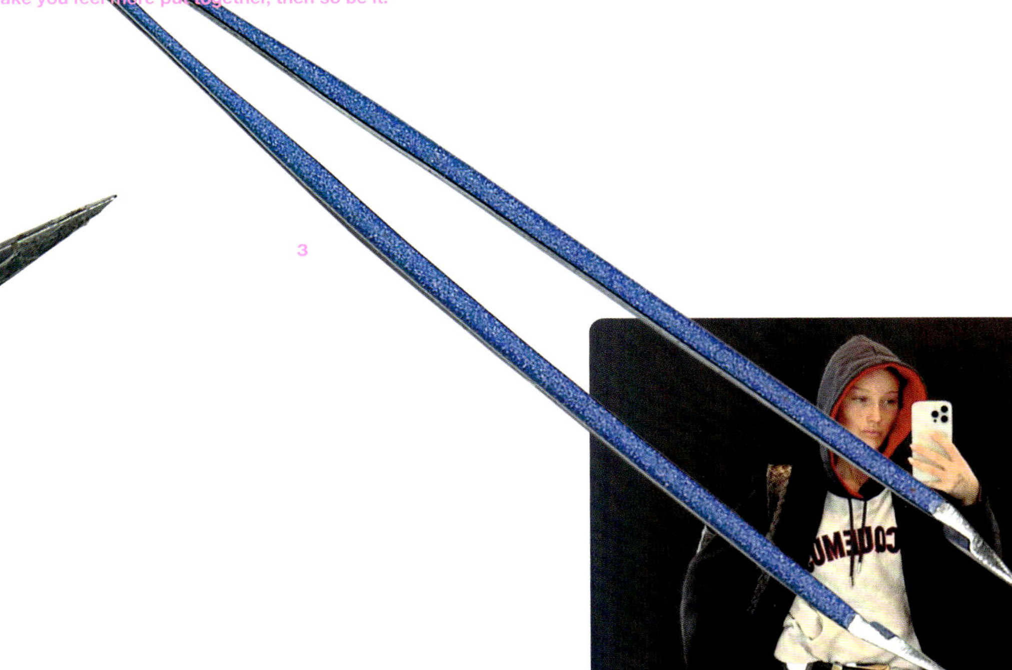

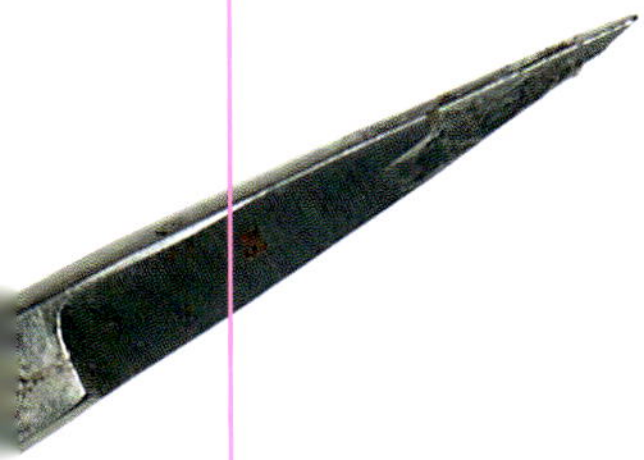

3

4

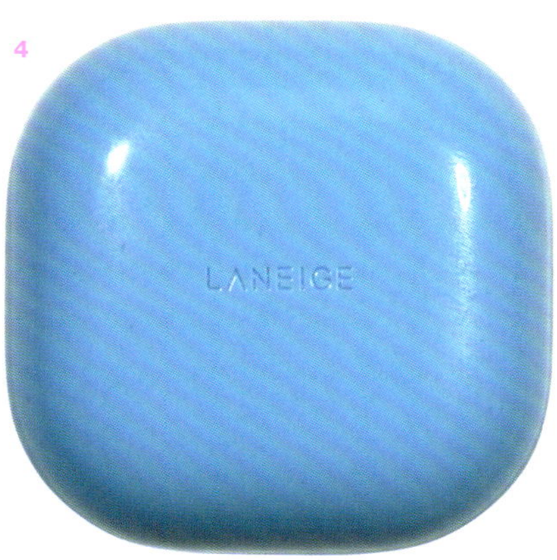

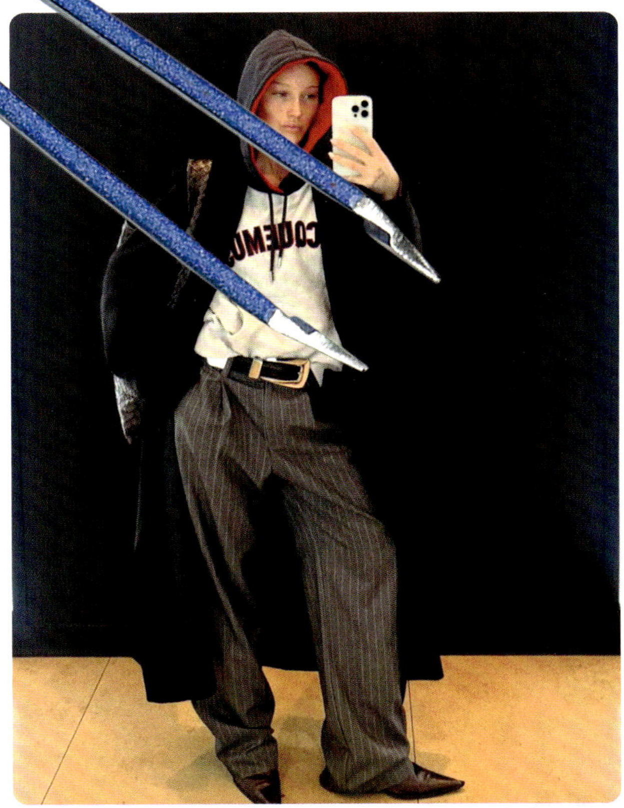

This was on my way to a casting! Modeling has truly pushed me to become more comfortable and confident in my own skin.

I love collecting pieces sent to me by brands. I have a special appreciation for them. Whenever I put this headband on, I feel so lucky that I get to work with brands like Dior Beauty.

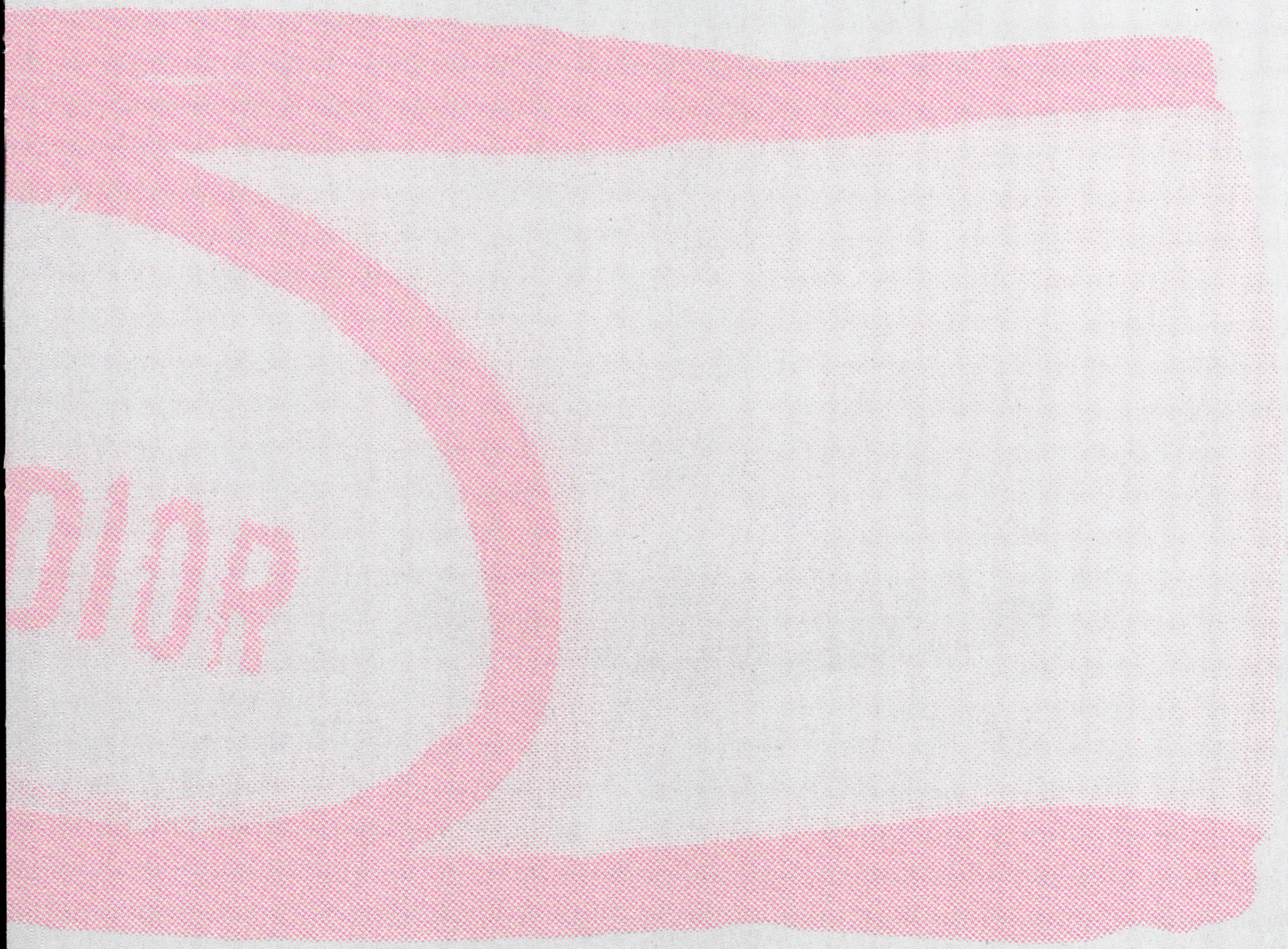
DIOR

Q At what point did you realize that you actually had too much filler?

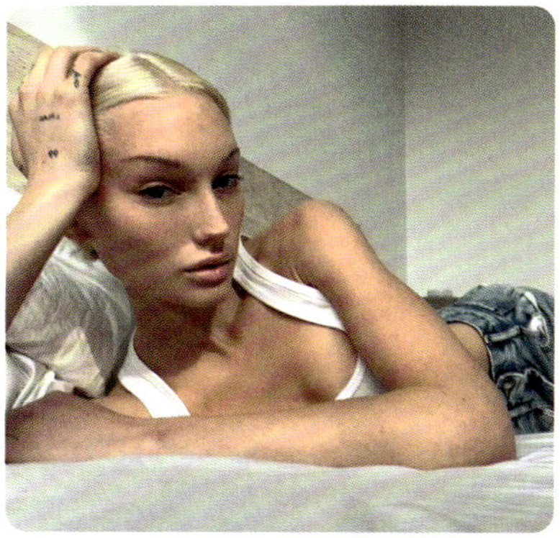

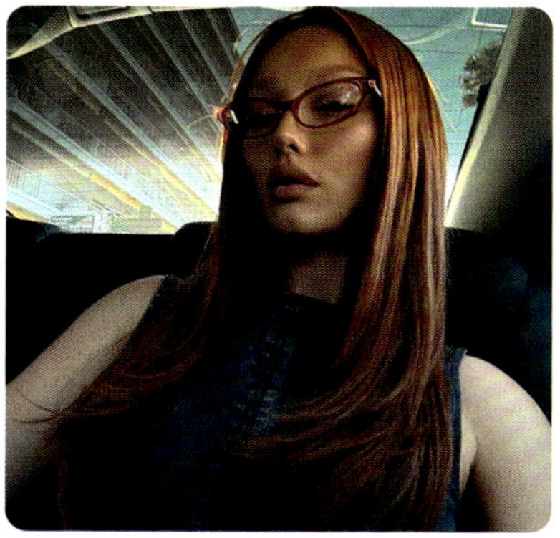

A face mask is an essential for me. It makes me feel cute while also doing good for my skin. I love popping one on while I'm cooking up dinner or chilling in bed with the pups! You can see above that I'm really in my natural era here, embracing my skin and letting my hair colors take the lead. Pay attention to your glam and how it lies on your skin after trying out new products! Not all products align well together. If you're not loving the way your makeup is turning out, look to your skincare products to see what the concern may be.

A I realized it when I started doing modeling and runway, and my team thought the more natural route was the way to go, especially in the European market. I thought, "Okay, I'll try it and see." I wanted to be successful and reach my goals, and I was willing to do anything to achieve them. It wasn't until after I dissolved the filler that I realized it was life-changing. I look back at it now and ask myself how I did not see how overfilled they were.

Q Have you ever looked at yourself or thought about a decision you were making and asked yourself, "Am I doing this for me, or am I doing this because I feel pressured to do it?"

A There are so many things that you look at in the mirror and might want changed. And you ask yourself, "But why do I want that done? Am I doing this for me or someone else?"

Q Throughout this whole conversation, we've talked about being comfortable in your own skin. Would you say that you feel comfortable in your skin now?

A Some days yes, some days no. It's a work in progress.

Q What days are harder than others?

A So many things in life and in our day-to-day affect our mood and emotions, and, of course, if we're having a bad day, we're going to feel more vulnerable about certain things, like our skin.

My community has contributed to making me feel a lot more confident in my skin, and that's exactly what I want to do for them as well.

Q Fill in the blank: I feel the most beautiful when…

A I'm happy.

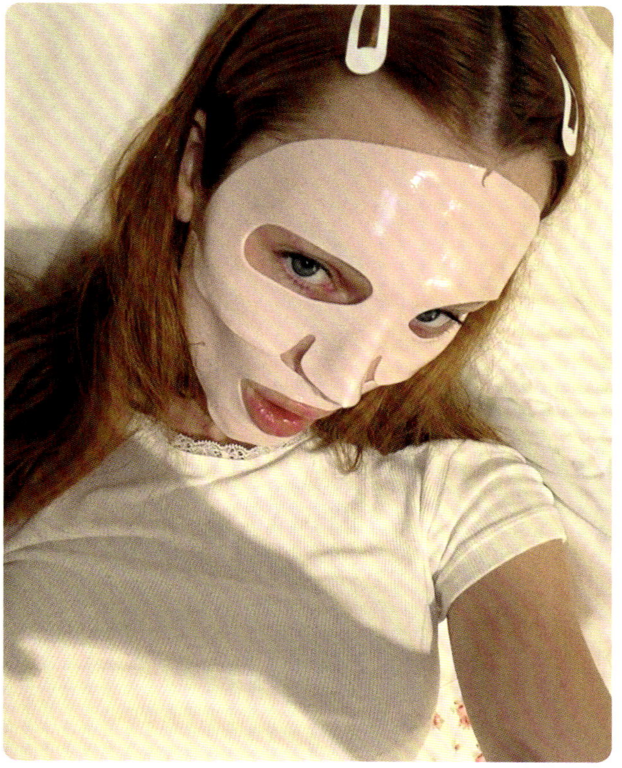

The Dr. Jart+ face masks...they're the cutest nighttime accessory to match your pj set, hehe! This is the Cryo Rubber Firming Peptide Mask. I think taking time out to do things for yourself is very important. We all deserve self-care. Using a face mask is one of my favorite ways to do that. Of course, it's even better when it's paired with a pint of Ben & Jerry's ice cream!

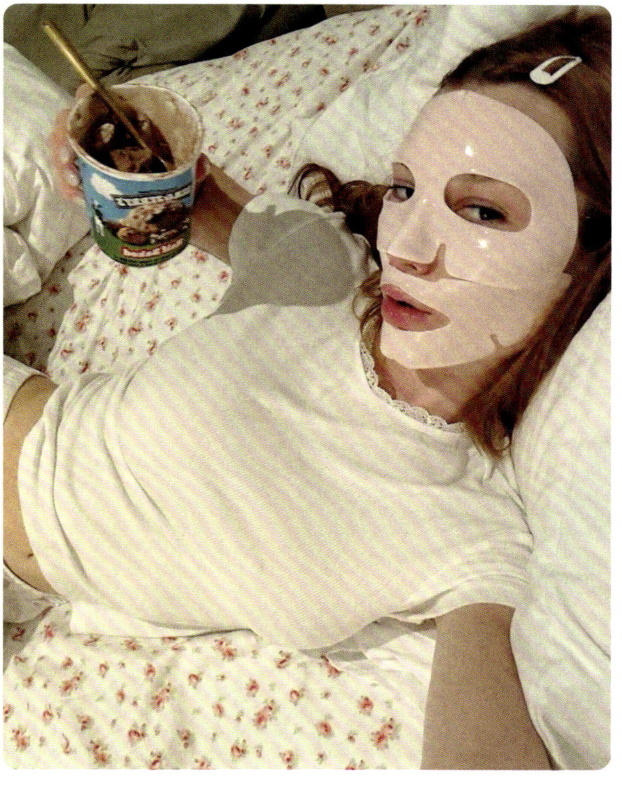

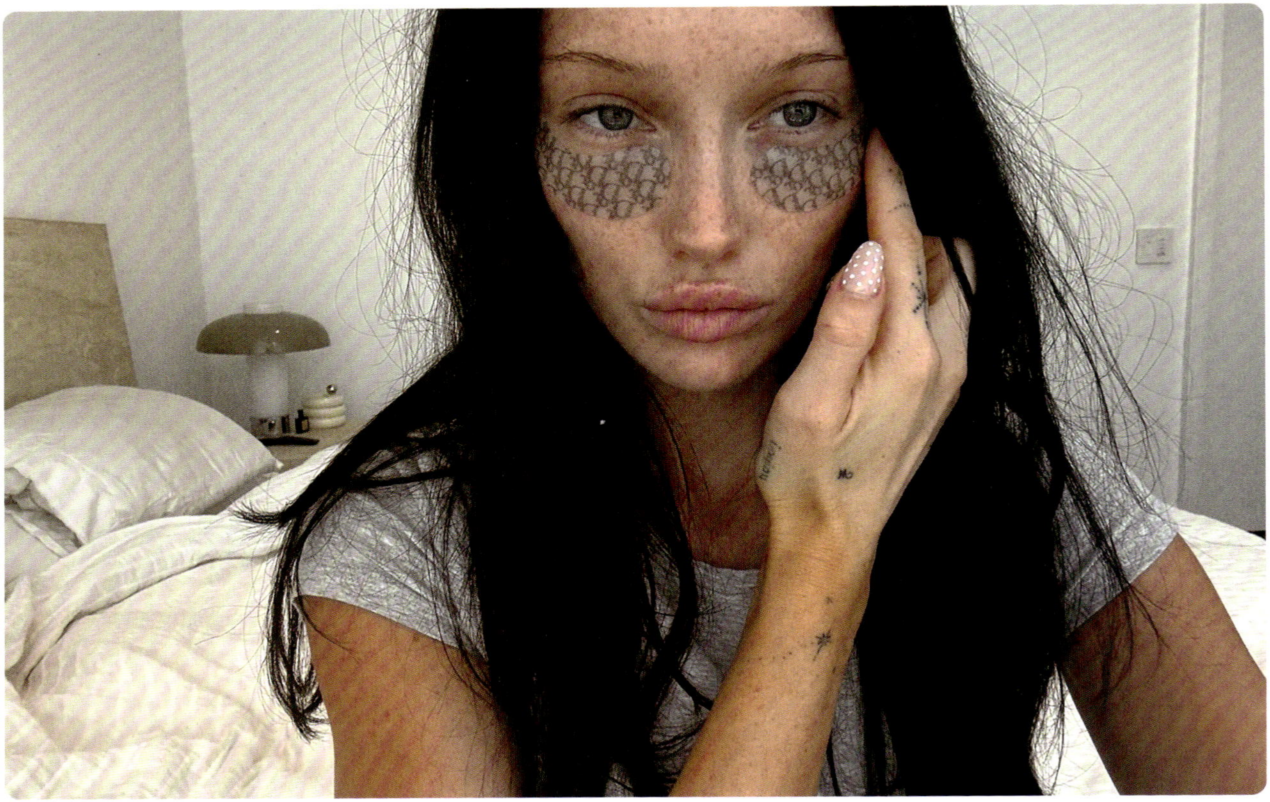

These Dior Beauty Eye Patches are so chic and a fun way to spoil yourself! It's easy to forget under-eye care, but your eyes deserve all the love, too! Plus, your concealer will lie so much smoother when you nourish those under eyes. Below is me in my super-natural era here! I let my hair play into this vibe with the beachy curls. Don't be afraid to really lean into a look!

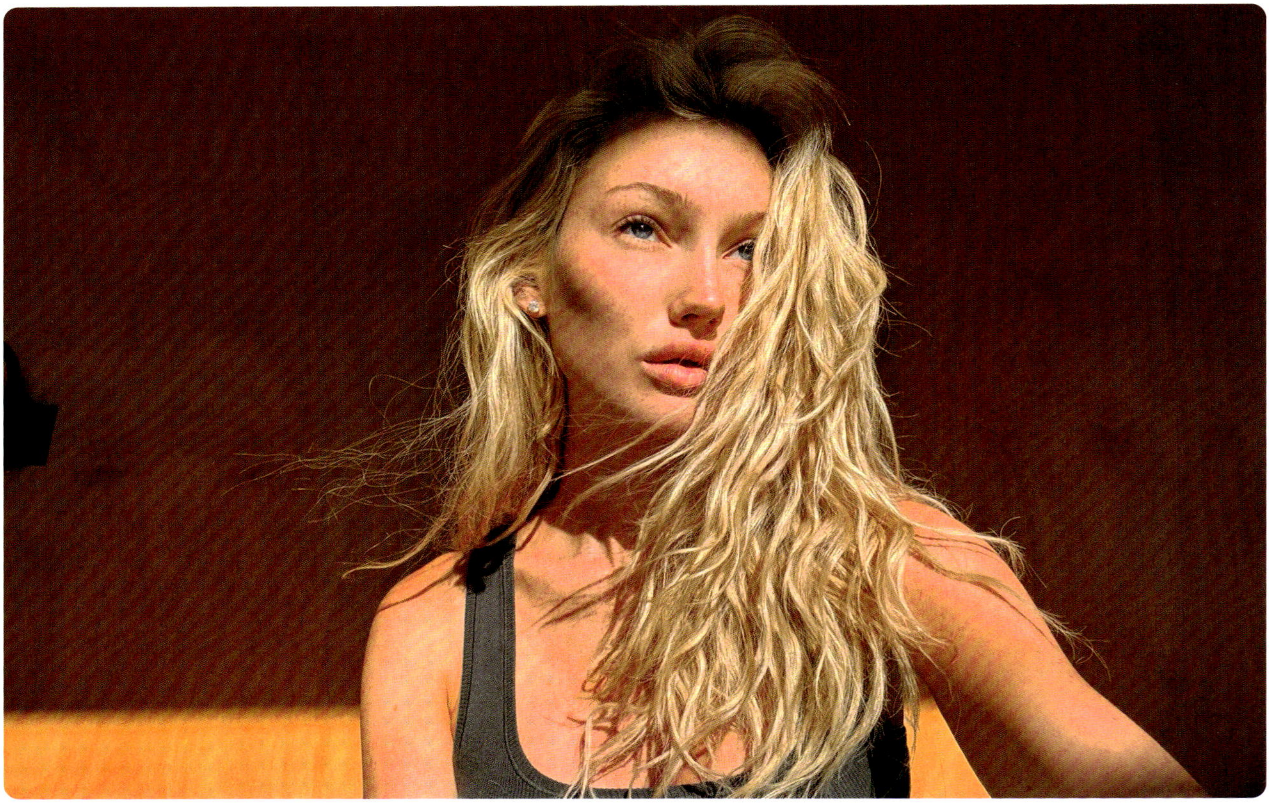

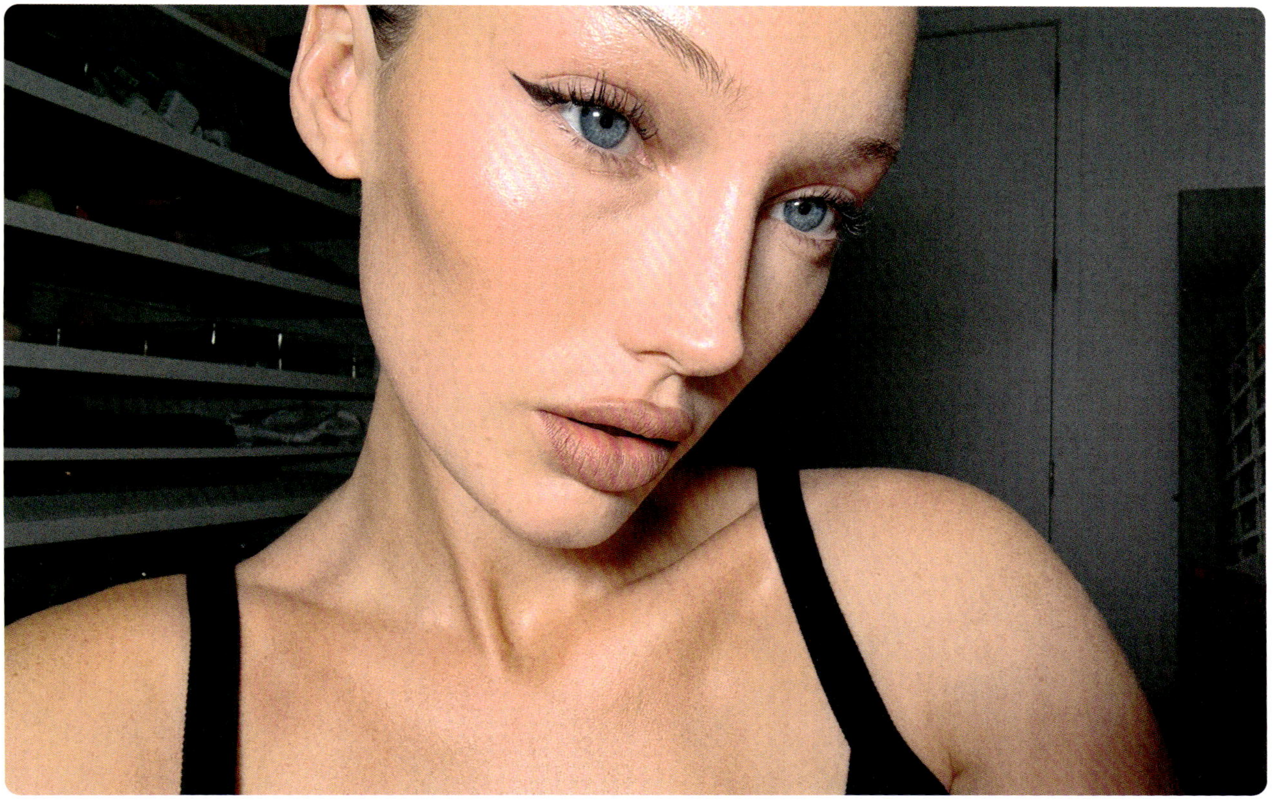

One of my favorite go-tos is a sleek, sharp eyeliner. I think there is something so angelic about it when paired with a fluttery or curled lash. I love seeing how my freckles look with each different hair color I try. I think the black hair brings the focus more to my eyes and makes my freckles appear a little softer. Food for thought: If you want to see a different version of yourself, try a new hair color or invest in a wig!

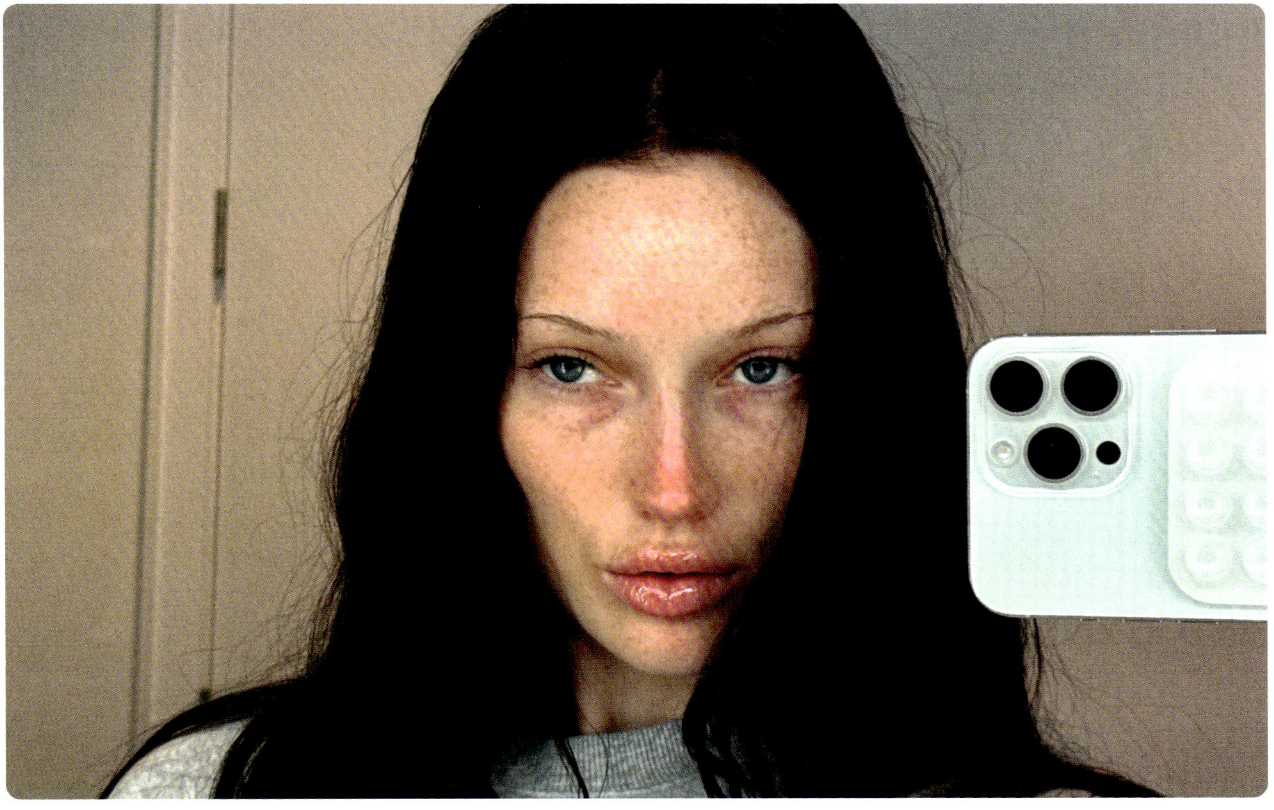

SKIN RAPID FIRE

Q If your freckles could talk, what would they say?
A We're kisses from the sun!

Q What is the first thing you do when you wake up and catch yourself in the mirror?
A Words of affirmation. I like to tell myself something I see that I'm liking in that moment, whether my hair looks good, my skin is glowing, or just simply that I'm looking hot!!

Q What is a skincare step that you will never skip, no matter how late it is?
A Moisturizer, my skin would hate me without it.

Q You have thirty seconds to leave the house. What is one thing you put on your face?
A Charlotte Tilbury Flawless Filter.

Q What is your delulu-but-it-works-for-me skincare belief?
A My toothpaste has a direct correlation with my skin.

Q If your skin had a personality, how would you describe her?
A She is just a girl trying to figure out her life.

Q What does aging gracefully mean to you?
A Aging how you please.

Q Which beauty trend makes you feel personally attacked?
A Clean-girl makeup.

Q What is one treatment you will never try?
A Snails crawling on my face. Never, ever, ever, ever.

Q What skincare product would have to be pried from your cold, dead hands?
A Kiehl's facial cleanser. I go through bottles of that.

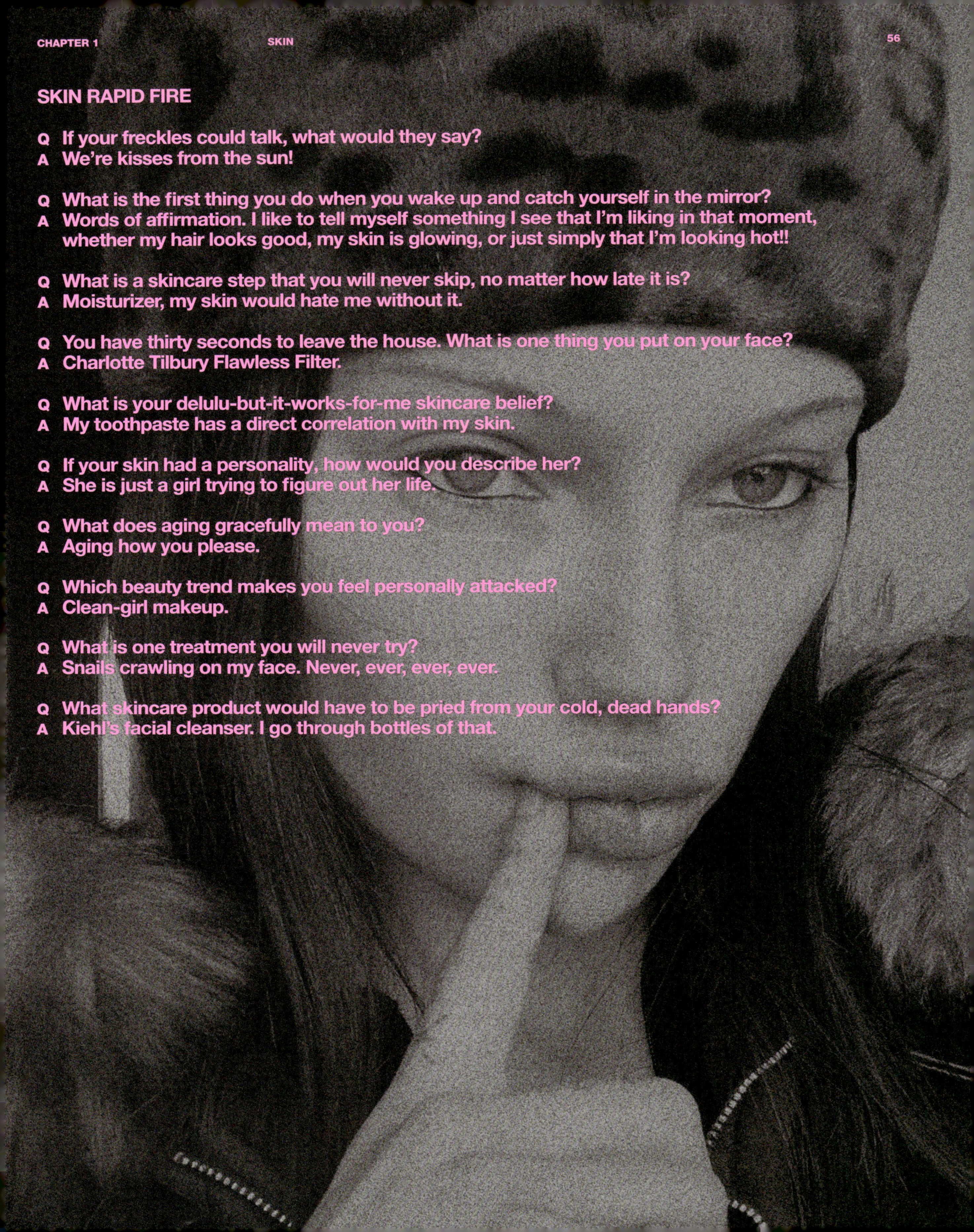

WOULD YOU RATHER

Q Botox or filler?
A Botox.

Q Perfect skin or perfect hair for life?
A Perfect hair.

Q A forehead that never shines or under eyes that never crease?
A Under eyes that never crease. Duh!

Q A breakout before a date or a sunburn before a photo shoot?
A A breakout before a date. I can fix that real quick.

Q Would you rather have glass skin in real life or airbrushed skin in photos?
A Airbrushed skin in photos—even if my skin is looking good, sometimes these photos like to trick us.

Q An SPF that magically appears on your face every two hours or a lip balm that reappears every time you lose it?
A A lip balm that appears every time I lose it. I've lost too many of them that have just disappeared into a black hole.

Q Under eyes that self-filter in every lighting situation, or a natural contour that always draws out your cheekbones?
A Under eyes that self-filter.

Q Do you want your derm on speed dial or a facialist who just knows what you need?
A A derm on speed dial. I never know when my skin is going to act out.

Q Skin that automatically clears overnight whenever you have a breakout or the ability to transfer your breakouts to your frenemies? You want to be chaotic. I know which one you can go with.
A Yeah, breakout to the frenemy! Ooop!

Q Hormonal acne that only shows up when you're in a good mood or dry patches that hit only on important days?
A Dry patches on important days. Let's let the good moods have their moment.

Q Which of these things do you bring to a desert island? Makeup or skincare…
A Makeup. At least I could take some glam shots in my free time there, lol.

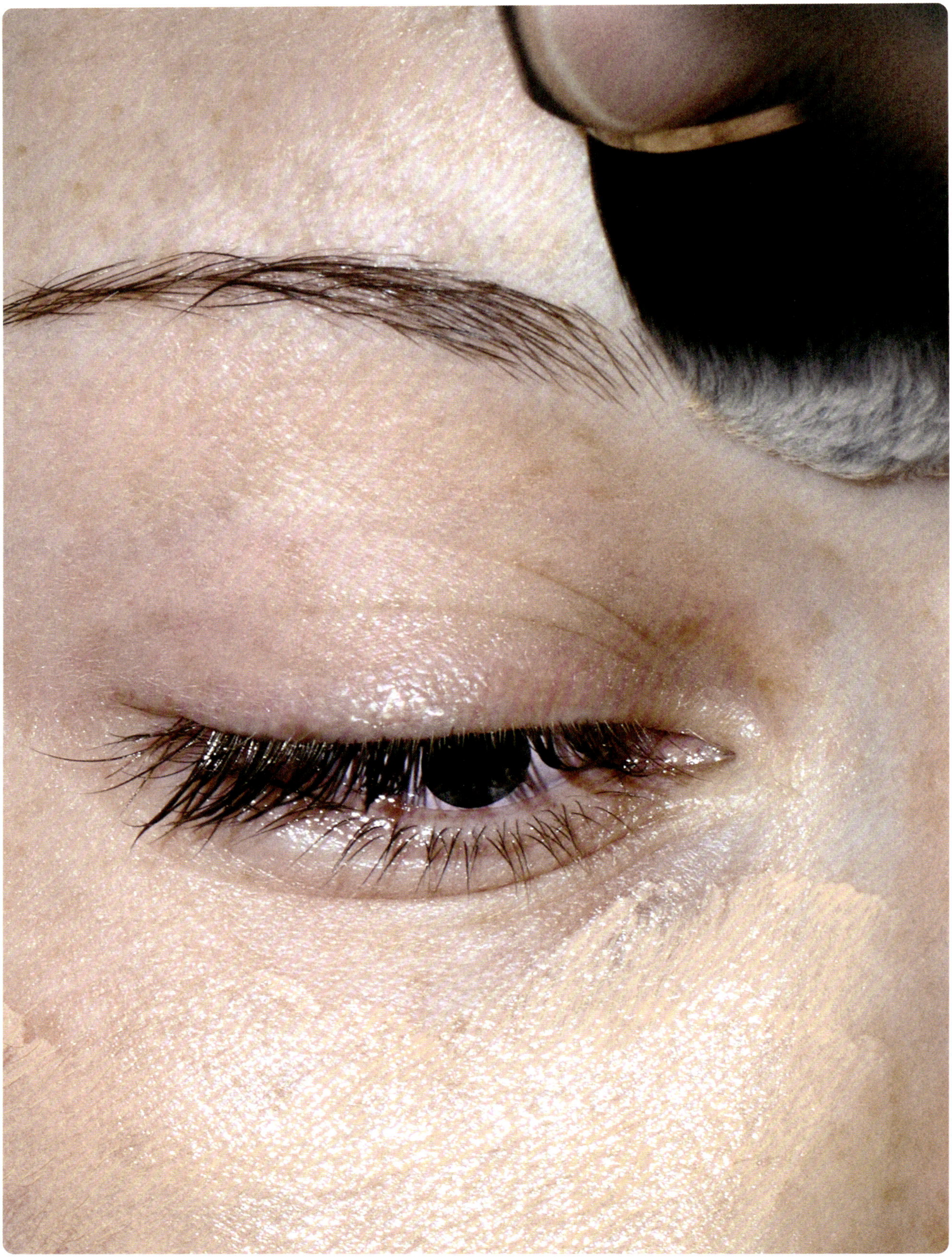

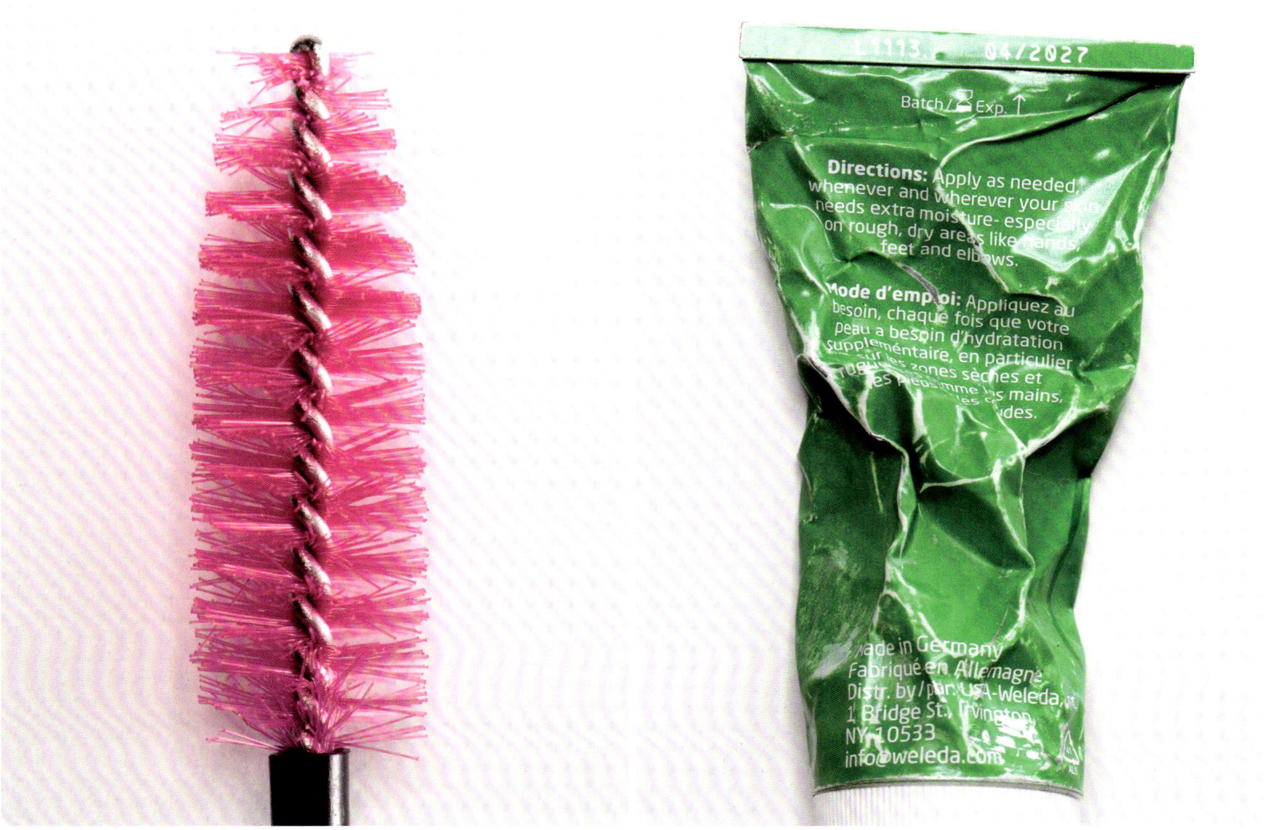
04/2027
Batch/ Exp.
Directions: Apply as needed,
whenever and wherever your skin
needs extra moisture- especially
on rough, dry areas like hands,
feet and elbows.
besoin, chaque fois que votre
peau a besoin d'hydratation
supplémentaire, en particulier
Fabriqué en Allemagne
NY 10533
info@weleda.com

GLAM

2

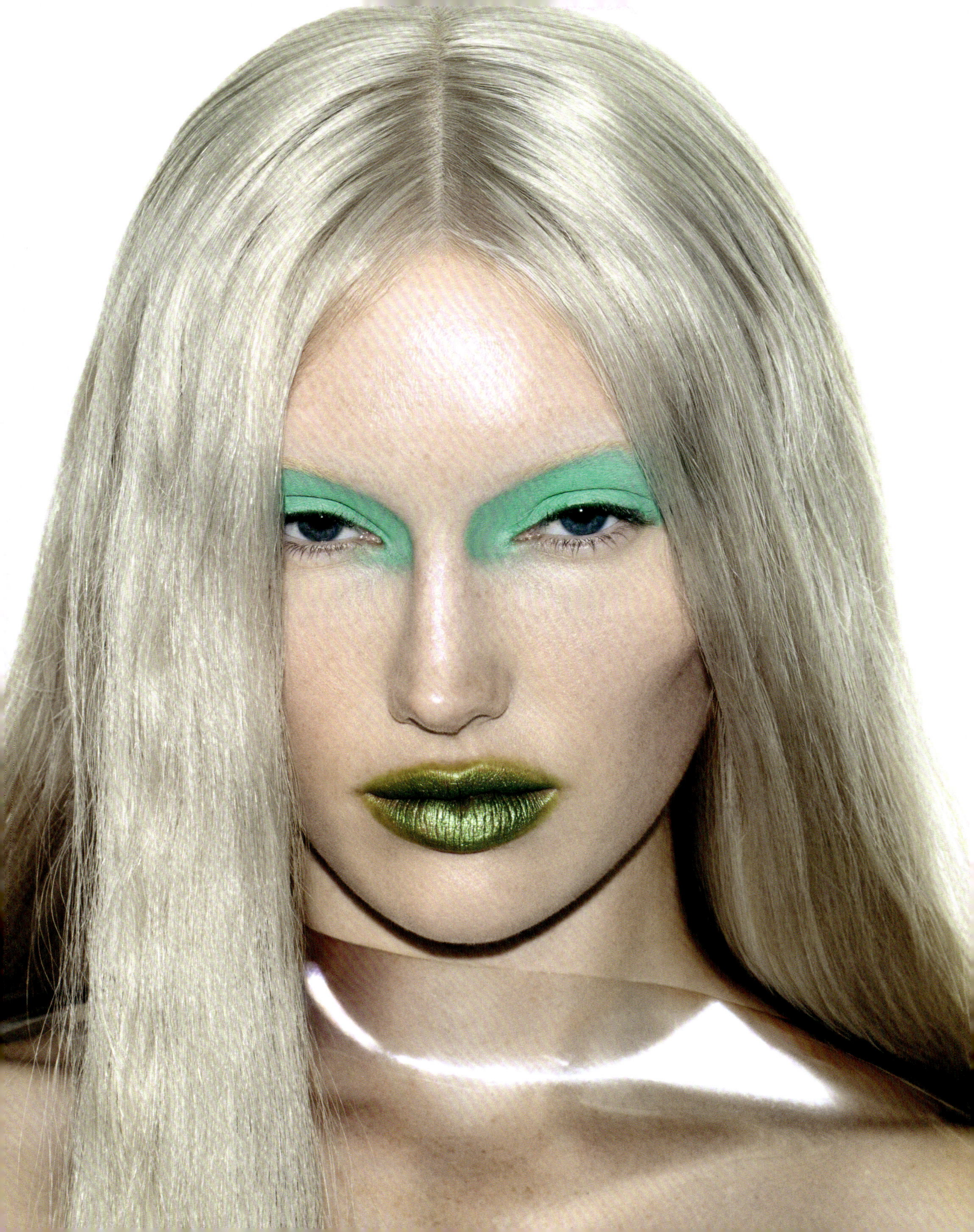

Makeup is meant to be fun! It's a way to express yourself, your creativity, and your passion. The reason makeup is such a form of art is because there are no rules; you're meant to color outside the lines! No two faces are the same, and that's what makes makeup so beautiful—each individual is going to have their own tips, tricks, and routine that works for them!

Glam, for me, has never been about looking perfect; it's about expressing yourself through a different lens. It's about slipping into a version of myself I haven't met yet, a new character I want to play, or simply just a louder version of myself. But that's the magic of glam: People can interpret it in any way they want.

When I'm in glam, I feel like there are no expectations or pressures of who I'm supposed to be. I can be whoever I want. Glam has always been my playground. The place where rules don't matter, mistakes turn into trends, and experimentation is the whole point.

This chapter is about that chaos. The freedom, the fun, the delusion, the reinvention. The haircuts that made me cry. The brows I shaved off on impulse. The ten pump technique that accidentally changed my life. Glam isn't about perfection. It's about the thrill of becoming the exaggerated, expressive, unapologetic version of myself I always knew was in there.

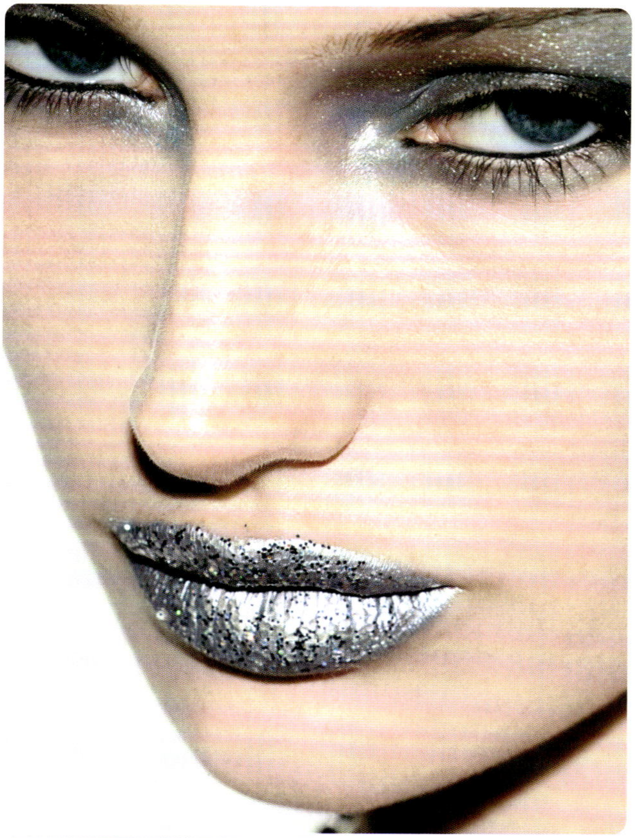

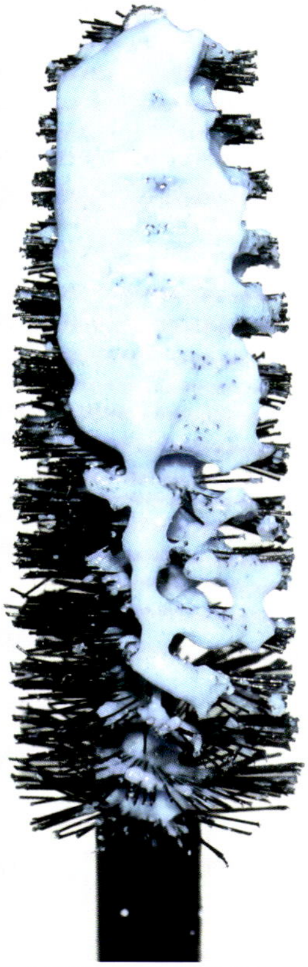

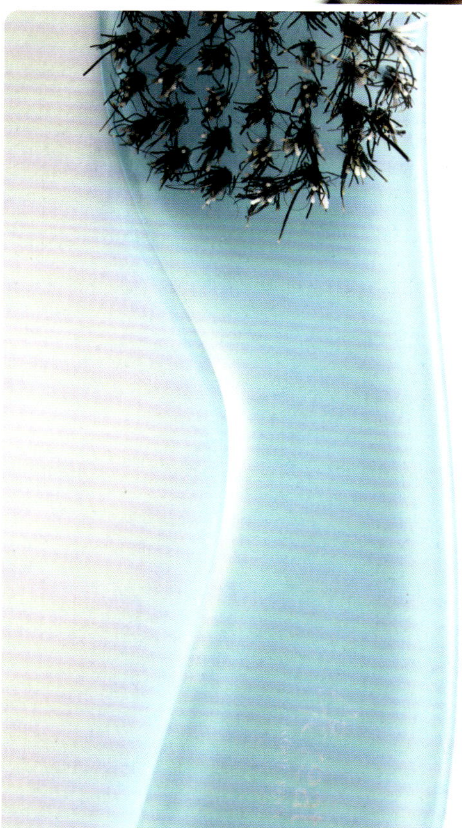

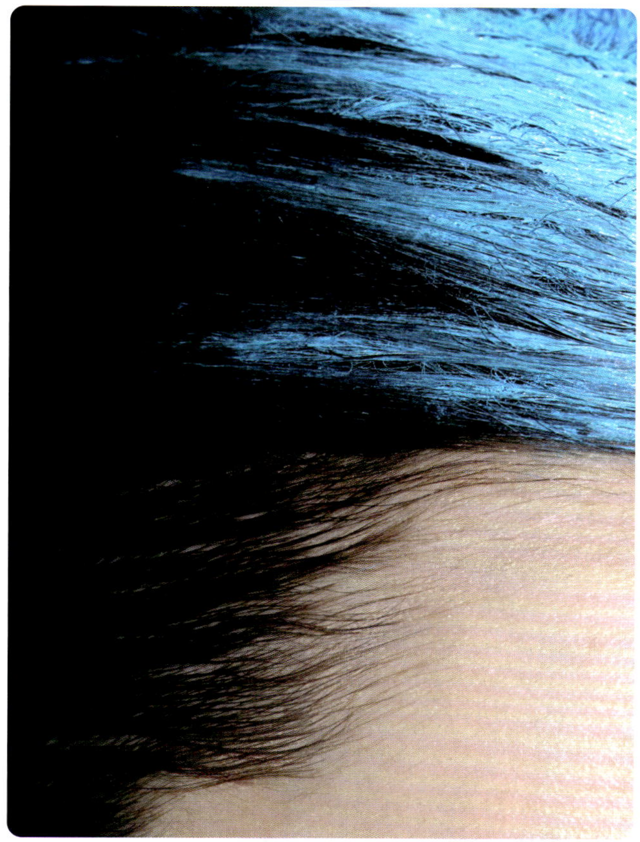

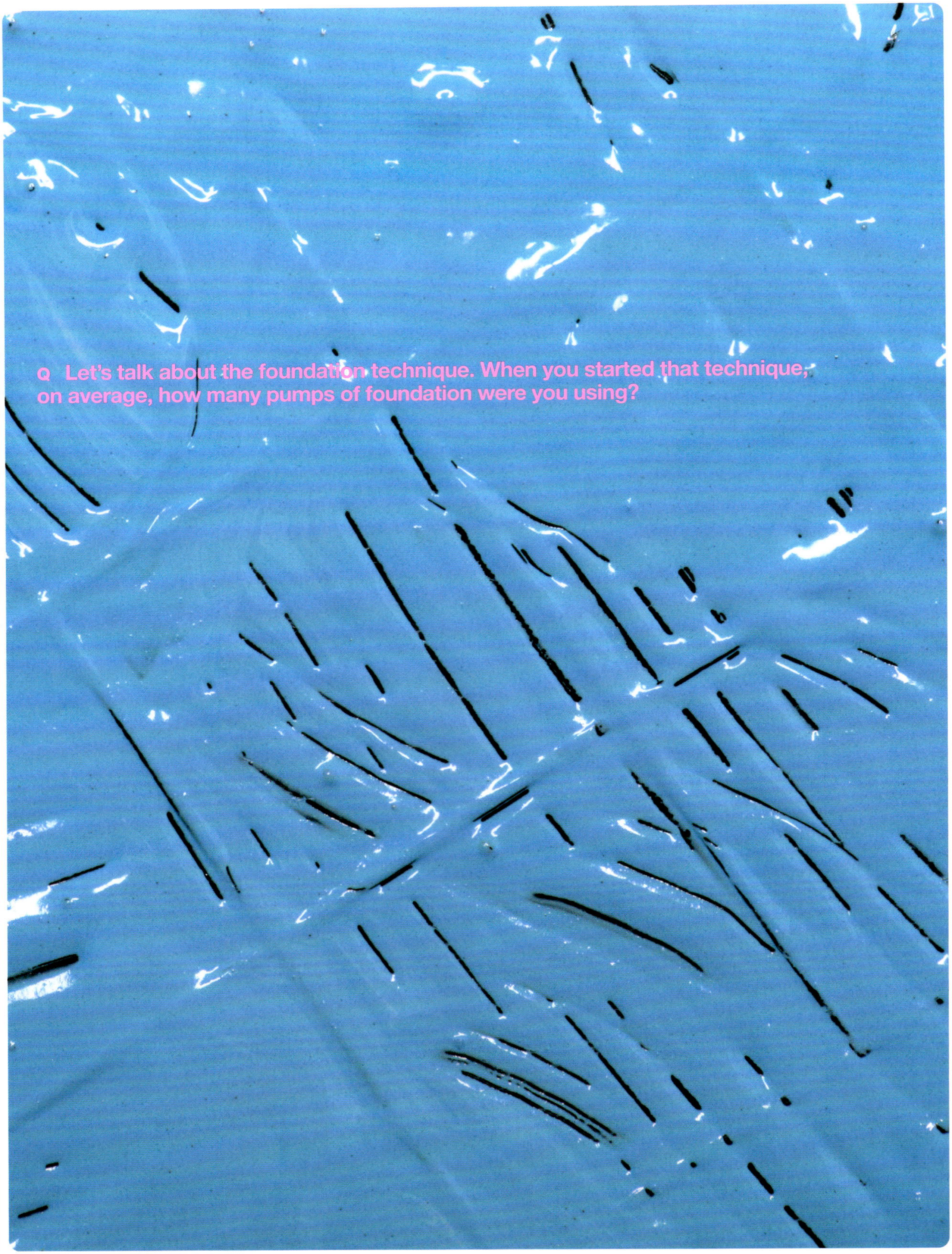

Q Let's talk about the foundation technique. When you started that technique, on average, how many pumps of foundation were you using?

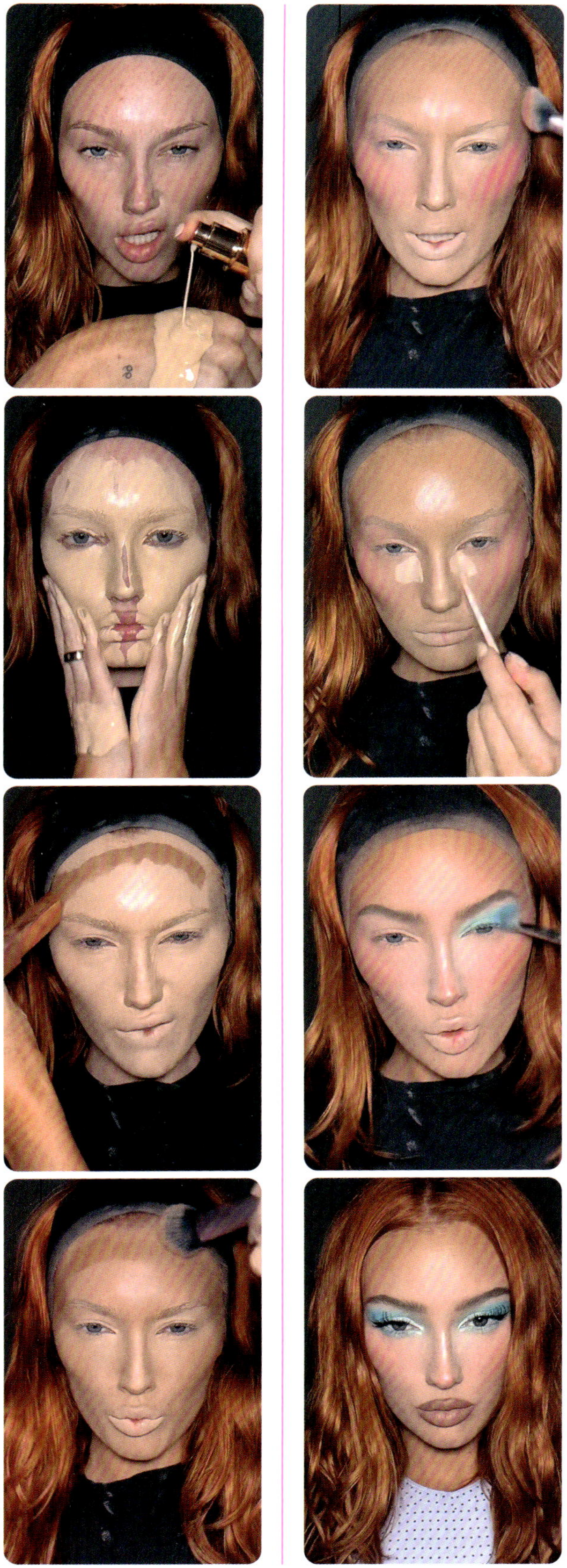

A Ooh, now the juicy stuff…ten pumps!

Q What made you decide that your hands were the tools as opposed to a makeup brush or a beauty brush?

A It really stemmed from the insecurity I had about my freckles when I was younger. I've grown to love and embrace them, but at the time, I wanted them totally covered, and no tools were doing that for me except my hands, because they didn't absorb the foundation. When I was cleaning my makeup brushes, so much product would come out of them that was just being wasted. As a college student, I didn't have much money, and I couldn't afford to waste $55 on a new foundation bottle every week. I also just loved the way my hands melted the foundation into my skin. Turns out many skilled makeup artists use this approach!

Q What was people's initial reaction?

A "What the f***????" "Are you crazy!?" "Why are you doing this?" They were shocked, lol.

People were convinced that I was wiping it off my face. It was kind of an accusation that I had to live with. There was nothing I could do about it. People were so shocked by the amount of product I put on my face that they couldn't believe that I would walk outside like that.

Q Well, they probably thought it was a nice attention-grabbing bit, right?

A Yeah, they thought it was clickbait!

Q Let's clear it up here once and for all, because you made a video saying you wiped off some of your foundation pumps. Is it true that you actually did that?

A The ten pumps is real. When TikTok was going to be banned in 2025, there was a trend where everyone was making these funny confessional videos—like, if TikTok is going away, I might as well reveal and share my deepest, darkest secrets. So I thought it would be funny to play into the whole conspiracy that people had about me, that I wipe off the foundation.

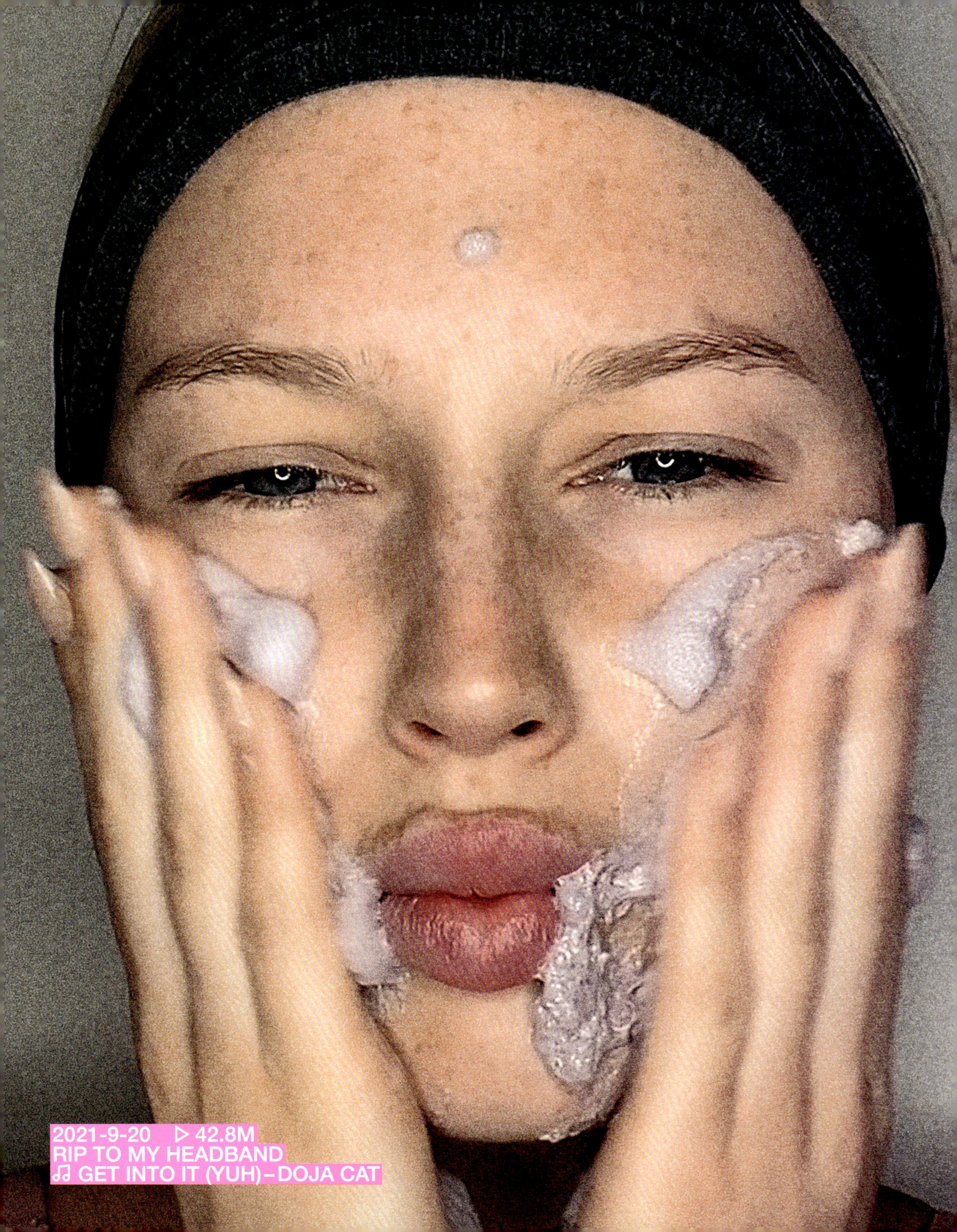
2021-9-20 ▷ 42.8M
RIP TO MY HEADBAND
♫ GET INTO IT (YUH)–DOJA CAT

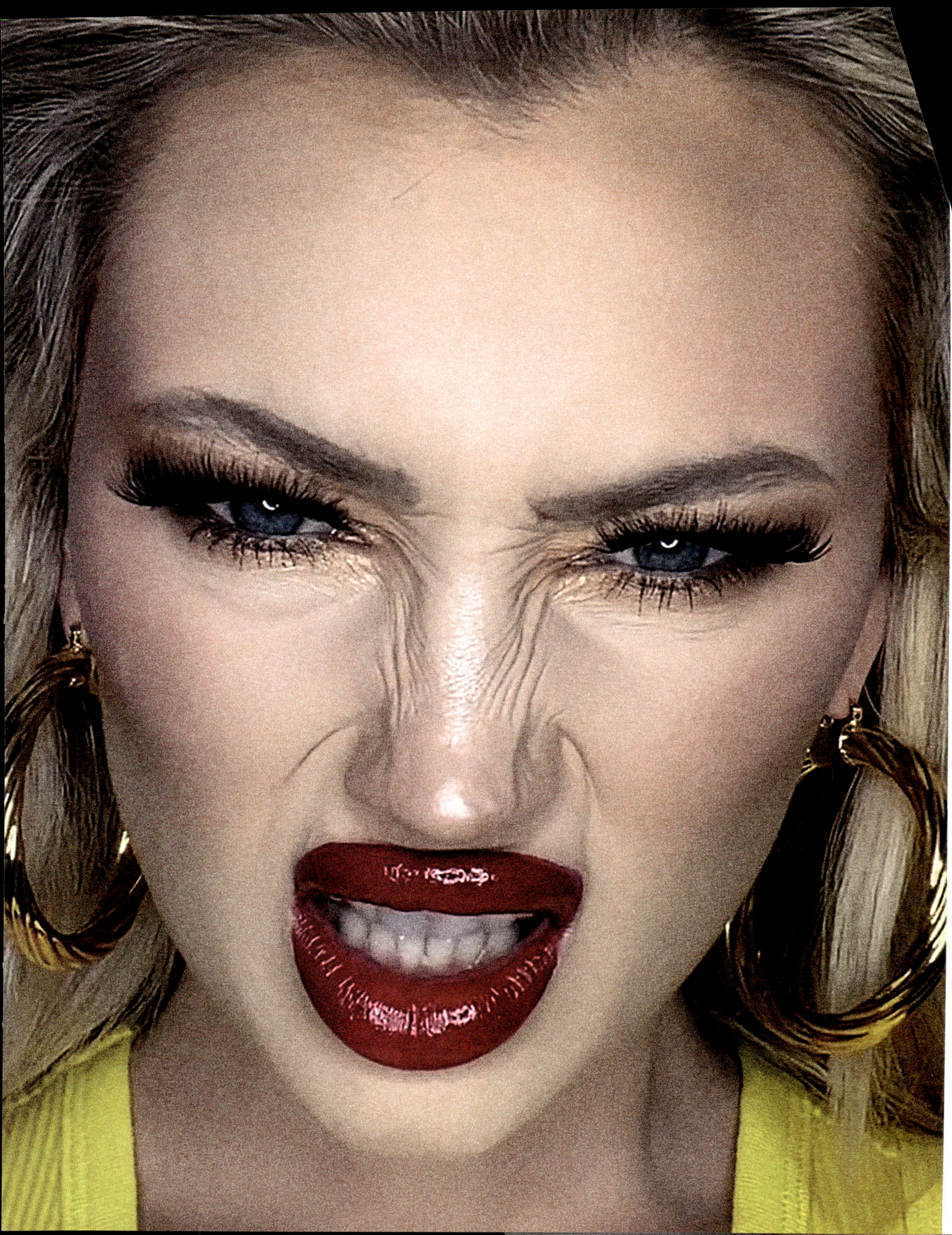

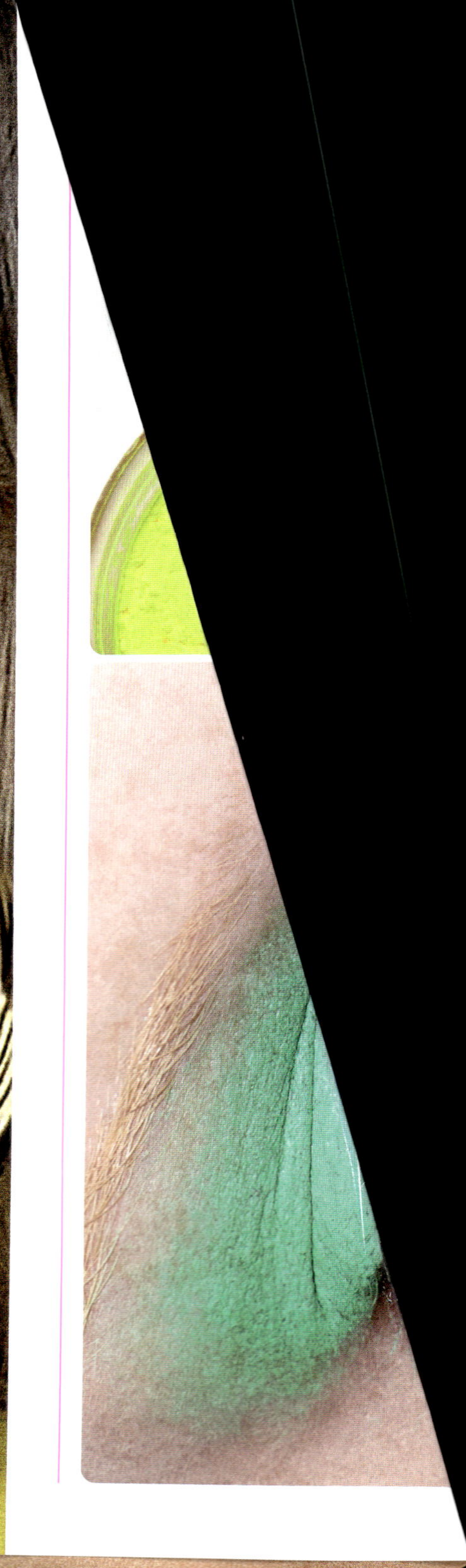

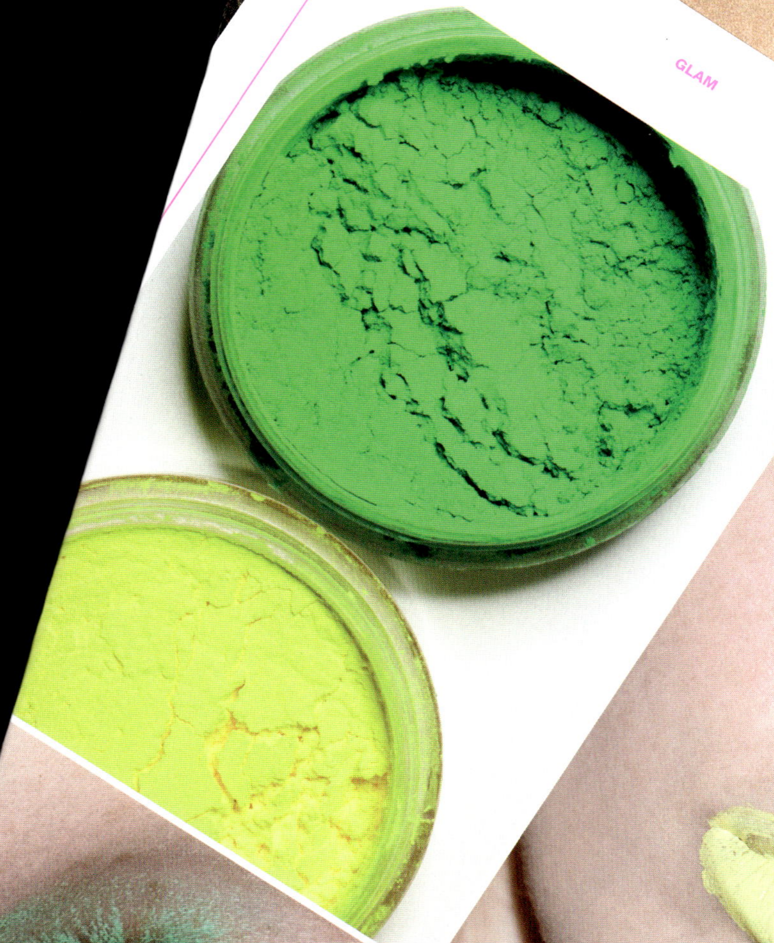

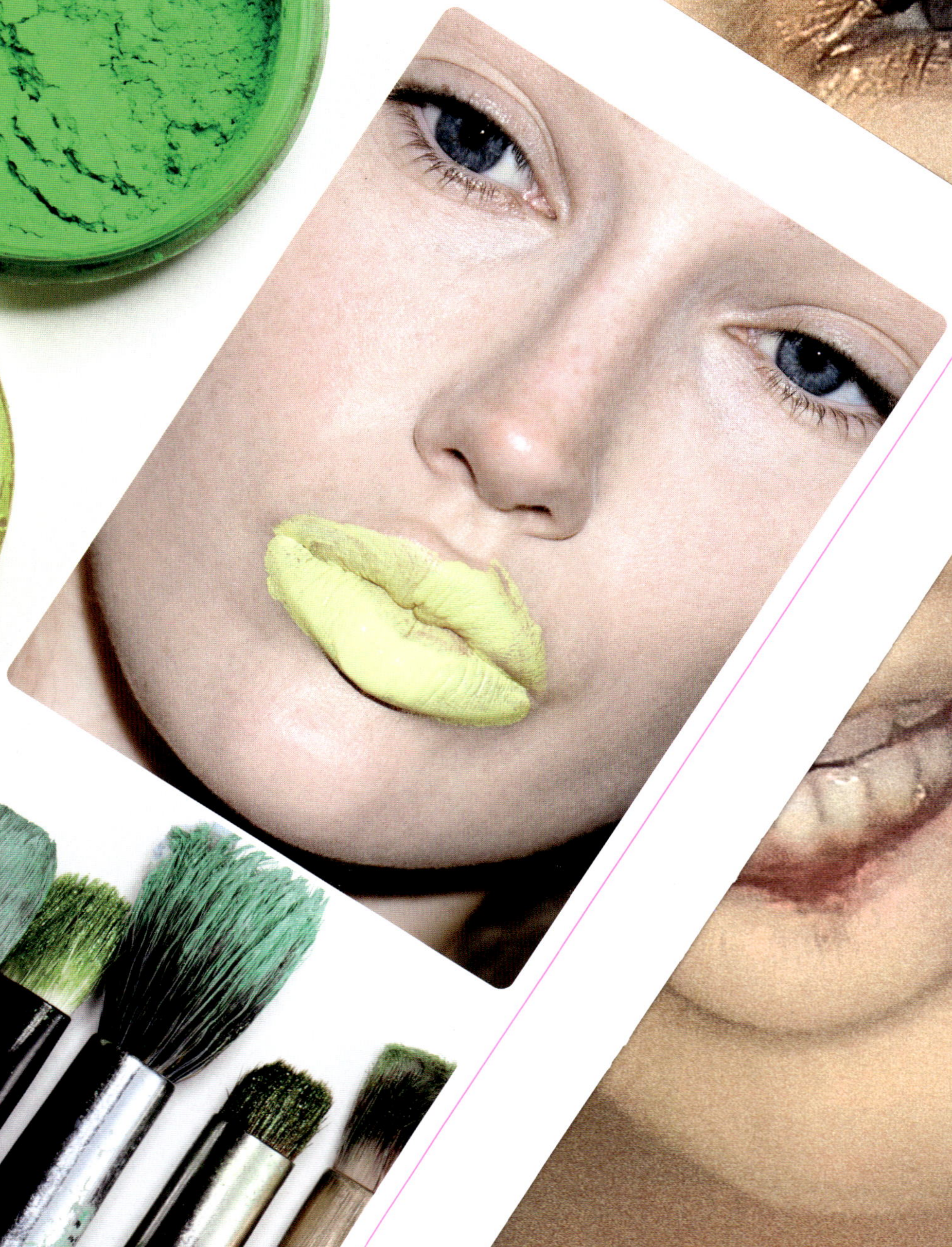

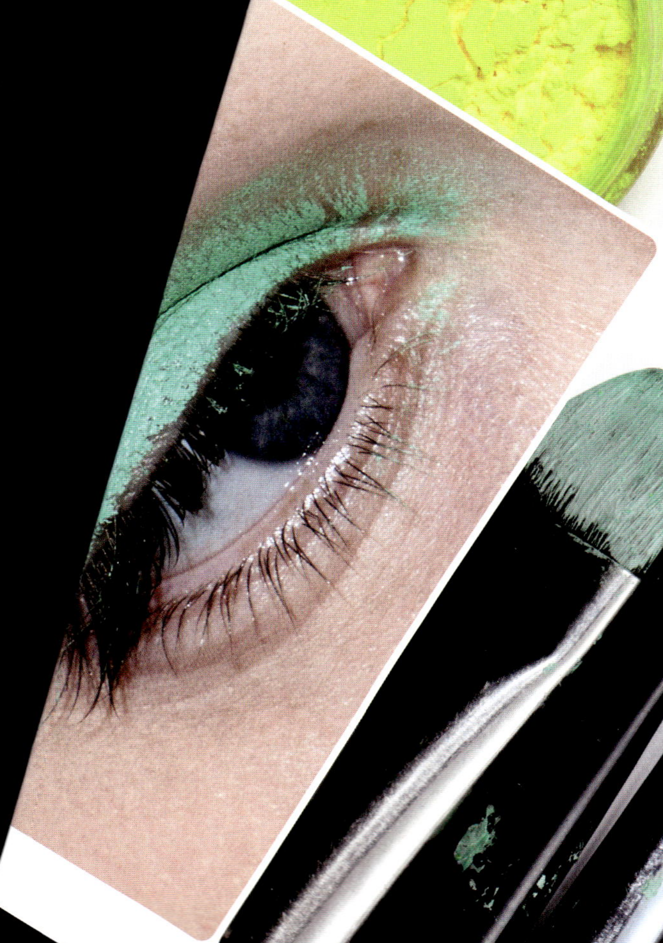

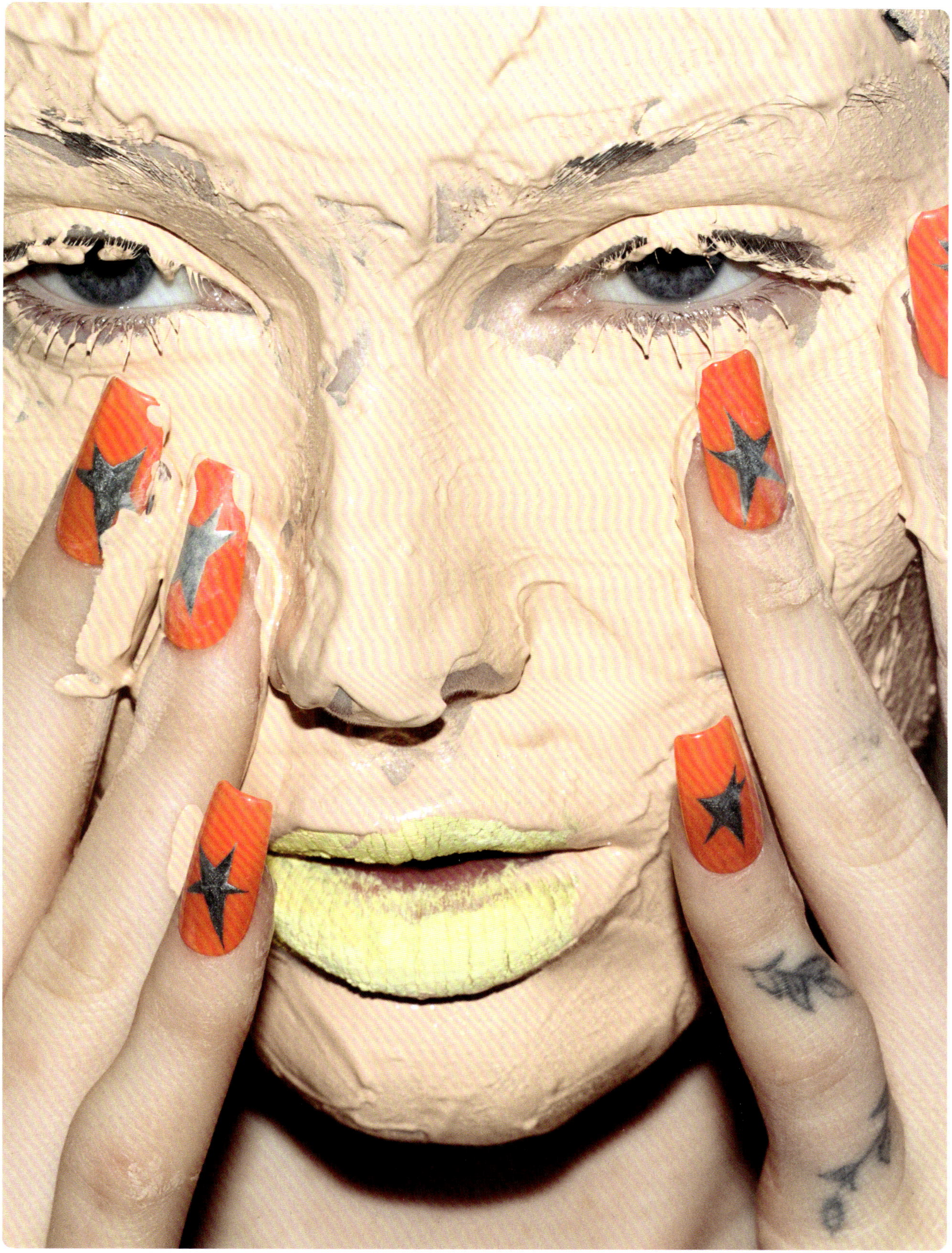

A I thought, "Okay, TikTok is ending. Let's create a little chaos." And then people ran with it and were like, "Oh, my God. I knew I was right!" and I was like, "Guys, it was a joke...."

I always get at least one comment saying, "She made a video confessing it. She wipes it off. It's true." It was hard because a lot of people didn't want to trust me after that, but I think people need to learn to play into trends because it's really not that serious.

Q Okay. Be honest. At any point, have you laughed your head off at some of the reactions to your foundation technique?

A Omg, of course. It's so entertaining when other people try the technique, and they're just so shocked by the texture and the feel of putting that much foundation on their face. It's hilarious because it was my norm, so it was fun to live vicariously through them all trying it for the first time.

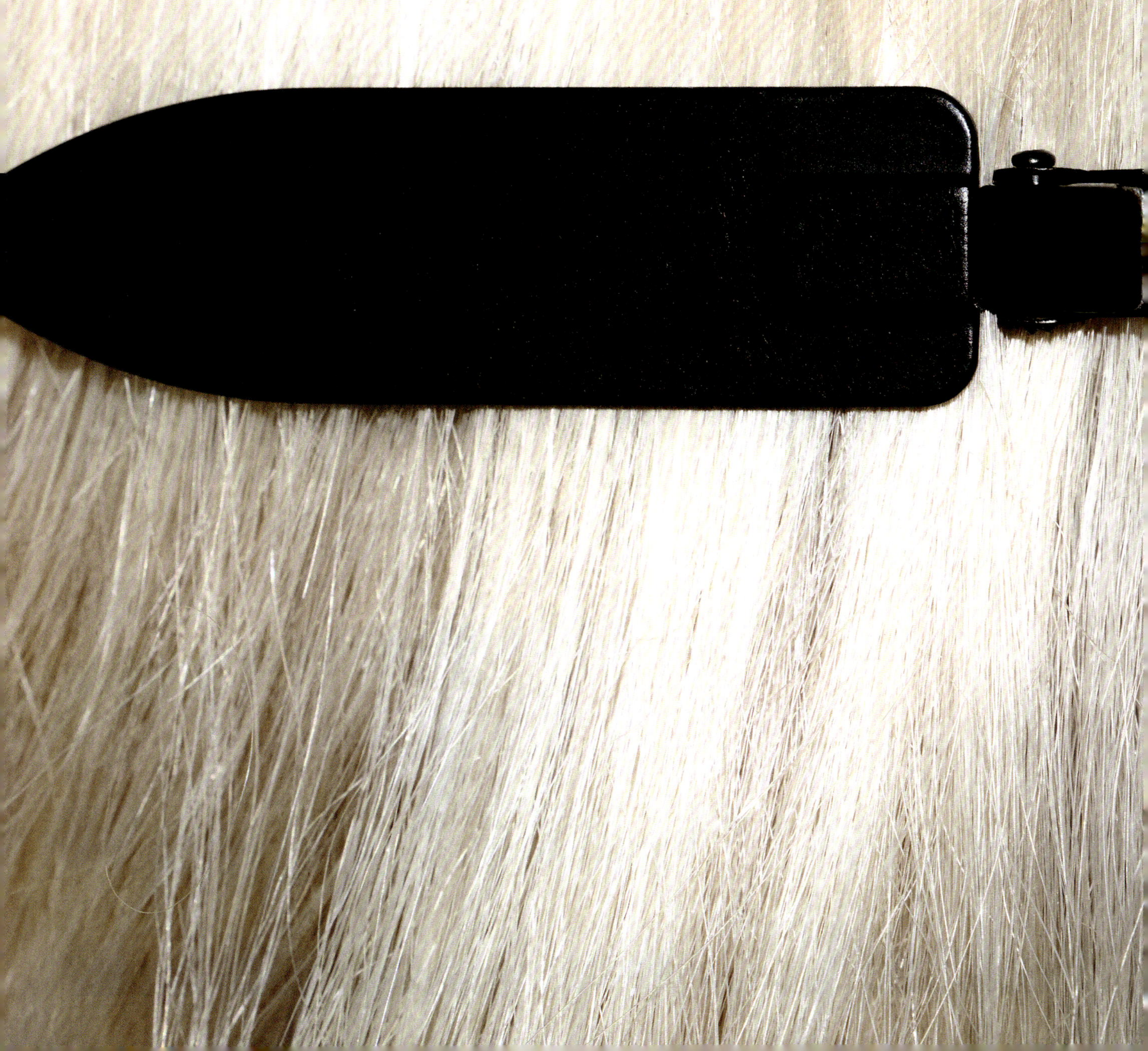

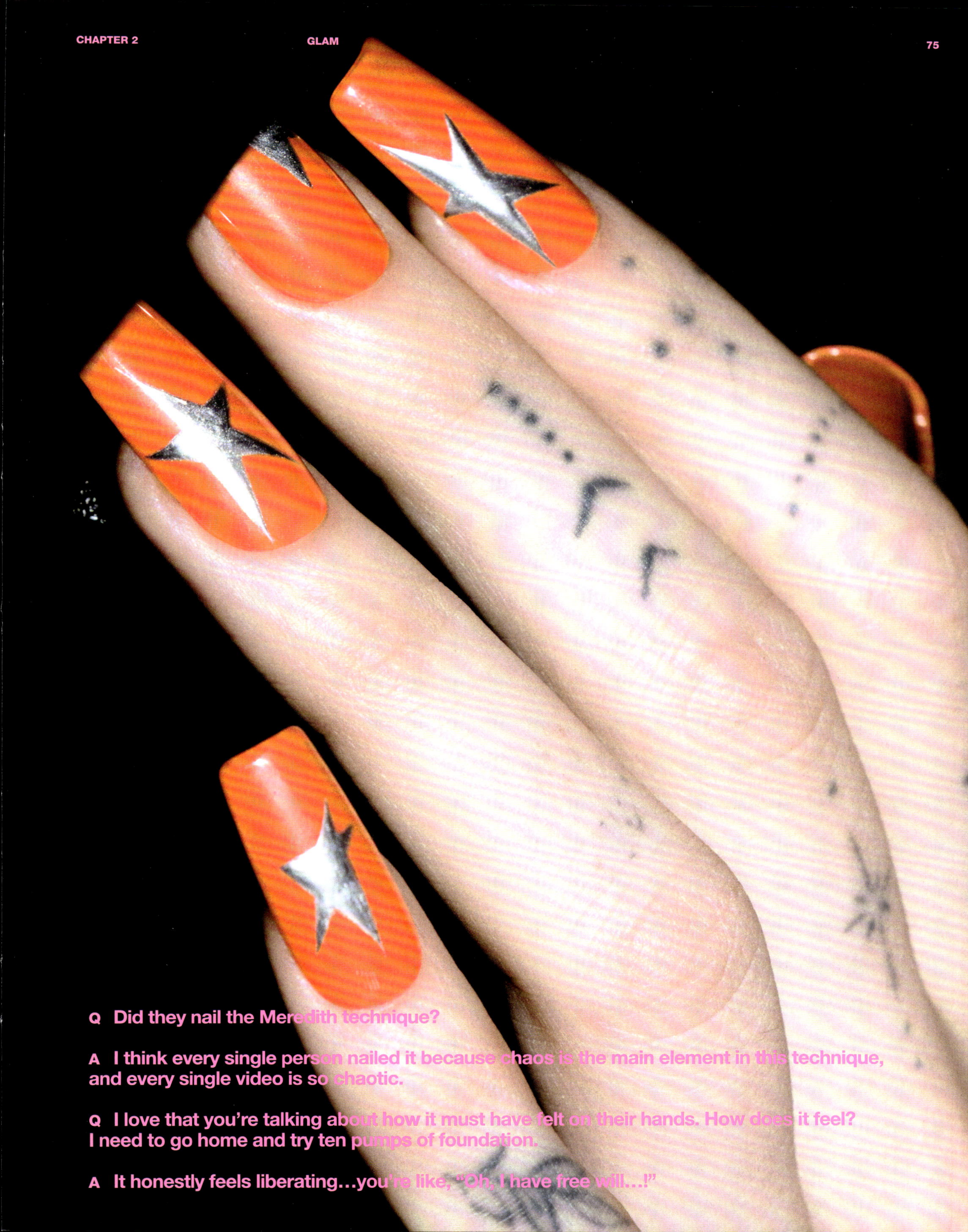

Q Did they nail the Meredith technique?

A I think every single person nailed it because chaos is the main element in this technique, and every single video is so chaotic.

Q I love that you're talking about how it must have felt on their hands. How does it feel? I need to go home and try ten pumps of foundation.

A It honestly feels liberating…you're like, "Oh, I have free will…!"

Q Looking back, is there something that you would do differently from when you first started?

A I would not change a thing because I'm so happy with the outcome, and I know that I have inspired a lot of people.

Q I love that you went viral lip-syncing to songs, like Nicki Minaj's "I'm Legit." What would the soundtrack of your glam be now? Three songs, no skips.

A "Sports Car" by Tate McRae, "Pussy Palace" by Lily Allen, and "Girls" by The Dare.

Q You previously told me you were in your soft-girl era. What era are you in now?

A Messy-girl era, for sure. Messy means no rules, no regulations, not thinking too hard, and just doing. It's important to show the imperfections and be as raw, real, and vulnerable as you can. I think we're coming out of the clean-girl era, and people really want to see relatable content.

Q How does your glam differ on a day-to-day basis from your everyday to the events? What do you do on the red carpet that is different than your everyday look? What are the commonalities?

A I would say my base is really the same for a lot of them now. What I change up the most is the eyes. The way you do your eye makeup can change a look so much—whether it's a cat eye or a doe eye, or if it's sparkly, matte, or smoky.

A look really comes together when you have both the hair and the outfit on as well. When you're sitting in your glam room with your pj's on, and you see this crazy glam, it doesn't always look right. But then when you see the full picture, it's like, *Ooooooh, okkkk!*

Q You recently said you are ready to move past the minimal space and get fun again. What does fun mean in Meredith World?

A Doing makeup as you please, add color, have fun! I hate rules, and I especially hate rules for makeup. That is not a thing to me.

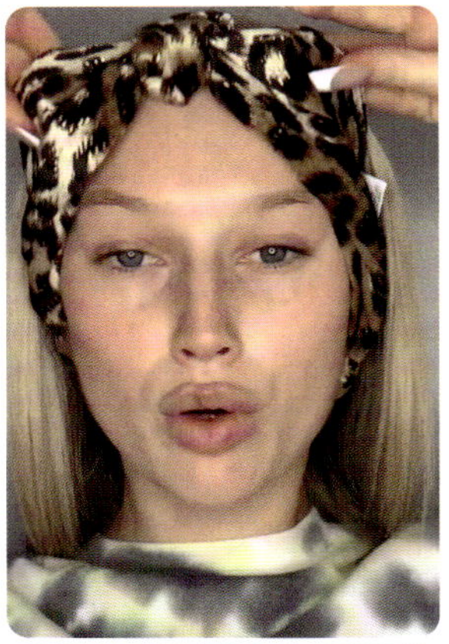
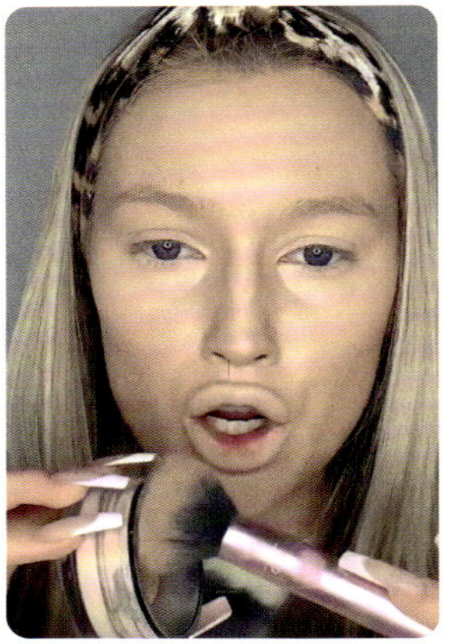
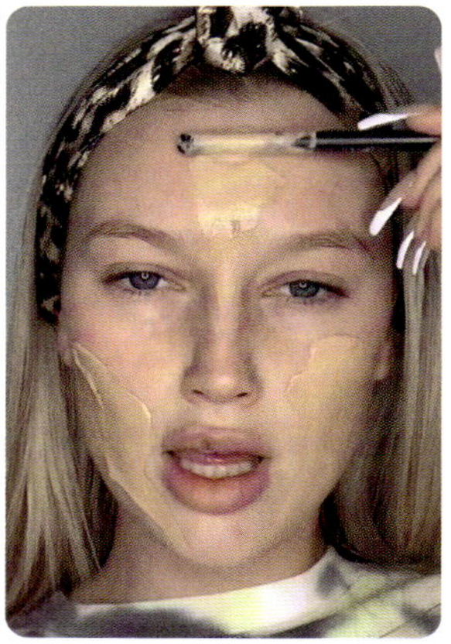
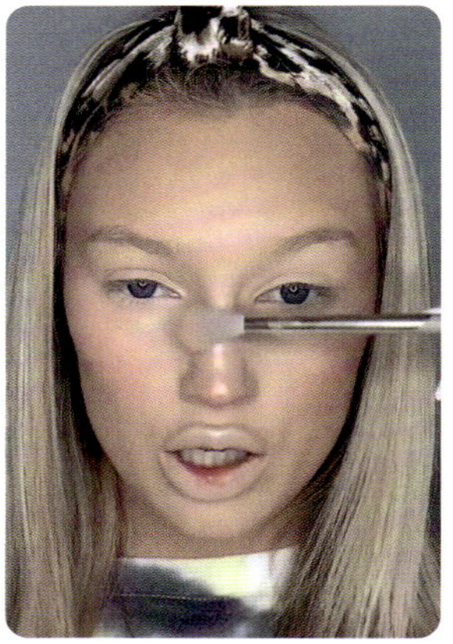
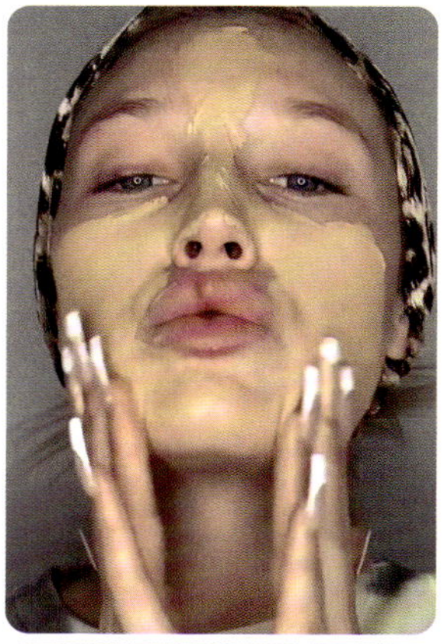
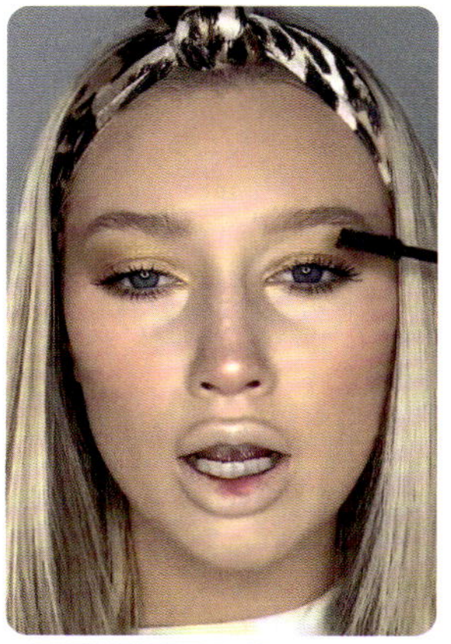
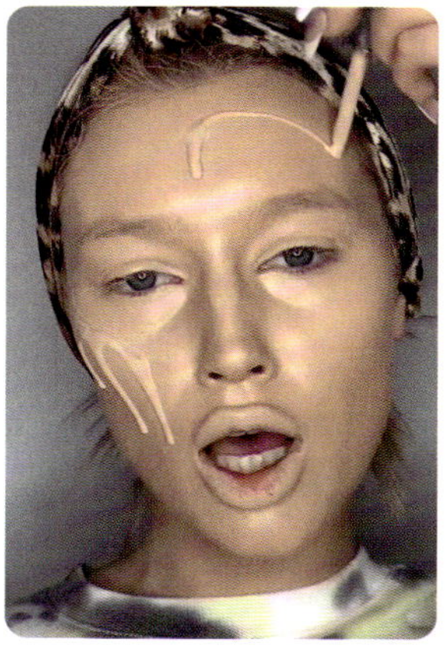
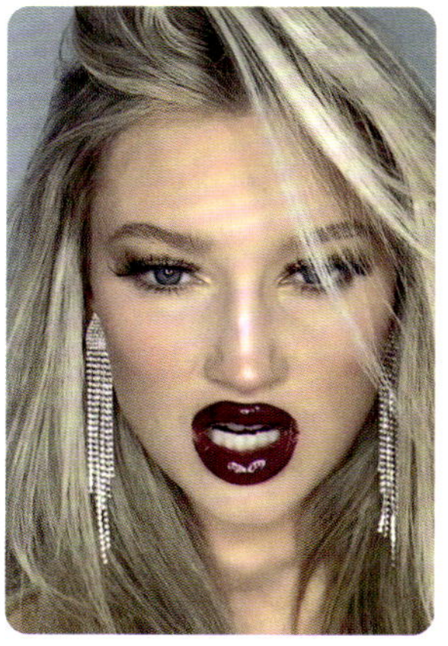

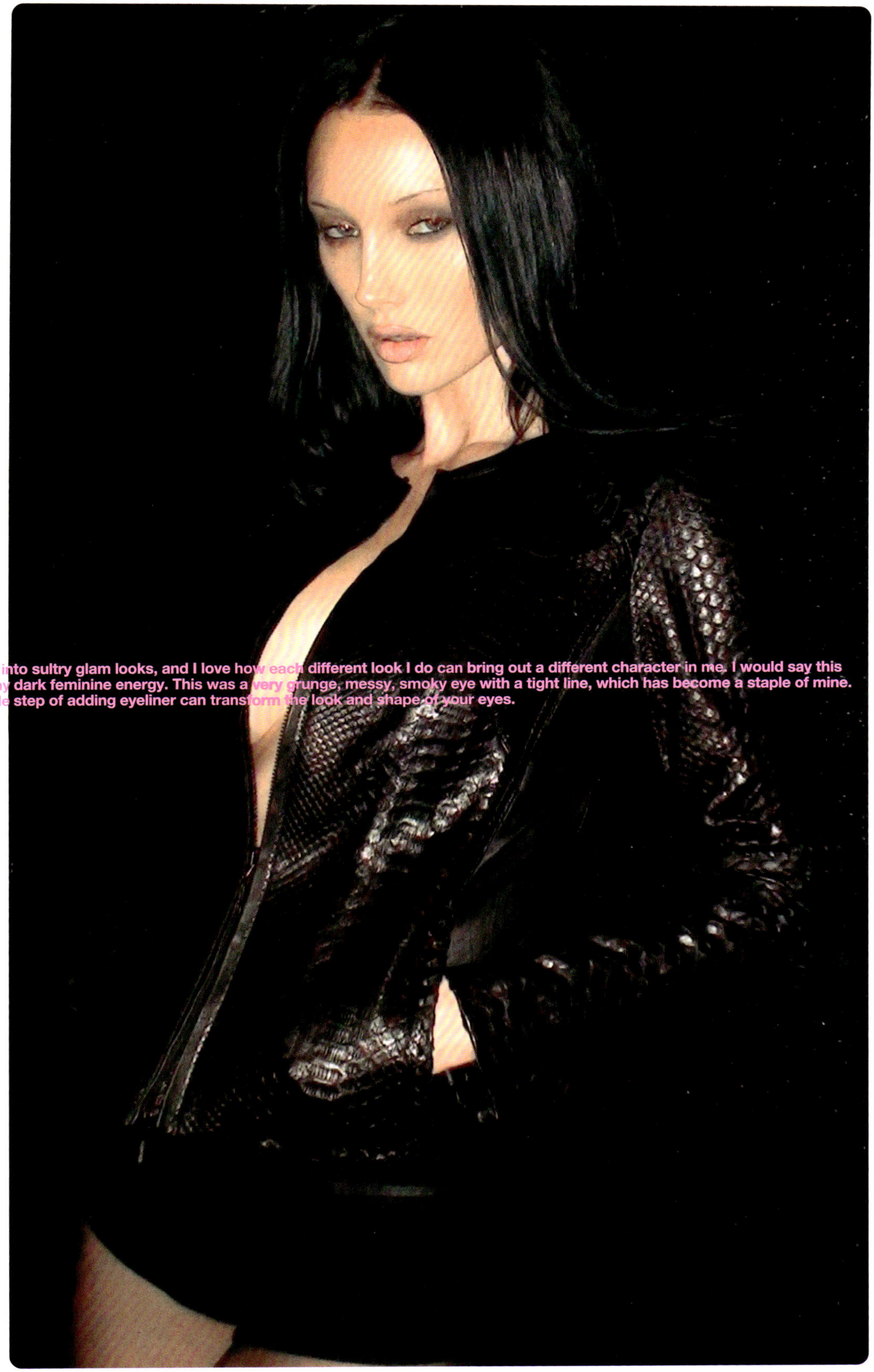

I've really been playing into sultry glam looks, and I love how each different look I do can bring out a different character in me. I would say this look really brings out my dark feminine energy. This was a very grunge, messy, smoky eye with a tight line, which has become a staple of mine. I love how such a simple step of adding eyeliner can transform the look and shape of your eyes.

Q **Complete the sentence. Clean-girl makeup is...**

A **Boring and over.**

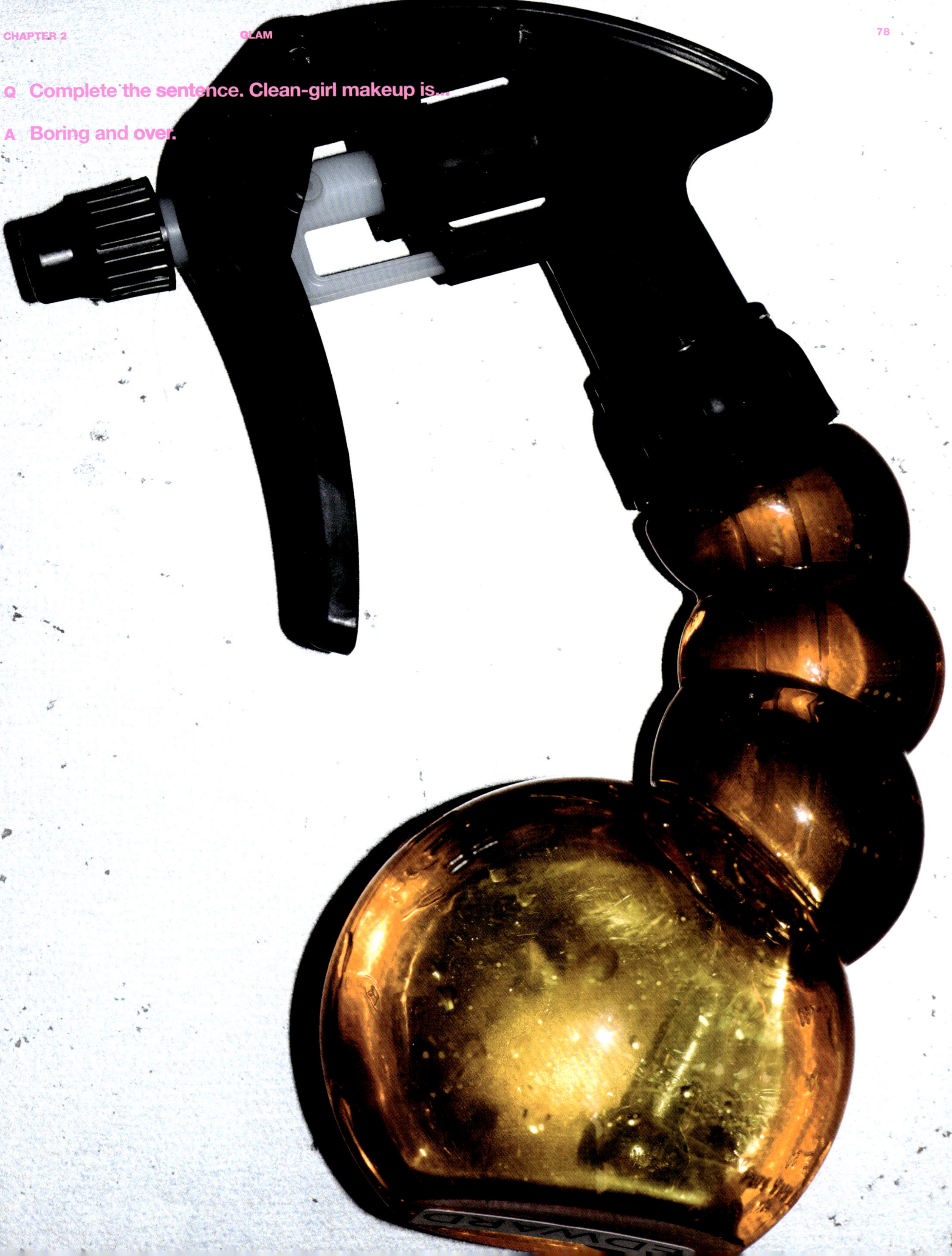

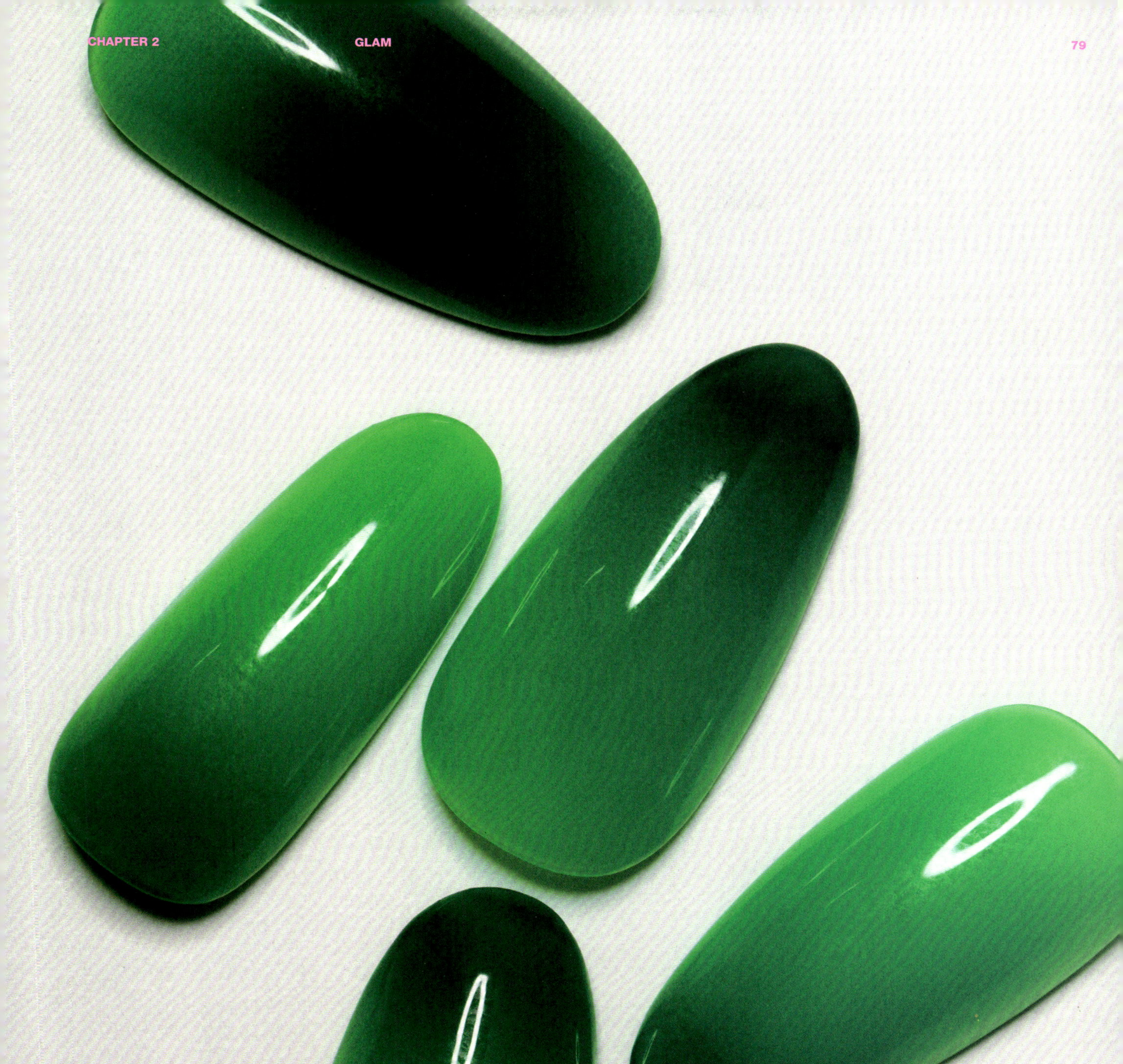

Q There was a time when people called your glam too much, too full coverage, too bold, too extra. How did you learn to stop shrinking yourself to make other people comfortable?

A Finding confidence in what I was doing, knowing I was following my passion, and recognizing that the art I was creating was helping me build towards a life I had always dreamt about.

Q What does that do for you emotionally? On an emotional level, how does it feel to finally realize that you are not going to shrink yourself for people?

A It's very freeing. There are a lot of opinions I feel I need to absorb, and I am trying to please a lot of people. But at the end of the day, when I cancel out that noise, I feel very invigorated.

One person's opinion is not going to matter to me in ten years' time. What is going to matter is that I have created the life I want for myself.

THE TOOLS

Tools and brushes are one of the most important parts of any beauty routine! They help define, sculpt, and shape each look! They can make or break how a product sits and blends onto the skin, so learning how to use and master these tools and brushes in the right way will help you achieve the most flawless glam! Tools and brushes serve a purpose more than just blending out a product onto the skin, it's what translates your inspiration and ideas into something real. Sometimes I find my emotions from the day can translate into the way that I use my brushes, whether I am more heavy-handed or just softly allowing my muscle memory to take over. These are some of my faves!

REAL TECHNIQUES
Expert Face Makeup Brush is such a gem find for me. This brush is an amazing tool for blending out your foundation or base layer. It has the perfect density, where it's soft enough to buff the product into your skin.

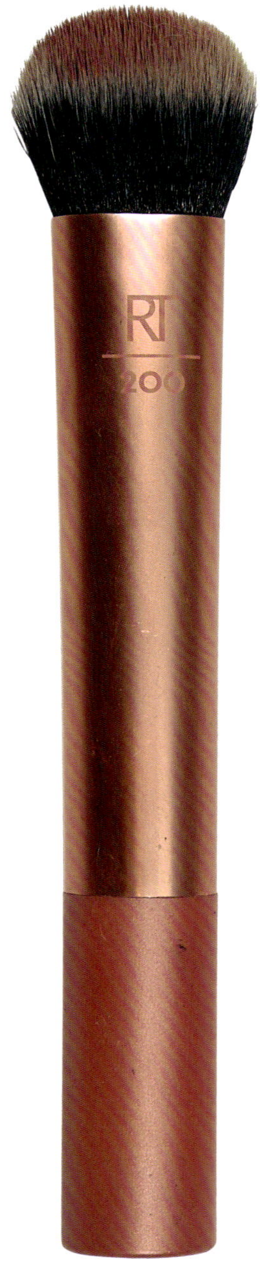

CHRISTIAN LOUBOUTIN
Teint Fétiche All-Over Me Foundation Brush.
I love a foundation brush that makes my foundation glide right on like melted butter, which is exactly what this Louboutin one does.

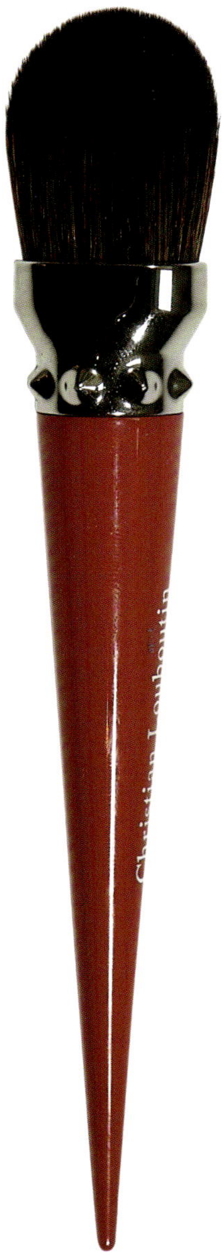

HOURGLASS
Ambient Soft Glow Foundation Brush.
I could have 100 of these hourglass brushes! It's mainly used for cream blush and contour, but I've recently fallen in love with it for blending in my liquid highlighter.

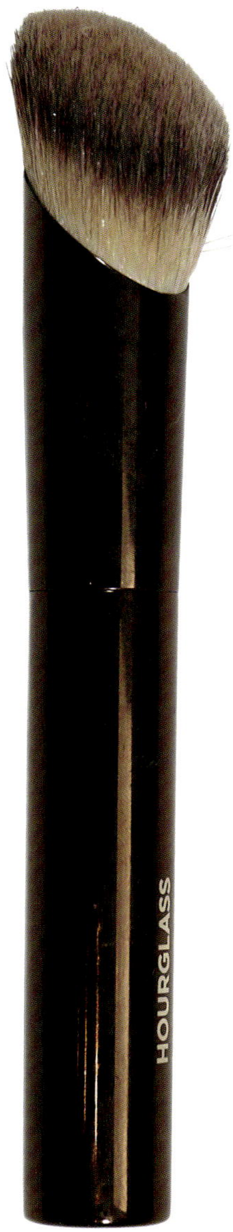

CHARLOTTE TILBURY
Hollywood Complexion Brush. This brush is definitely a top-ten favorite brush—of course, another Charlotte Tilbury find. I love the dual ends for precision and multiuse. I use this brush most often for blending in liquid highlighter. It gets the job done perfectly!

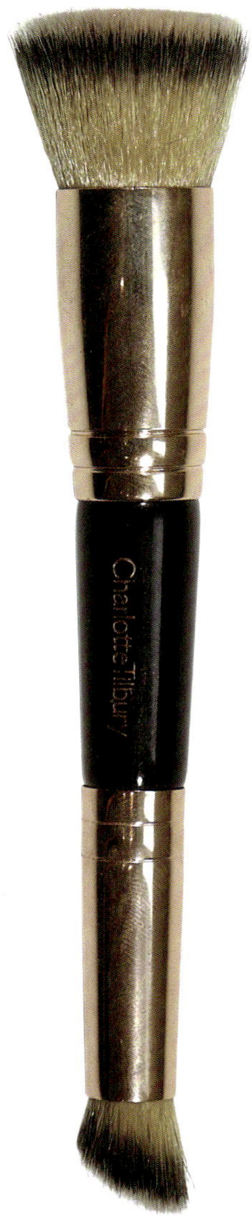

MORPHE X ARIEL
A58 Signature Cream Contour Brush. Morphe is known for its amazing brushes. One collection I really fell in love with was the Morphe x Ariel collection. I love the minimalistic style and packing of the brushes, as well as the quality and softness of the bristles! This is a perfect staple powdered bronzer or blush brush.

PATRICK TA
Major Sculpt Dual-Ended Sculpting Brush. Another favorite dual-ended brush! I specifically use this one when I'm contouring. It will get you snatched!

CAIA
F04 Paddle Powder Brush. CAIA Cosmetics is such a gem find. This brush is perfect for blending in cream contour or blush! It's dense but just the perfect amount to gently blend in those creamier products!

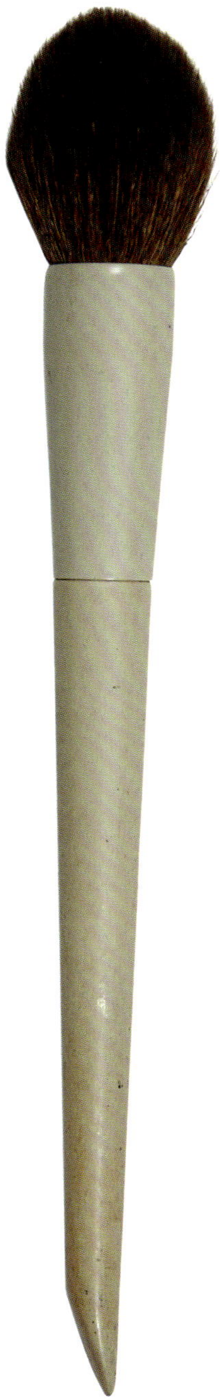

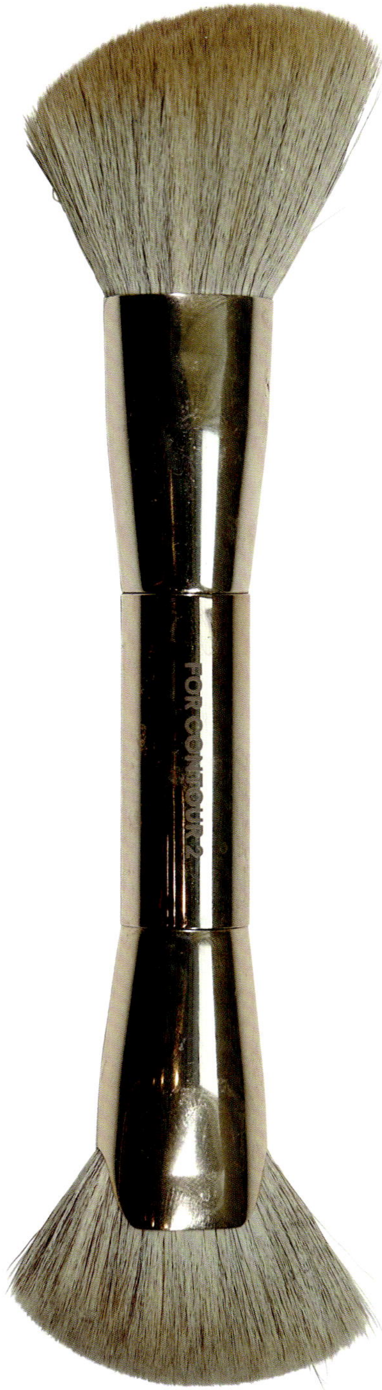

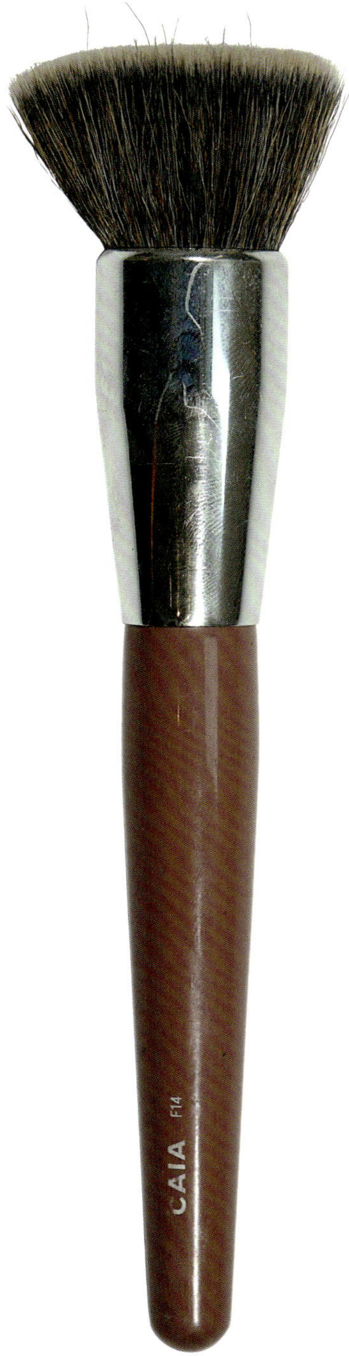

SEPHORA COLLECTION
PRO Brush #93. This specific brush is really great if you're bronzing and want very precise placement. The angle of the bristles allows for perfectly snatched cheekbones.

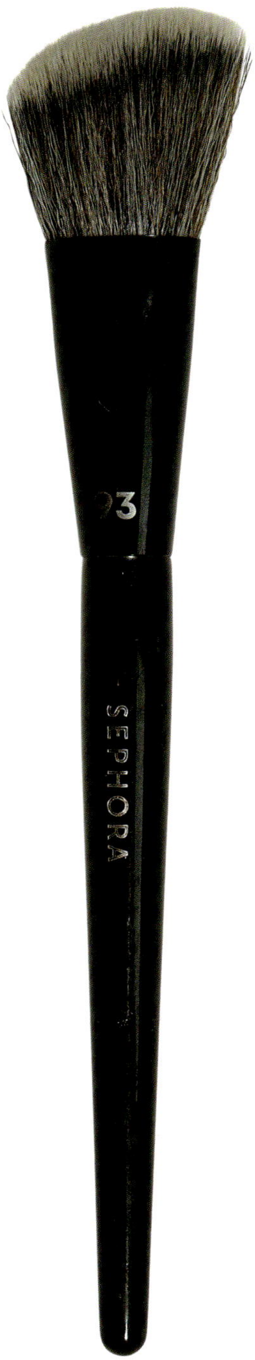

CHARLOTTE TILBURY
Bronzer and Blusher Brush. Another staple powdered bronzer or blush brush from Charlotte Tilbury! I like that this one is a little wider, so that you can target a larger area if you want!

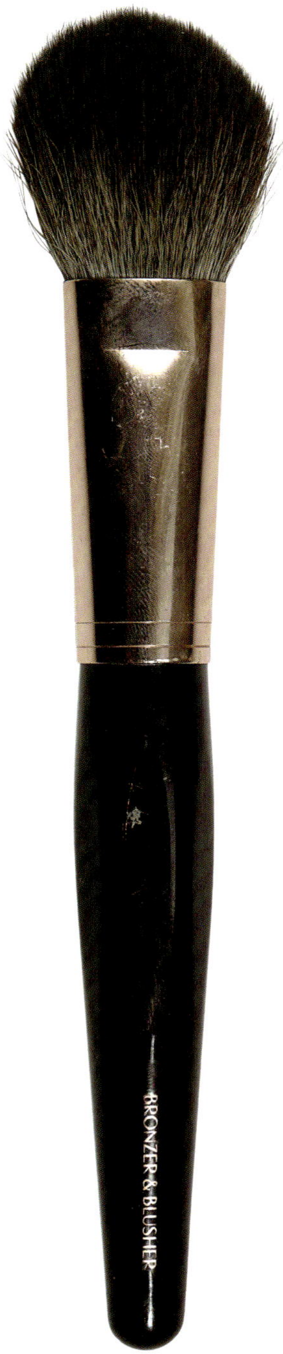

CHARLOTTE TILBURY
Powder and Sculpt Brush. Charlotte Tilbury has some of my favorite brushes. They're so soft and buttery, but also durable. I reach for this one when I'm going in with a powered bronzer or blush. It's the perfect shape and size for creating that contoured, lifted look.

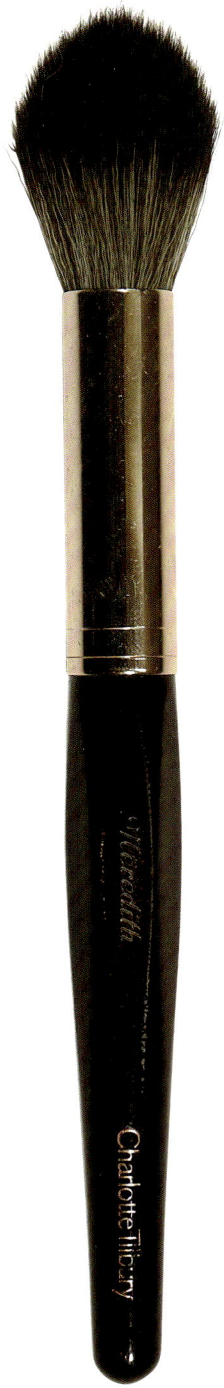

RABANNE BEAUTY
1969 Makeup Clutch in Antique Gold. How cool is this!?!? Rabanne Beauty has *the* eye for fashionable packaging! I mean, are we surprised? This is a highlighter in a purse. She's definitely going in the archive to show my kids one day.

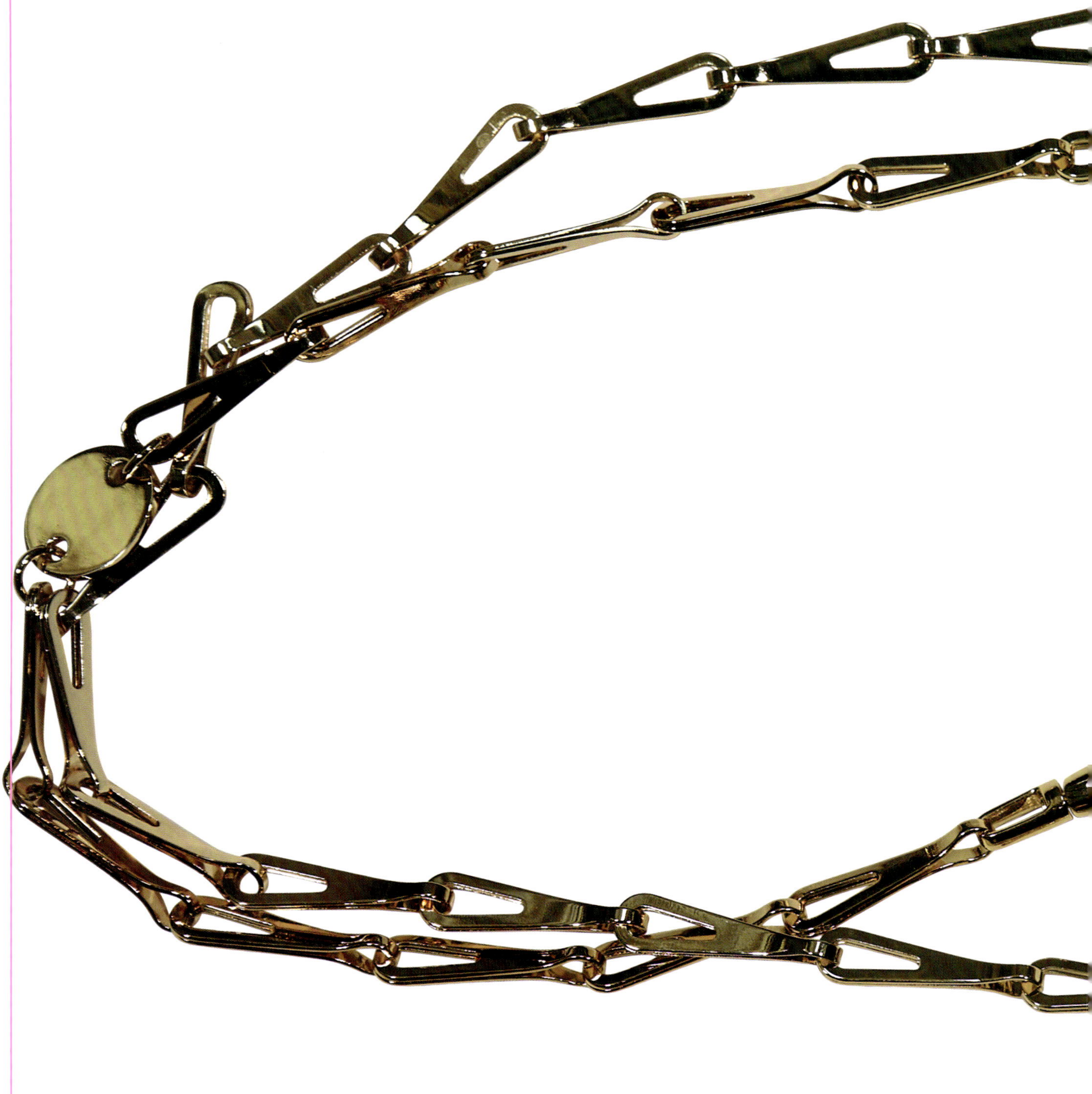

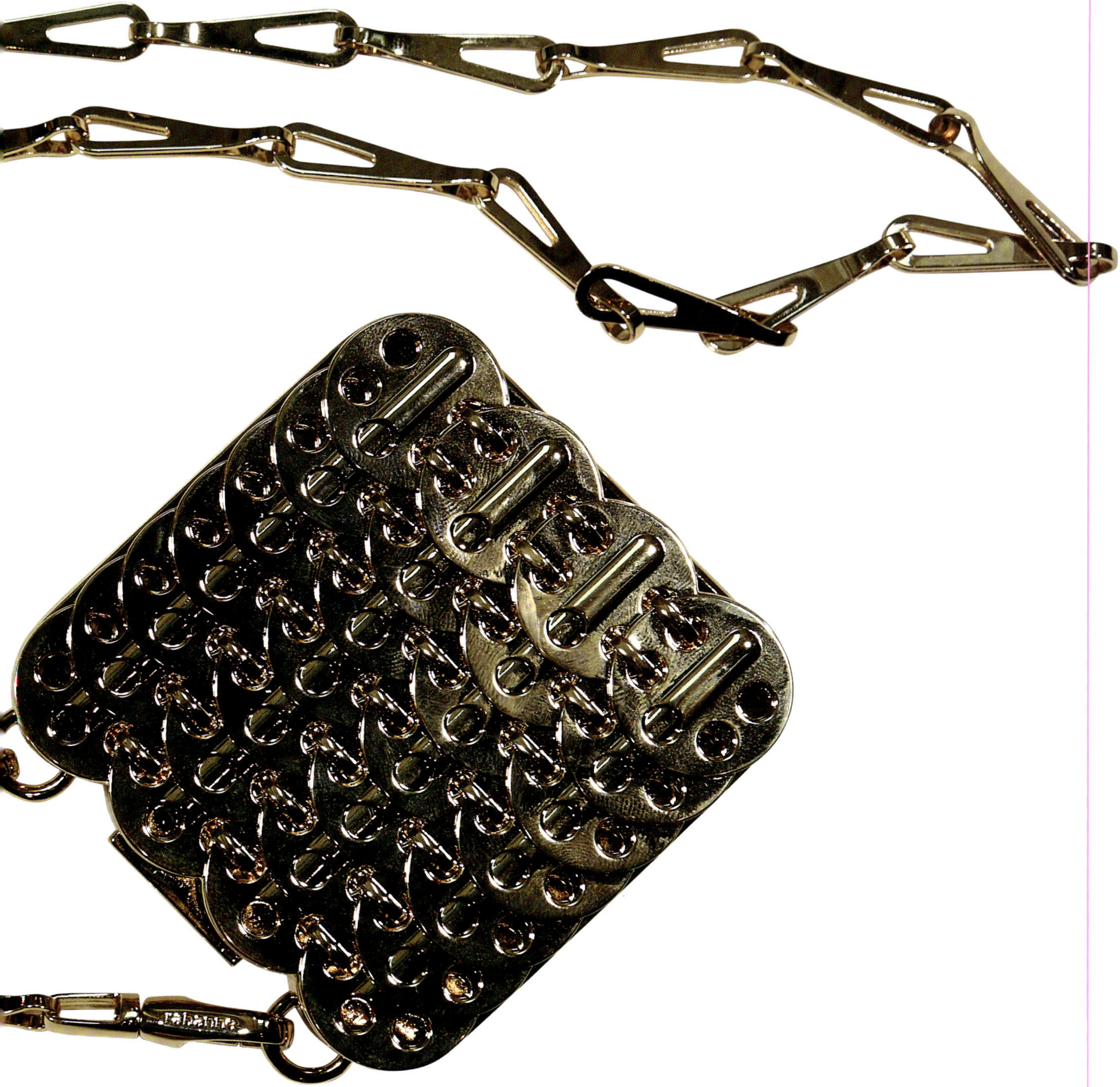
rabanne

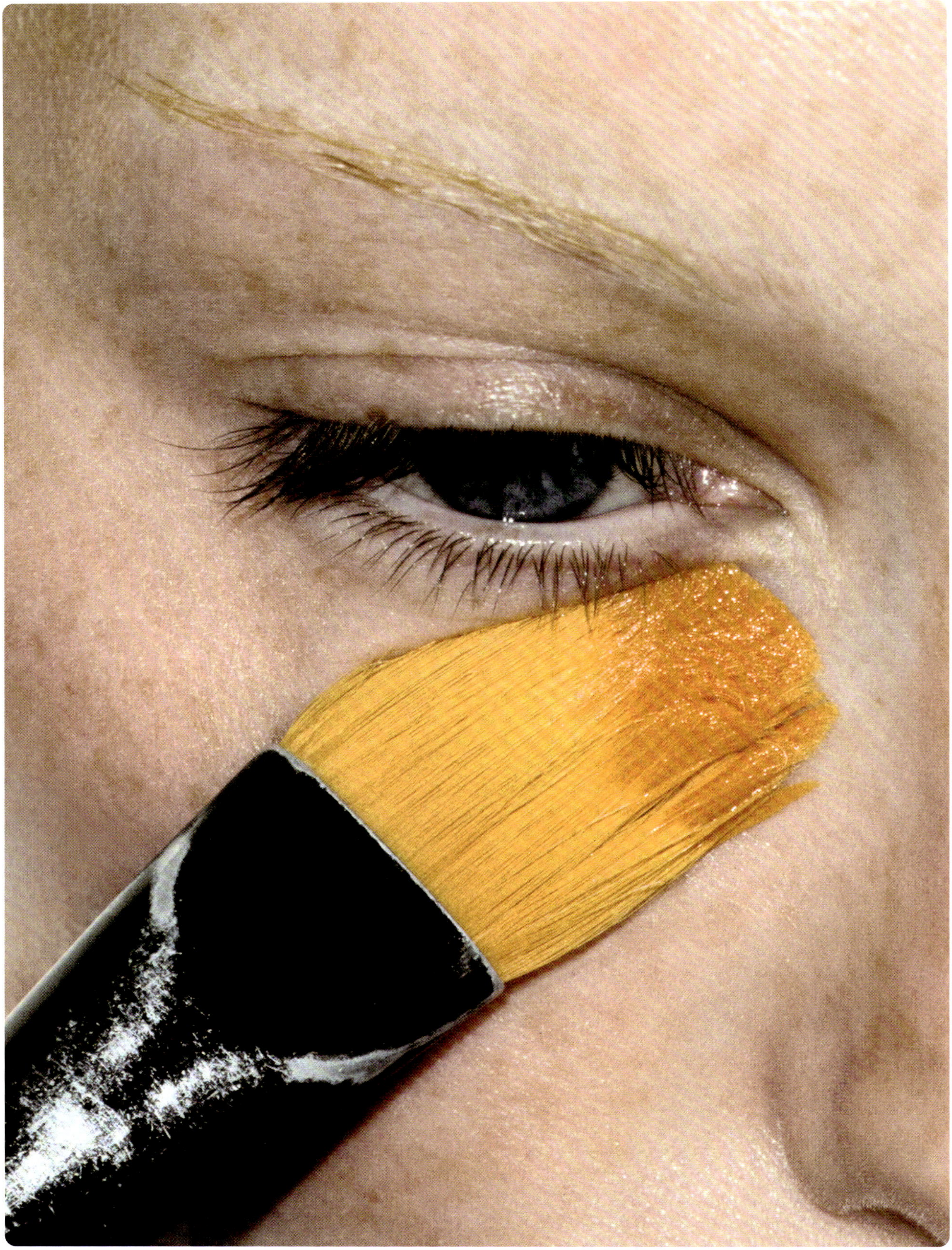

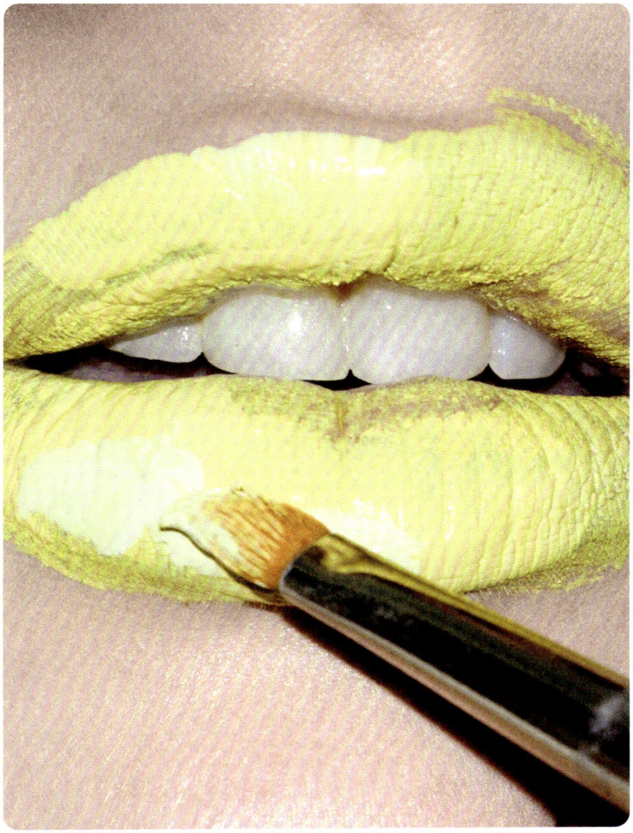

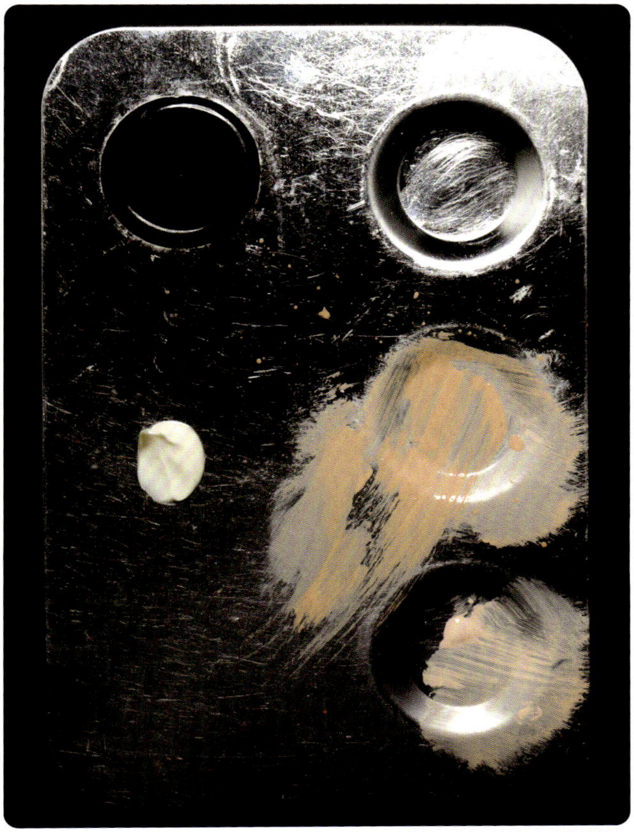

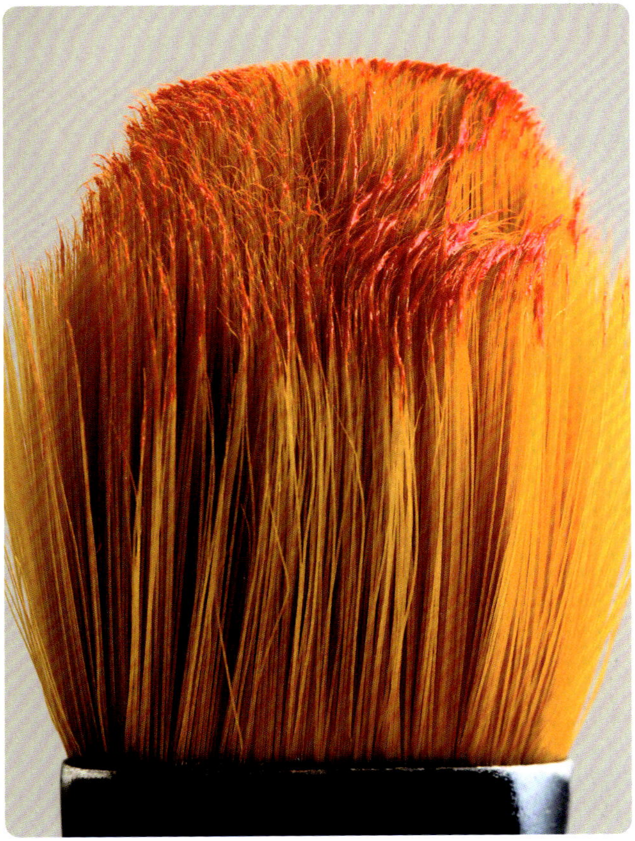

MAKEUP BY MARIO
F2 Dual-Ended Powder Brush. Makeup by Mario has amazing brushes. This one is great for powdered blush and bronzer. I like it specifically when traveling because of its dual ends, so it's one less brush to have to pack!

PATRICK TA
Dual-Ended Blush Brush. This is my favorite blush brush. One side is for cream, the other side for powder. Are we surprised it's Patrick Ta? He's the master of blushes!

IT COSMETICS
Love Beauty Fully All-Over Powder Brush #211. A big fluffy brush should be an essential in anyone's makeup kit. This one is the perfect finisher brush! I always reach for it either when I want to warm up my face with more bronzer and just want to cover a large area, or when my look is all complete but I want to touch up with one last dusting of powder.

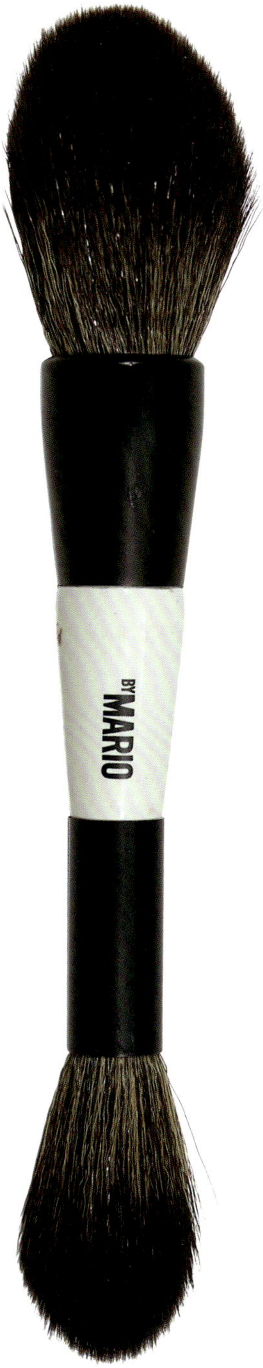

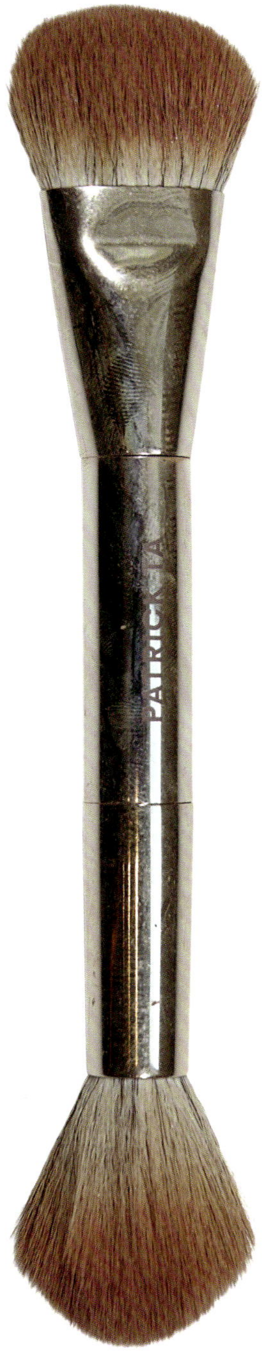

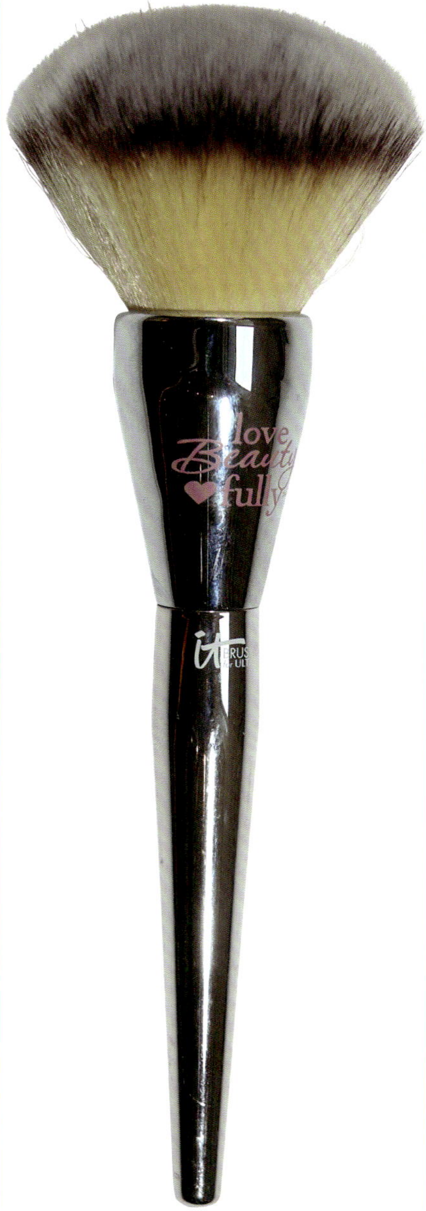

SEPHORA COLLECTION
PRO Fan Highlight Brush #62. If you're dipping into a powdered highlighter, a fan brush is always a must-have! This one is more condensed, which I personally like because I feel I get more pigment payoff. The smaller shape of this highlighter brush allows for a supersmooth, precise application on the high points of the cheekbone or on the bridge of the nose.

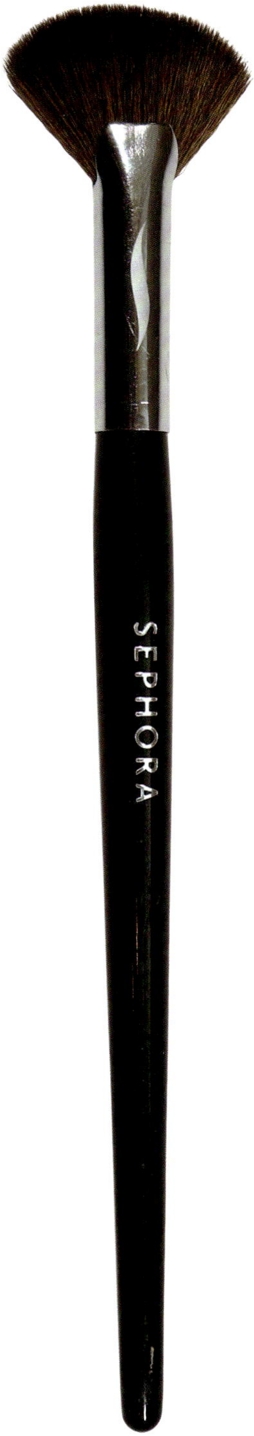

MAC
204 Lash Brush. Who doesn't love a spoolie? She's crucial. You can't forget to take care of those brows! I love to use this tool to tame them and get them in place. PRO TIP: If you smudge your mascara anywhere on your face after you've applied your makeup, wait for it to dry, then lightly brush it off with a spoolie. Voilà, it's gone!

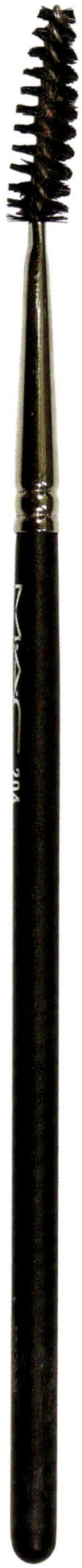

E.L.F. COSMETICS
Dual-Sided Eyebrow Brush. I love a dual-ended spoolie! The brush tip can be used either for filling in your brows or creating a sultry, sharp liner!

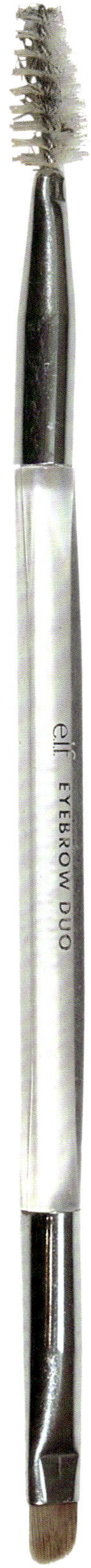

PALETTES, PALETTES, PALETTES!

Product packaging is a really big inspiration for me when creating my makeup looks. I always like to take in the things around me for inspiration, whether that's certain colors, textures, or shapes. These are a mix of some of my favorites. Some days, I'm feeling more sleek and minimal, and other days I'm feeling eccentric and want color, boldness, and fun!

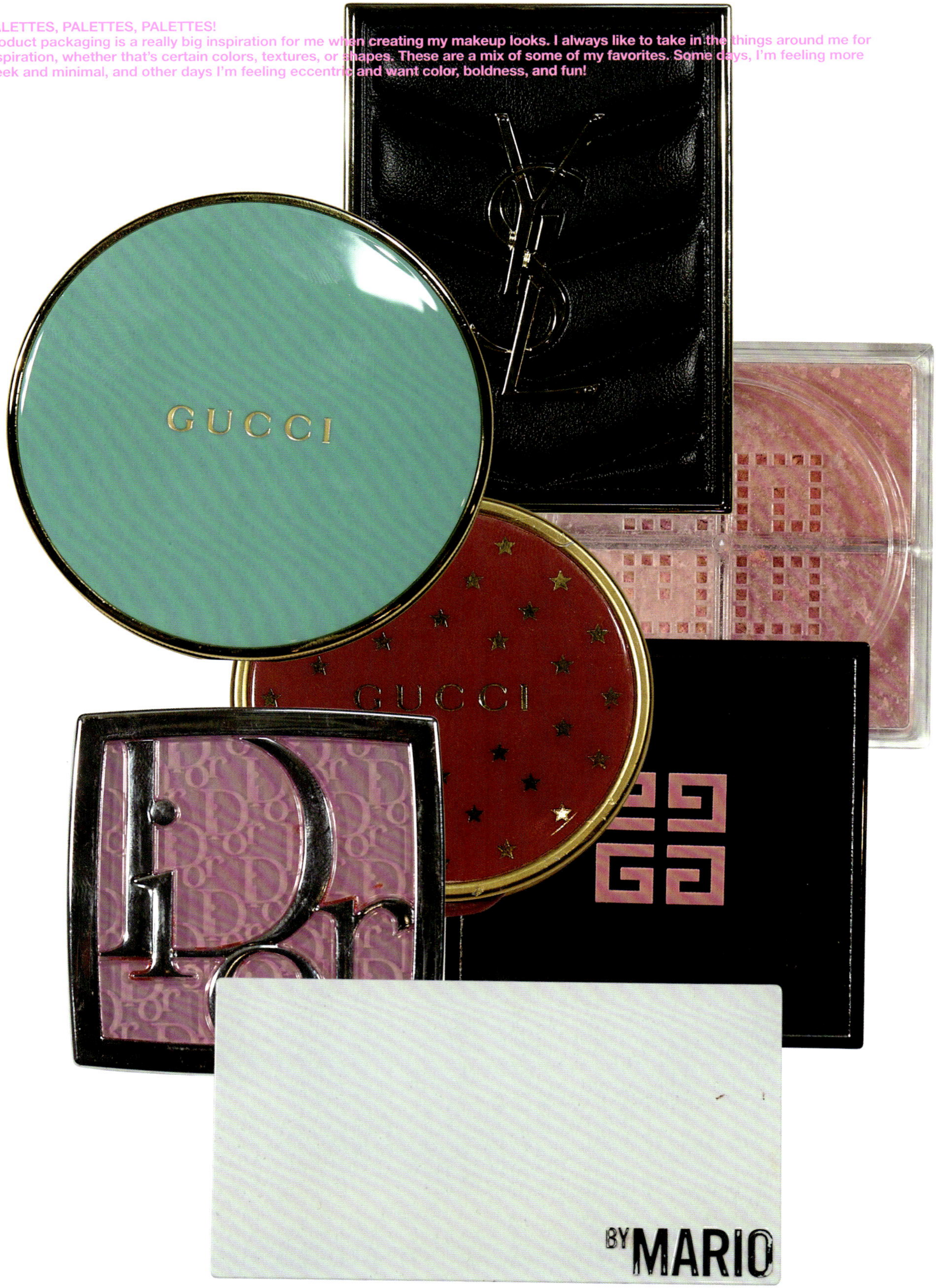

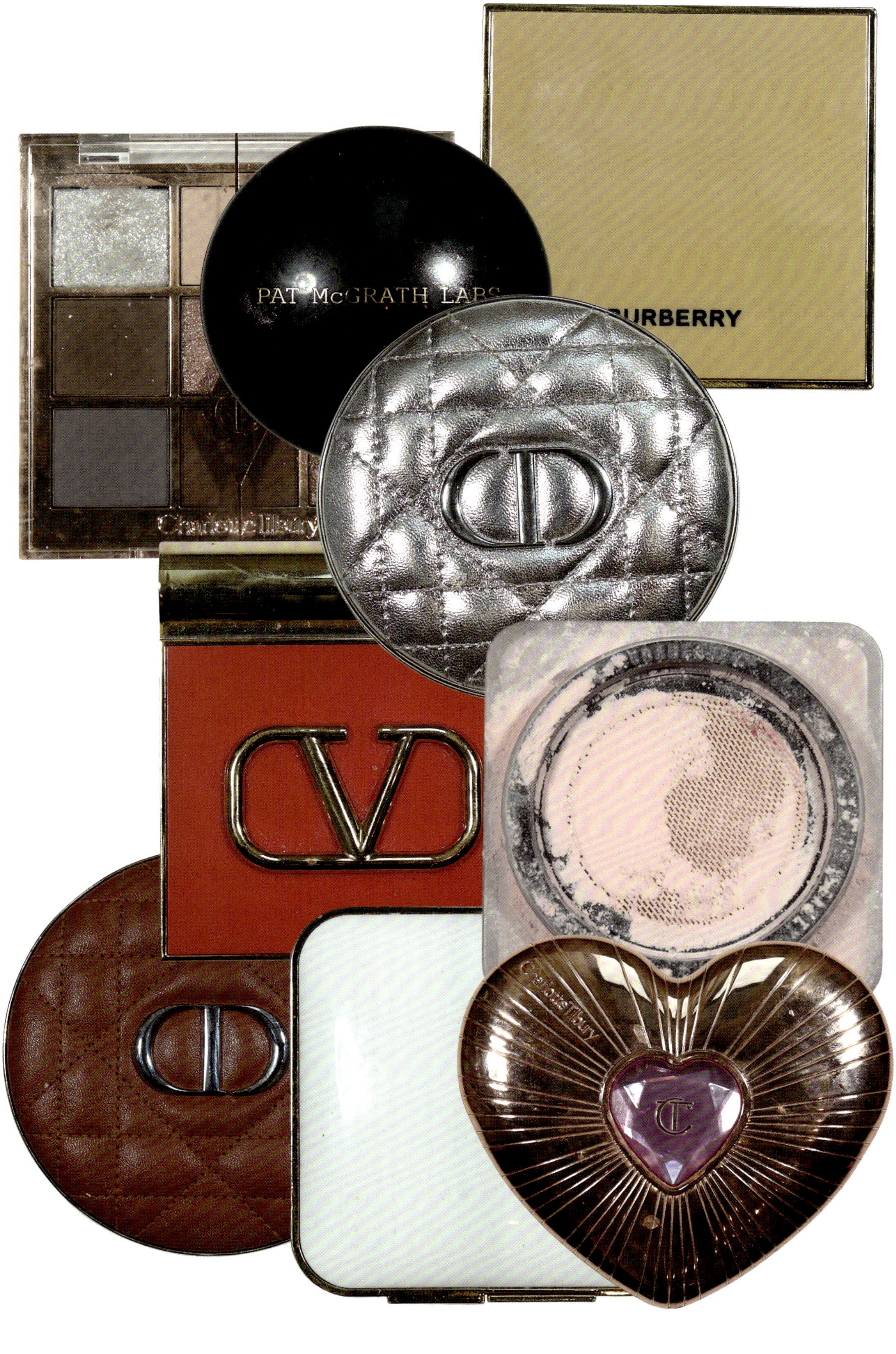
PAT McGRATH LABS
BURBERRY

PATRICK TA

Major Dimension II Rose Eye Shadow Palette. If you're a pink, rose-toned kind of makeup girl, this palette is for you! I love this for when I want to tap into my superfeminine side and create a glittery pink glam. I love how versatile the palette is with two cream shades for building up a nice base. There are also some smokier shades if you want to go in a more glam direction and pair it with a shimmer.

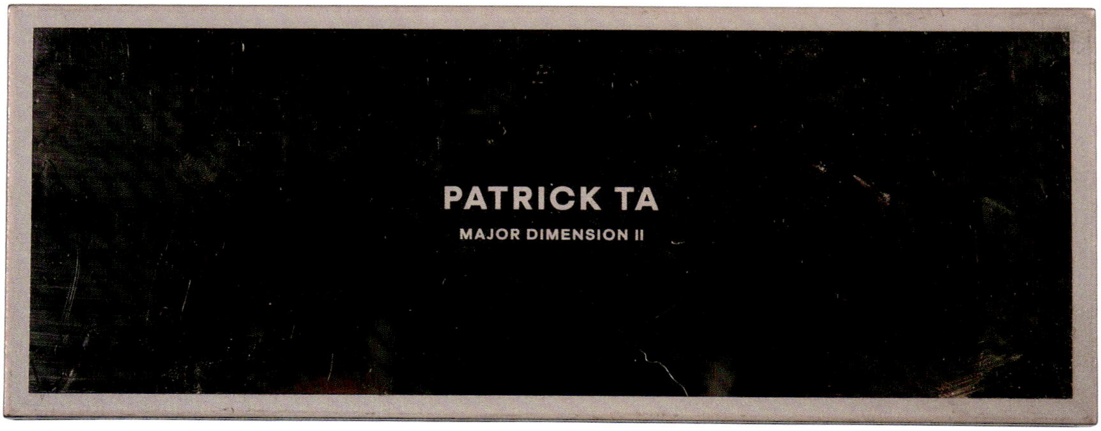

PAT MCGRATH LABS MTHRSHP

Mega: Celestial Nirvana Eye Shadow Palette. MOTHER! We all know how iconic Pat McGrath is, and if anyone is going to have a killer formula, it's going to be her! She has mastered so many things, but I *love* her eye shadow palettes. This specific one is very meaningful to me because it is a limited edition, and I really feel grateful to be able to hold onto and experiment with such a special launch. I love the color story of this too; there is a perfect mix of neutrals, fun pops of color, and deeper tones.

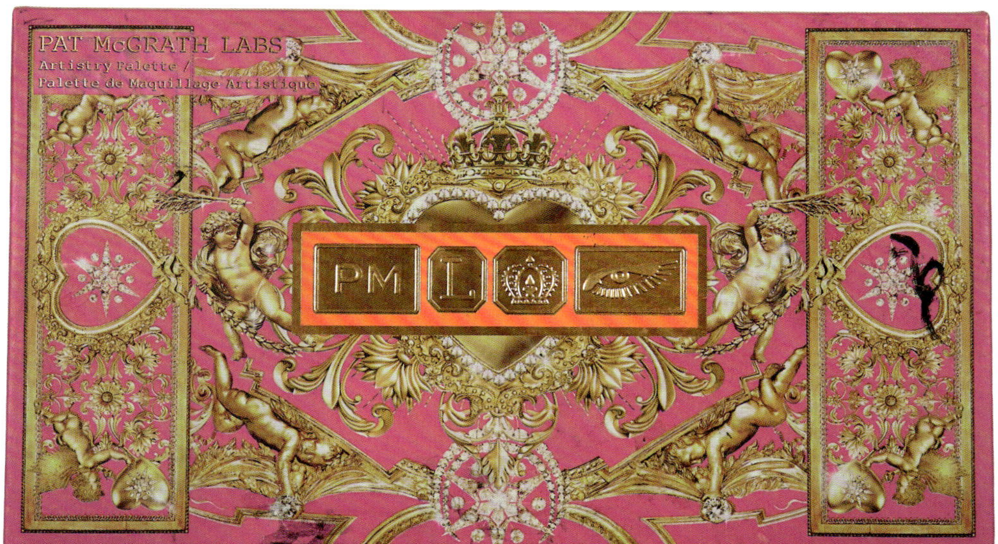

PAT MCGRATH LABS

Mothership IX: Huetopian Dream Palette. I reach for this palette when I want to *shine*! Pat McGrath's shimmers are like no others. All you need is a finger swatch, and you have the deepest pigment!

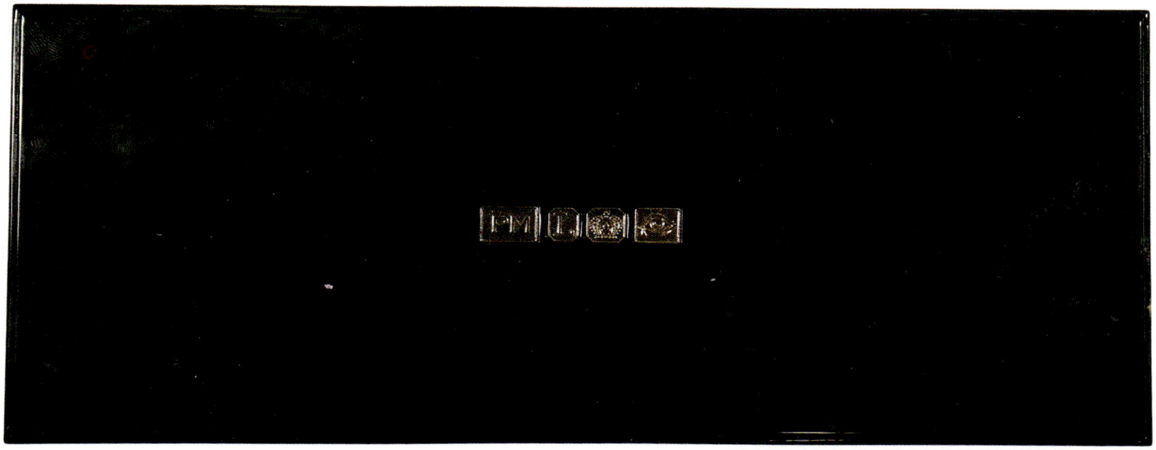

MORPHE X MEREDITH DUXBURY

Power Multi-Effects Palette. This palette is part of a collection that I co-created and designed with Morphe. It represents so much to me: my creativity, passion, and hard work. It's an incredible feeling to hold something tangible that I poured my ideas into. I use it all the time, and I love how multipurpose it is. Of course, it's great for a rosy shimmer eye look, but I also love to dip into it and use it as a highlighter!

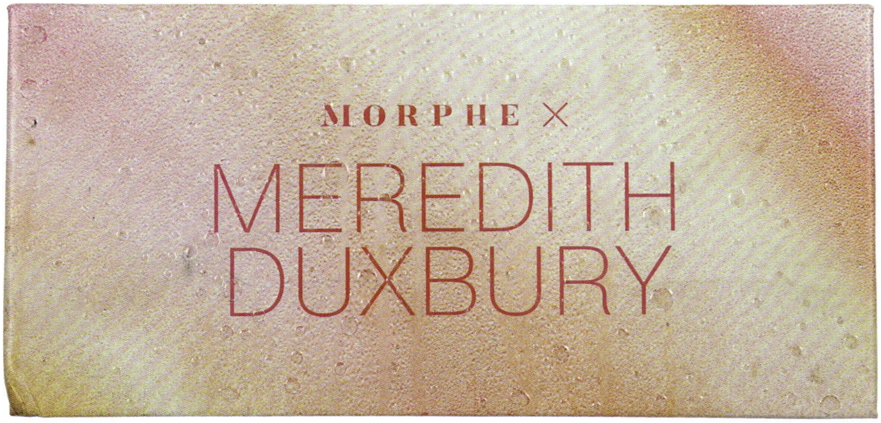

LA ROCHE-POSAY
Anthelios Melt-in Milk Sunscreen for Face and Body SPF 100. Those with freckles get it: SPF is our bestie in the summer. I always go for SPF 50 or above, so when I found out SPF 100 existed, I knew it was something I couldn't live without in the summer.

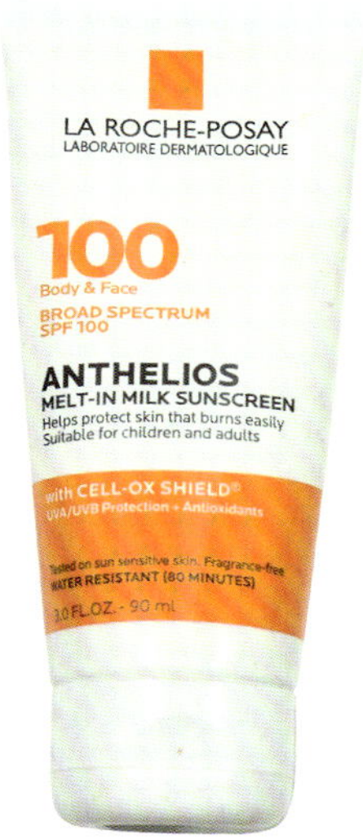

KIEHL'S
Ultra Facial Cleanser. I go through bottles of this cleanser. I have super-sensitive skin and struggle with perioral dermatitis. I found this cleanser helped to calm my skin while still removing my makeup. The formula is non-stripping and leaves your face super-hydrated and feeling soft like baby skin.

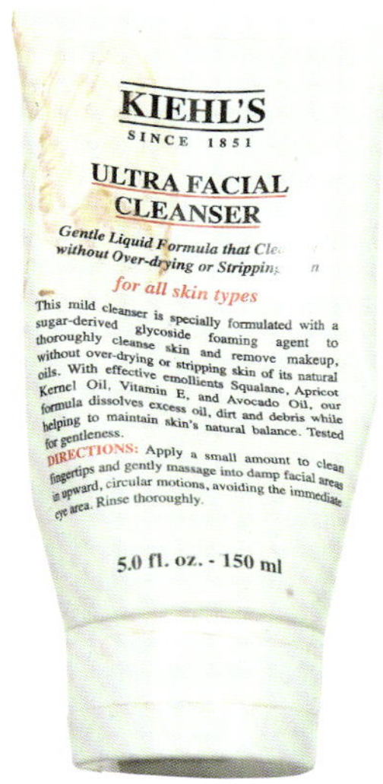

CHARLOTTE TILBURY
Magic Hydrator Mist. Let's talk about the glow...you know, that feeling after powder where you feel like you've lost all the glow you worked so hard to create during those base steps? Well, this product is going to bring that glow right back. I promise you it won't disappoint. PRO TIP: Drench your face in this after powdering and then use a fan to dry it.

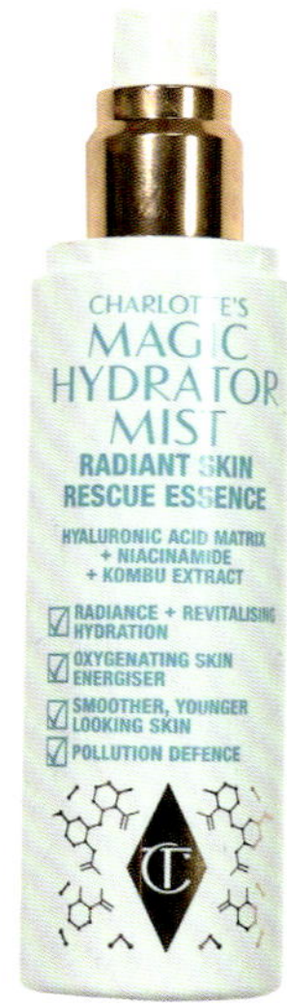

L'ORÉAL
EverPure Glossing Shampoo. This has drastically helped change the texture of my hair. I used to wonder why my hair wasn't shiny and smooth. The reason was that I wasn't feeding it the right ingredients.

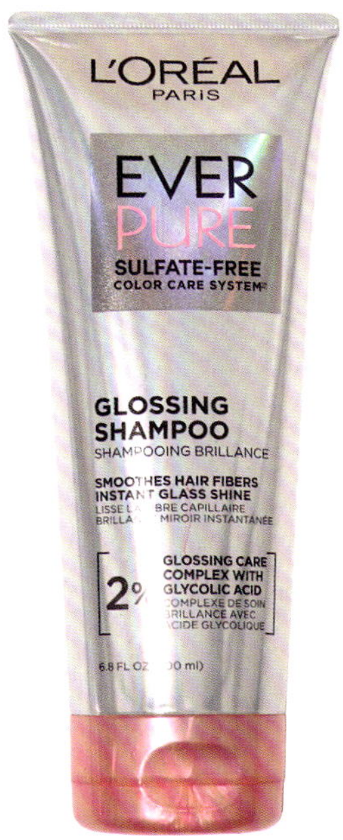

L'ORÉAL
EverPure Glossing Conditioner. These products help to smooth hair fibers and are perfect for girlies with color-treated hair.

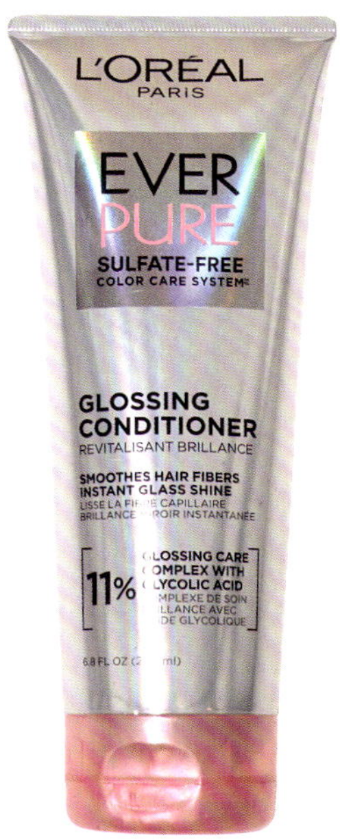

HEADBAND
What's a Meredith Duxbury makeup look without the iconic headband????

MAYBELLINE
Grippy Serum Primer. If you have a date night planned, you'd better be using this before doing your glam. You could wake up the next day, and your makeup will still be intact...no matter what you got up to on that date.

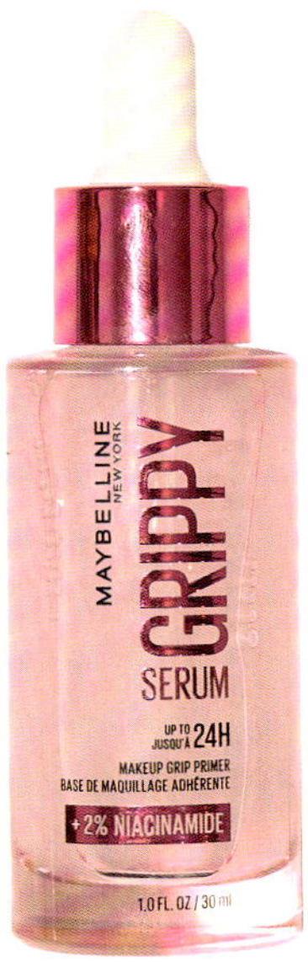

LA PRAIRIE
Skin Caviar Concealer Foundation SPF 15. If you want to splurge, go for this product. It's a two-in-one foundation and a concealer. It offers super high coverage but is still dewy. It also contains caviar extract, if you feel like being extra bougie.

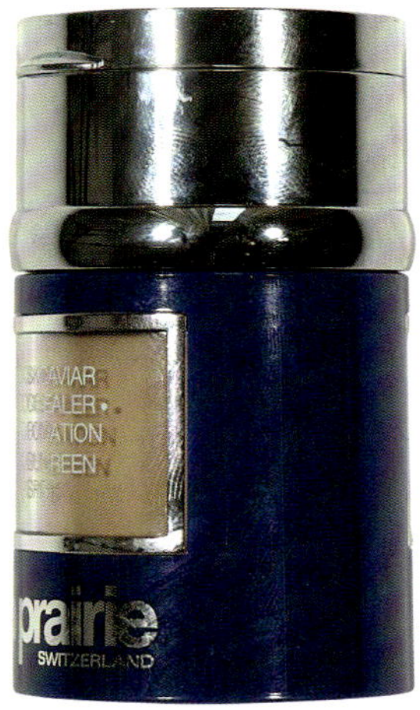

GUERLAIN
Terracotta Le Teint Healthy Glow Foundation. This is one of my favorite full-coverage foundations. It's for the girls who want a very matte look. The final result gives a very airbrushed, matte feeling and look. PRO TIP: Make sure to moisturize and do a really great skincare routine before applying for the best results.

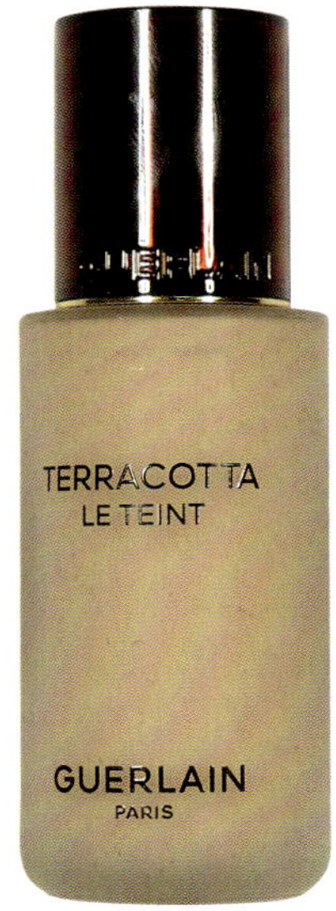

CHARLOTTE TILBURY
Airbrush Flawless Foundation. Charlotte Tilbury is known for her magical makeup results, and let me say that's what you're going to get with this foundation. It is a soft, matte full-coverage, long-wearing foundation (my fave for a night out). With a lot of full-coverage foundations, you tend to feel it lying on top of your skin, but with this one, it honestly feels like a second layer of skin.

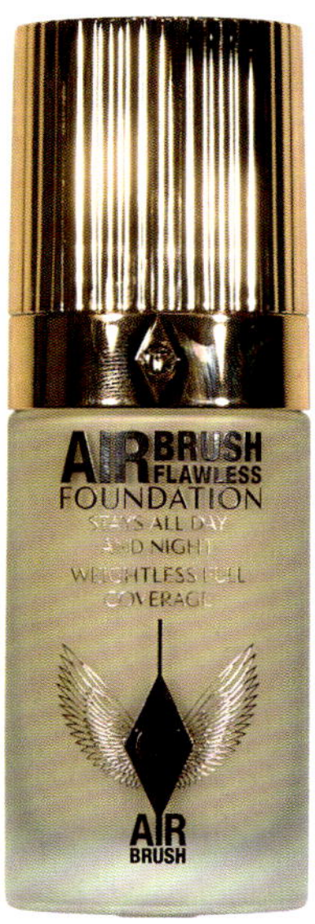

E.L.F. COSMETICS
Halo Glow Skin Tint SPF 50. This skin tint is perfect to throw on for a super-natural look. It makes the skin glow. I have personally used it as a full-coverage foundation and *love* it. It has SPF 50 in it, so it's a great summer staple!

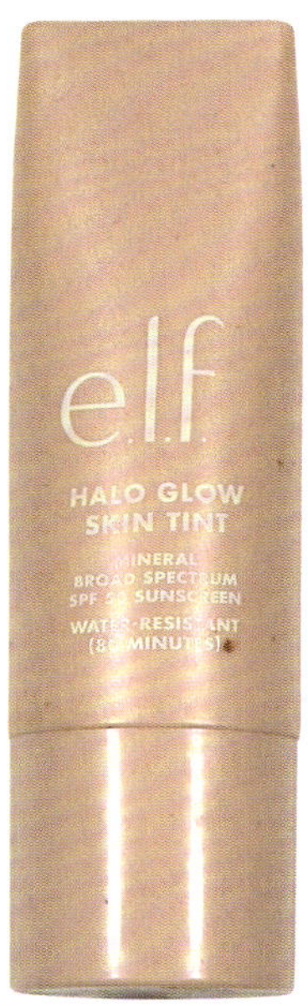

CATRICE
HD Liquid Coverage Foundation. We all know this product. It is the iconic dripper foundation that you see in all my most viral foundation videos. The formula is beautiful and builds so seamlessly.

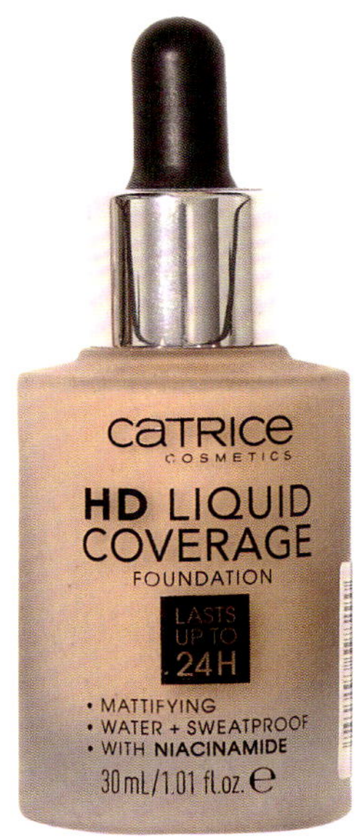

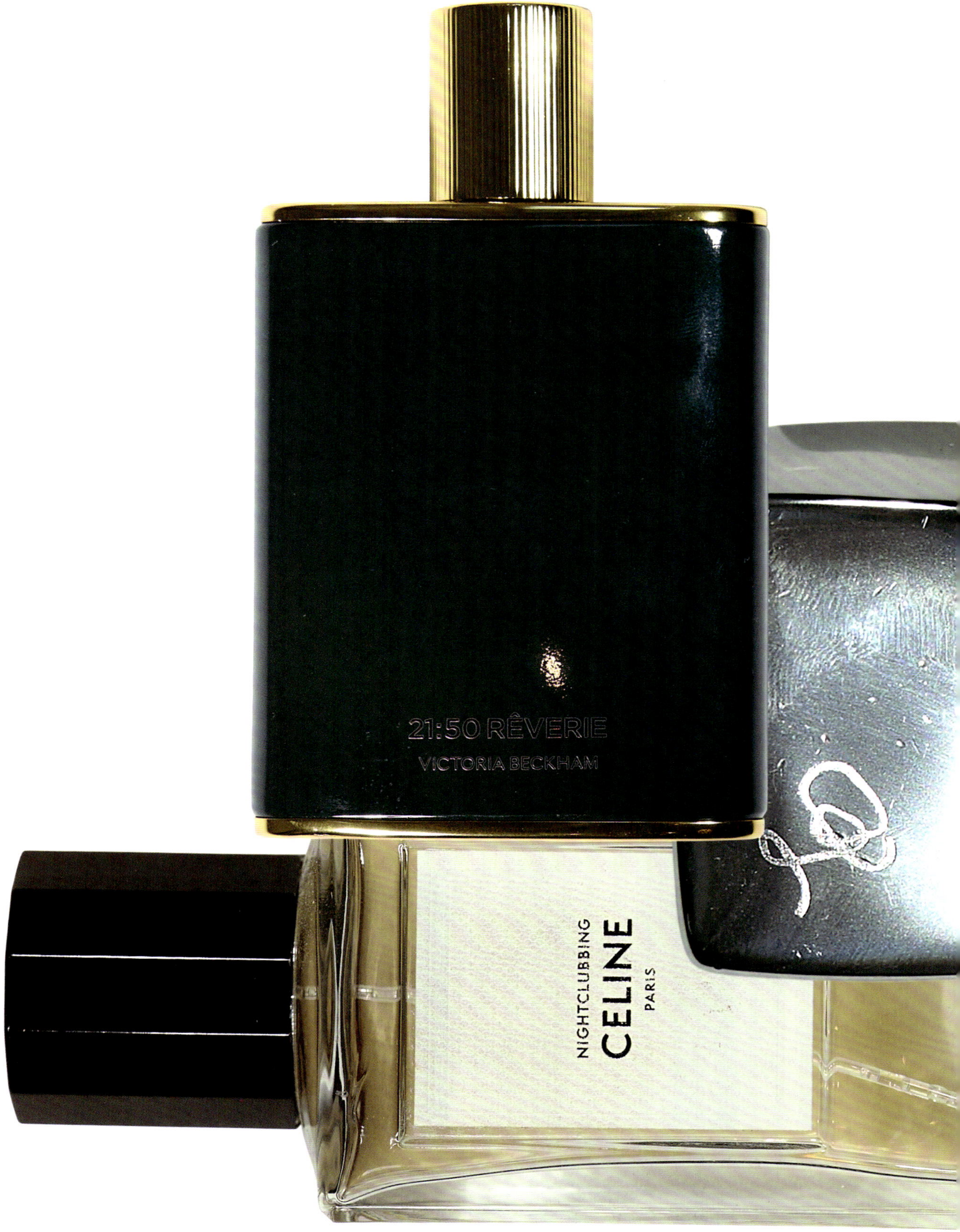
21:50 RÊVERIE
VICTORIA BECKHAM
NIGHTCLUBBING
CELINE
PARIS

PERFUME, PERFUME, PERFUME!
VICTORIA BECKHAM BEAUTY *21:50 Rêverie Eau de Parfum*. This is one of my absolute all-time favorite scents. It's sweet and smoky. **CELINE** *Nightclubbing Eau de Parfum*…the name says it all. **LORE DISFRUTA** *Eau de Parfum with Mezcal*. Lore is another all-time favorite. When I discovered these fragrances, I felt like I was taken into a whole other universe. Each smell has a world of its own. Like I always say, packaging has a huge impact on how I view products, and I love the tops of these. For Lore, the bottle's cap can also be used as a candlestick holder...how genius.

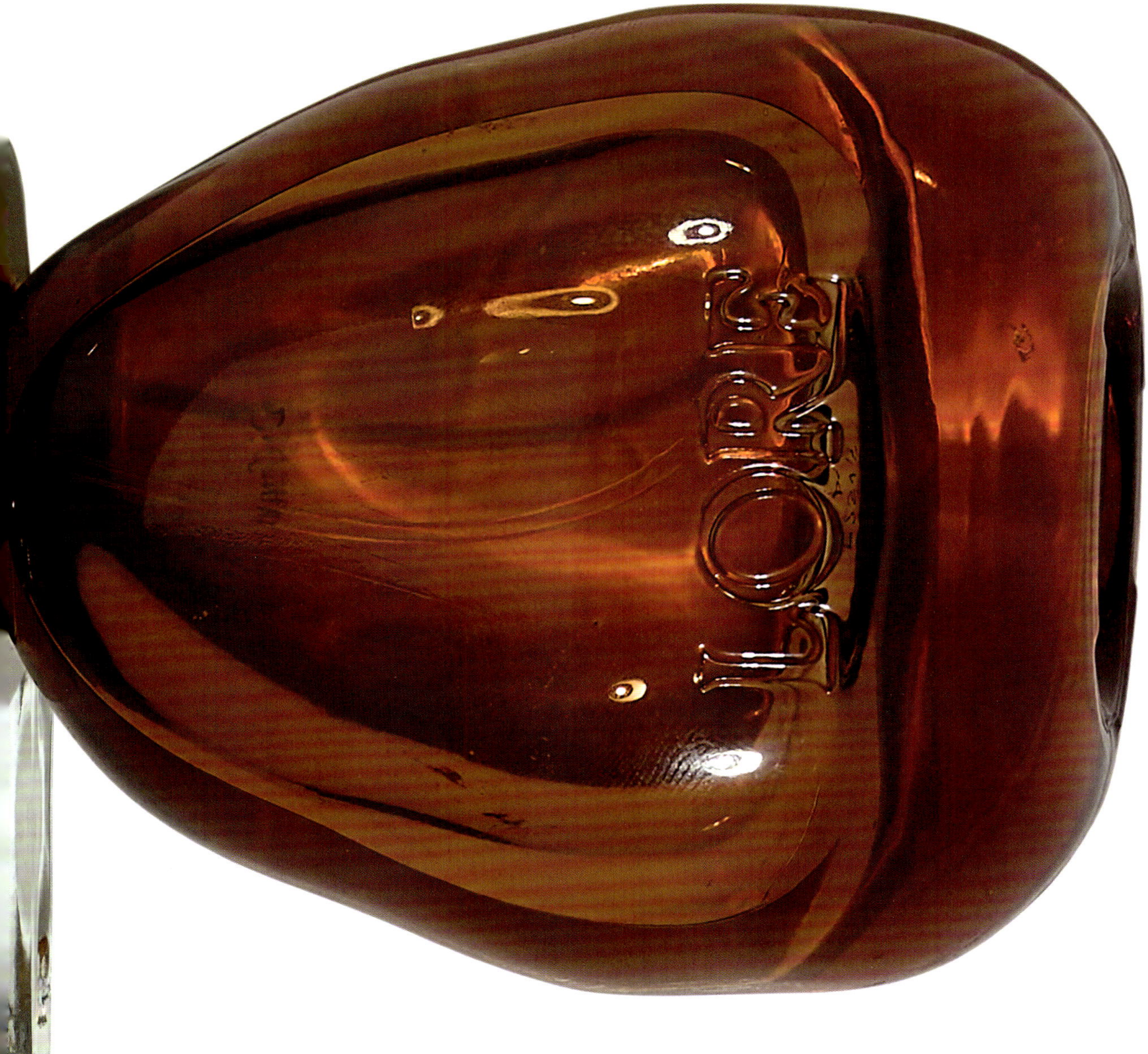

ARMANI BEAUTY
Luminous Silk Cheek Tint Blush (shade Delicate Mauve). Armani Beauty blushes are chef's kiss! The applicator is great for precise application, and it gives off the most natural glow!

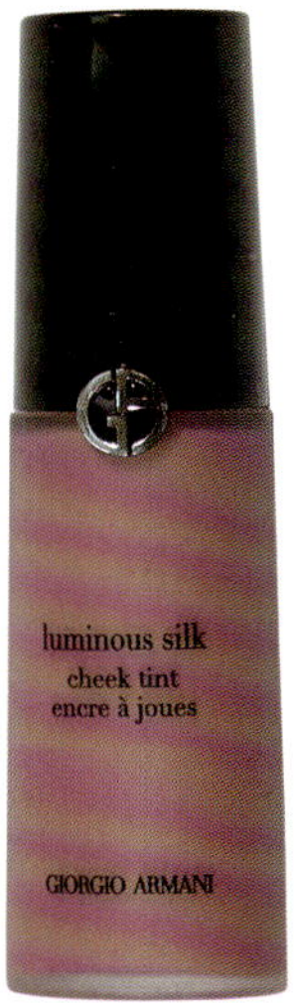

ARMANI BEAUTY
Luminous Silk Cheek Tint Blush (shade Rosy Peach). This is one of my favorite peachy liquid blush shades. You just have to try it!

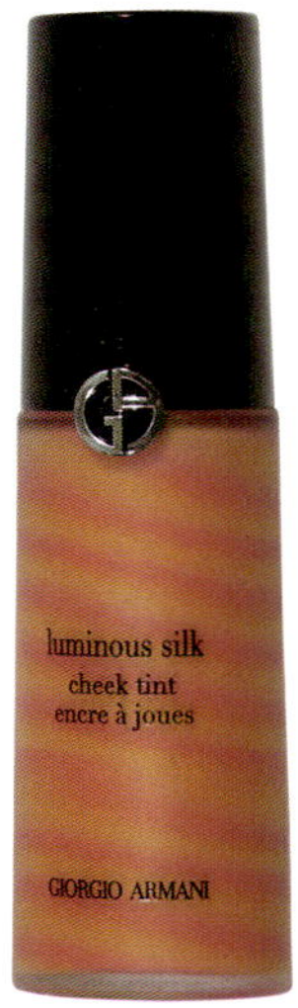

CHARLOTTE TILBURY
Unreal Blush Healthy Glow Stick (shade Rosy Glow). If you want glowy skin, this is your girl. Charlotte Tilbury is the queen of glowy, flawless skin. When this launched, I gasped because I absolutely love the foundation stick, so to have it available in a blush formula now, I could only imagine how smooth and airbrushed the formula would be.

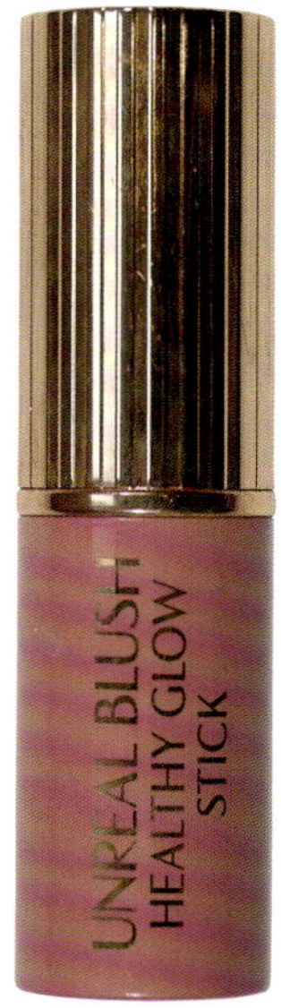

RHODE
Pocket Blush (shade Tan Line). I really love a portable beauty product, and rhode has perfected this! It's easy to throw this in a bag and bring it to the beach. The formula is easy to blend in with your fingers and natural enough to pop onto your cheeks without needing a mirror for application.

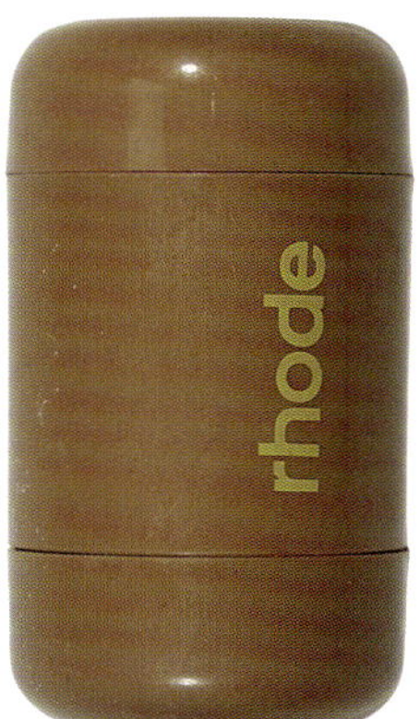

CHARLOTTE TILBURY
Hollywood Beauty Light Wand (*shade Spotlight*). My holy grail! I don't think I've created a makeup look without using this product in a long, long time. It is the perfect liquid highlighter, leaving the most natural glow.

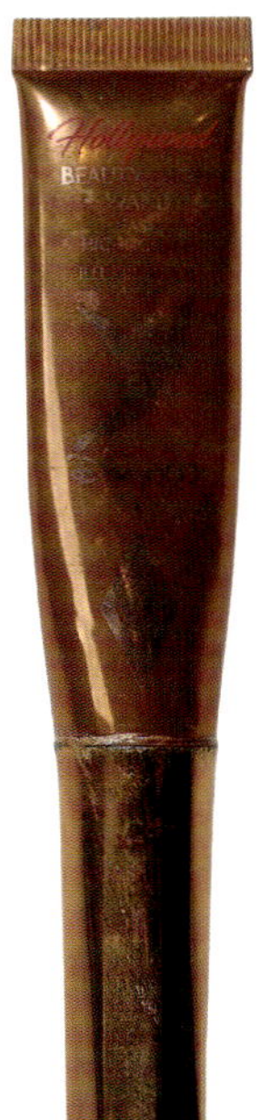

CHARLOTTE TILBURY
Beauty Light Wand (shade Pillow Talk). This is another shade of the Charlotte Tilbury Beauty Light Wand for when you want a more rosy-pink tone highlighter!

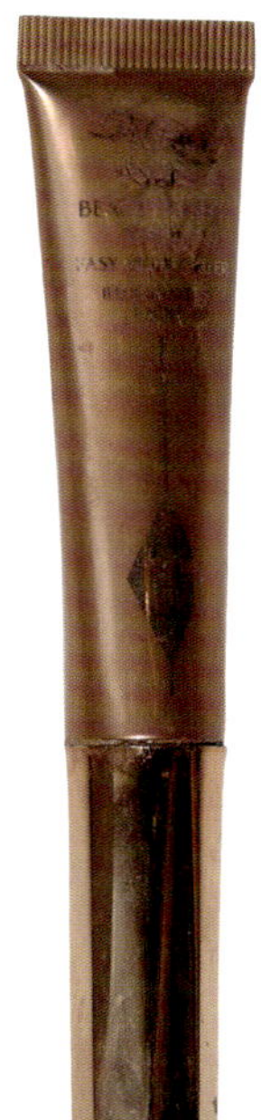

PRADA BEAUTY

Monochrome Soft Matte Blur Lipstick (shade Alabaster). Prada Beauty has amazing lipsticks. I love the variety of finishes. The matte ones are my faves! There's something about the way they smell delicious.

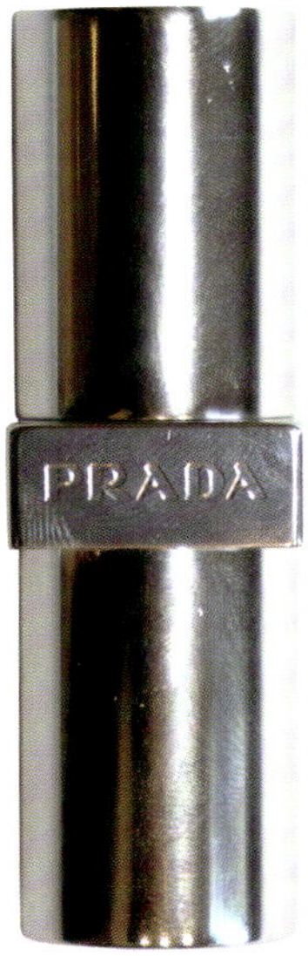

MAC COSMETICS

M·A·CXIMAL Silky Matte Lipstick (shade Yash). MAC has some of the most iconic lip shades. Ever. They are trusty, and the formula is always killer. This shade is for the nude-lip lovers, like me.

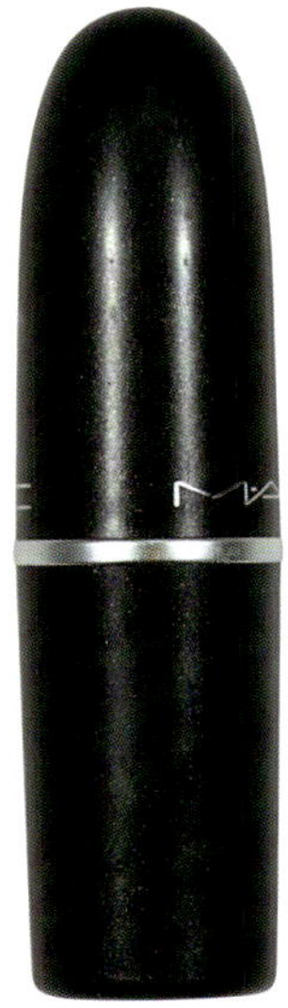

CHRISTIAN LOUBOUTIN BEAUTY

Rouge Louboutin Silky Satin Lipstick (shade Dune Kiss). The packaging is 10/10. I want to frame this...how iconic!?

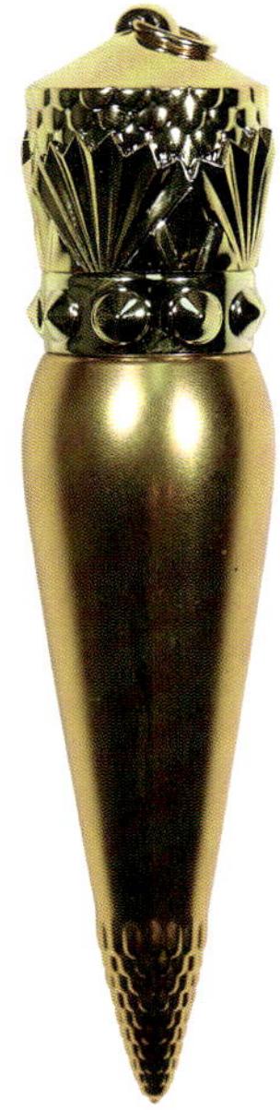

PAT MCGRATH LABS

SatinAllure Lipstick (shade Nude Fantasia). Pretty in pink with a cute little bow! I love Pat McGrath for this one. Her lip formulas are tip-top! I love how natural the shades can be—almost like it's your own natural lip color with a little flush to it.

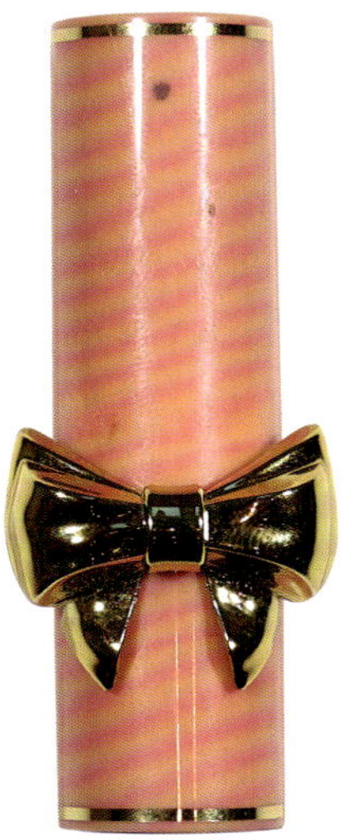

FENTY BEAUTY

Gloss Bomb Stix High-Shine Gloss Stick (shade Shimmering Hot Chocolit). This is the perfect brown lippie if you're going for a bolder lip and want to add some shine.

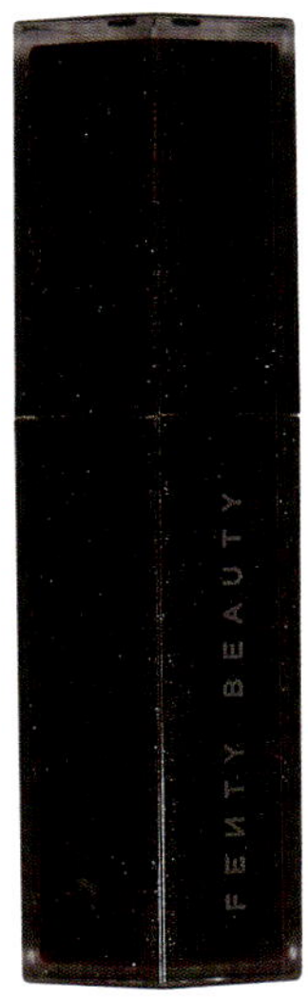

TOM FORD

Lip Color Matte Lipstick (shade Scarlet Rouge). Tom Ford Beauty is definitely a splurge, but it's a nice little treat. The packaging is so chic and durable. I love the range of shades. If you're a red-lip girl...Tom Ford Beauty is where you're going to find your perfect red.

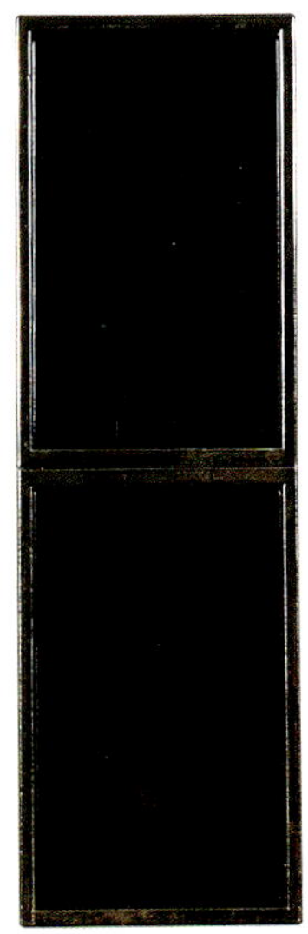

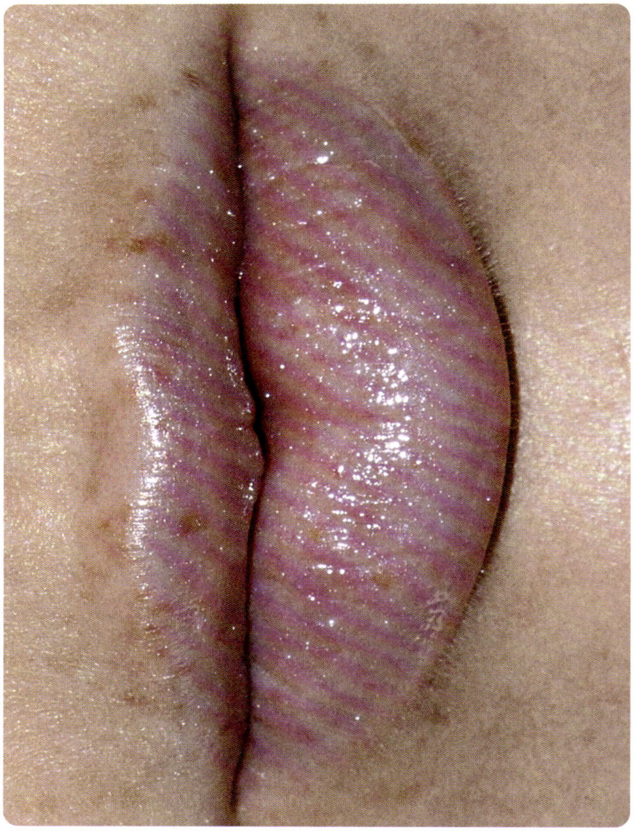
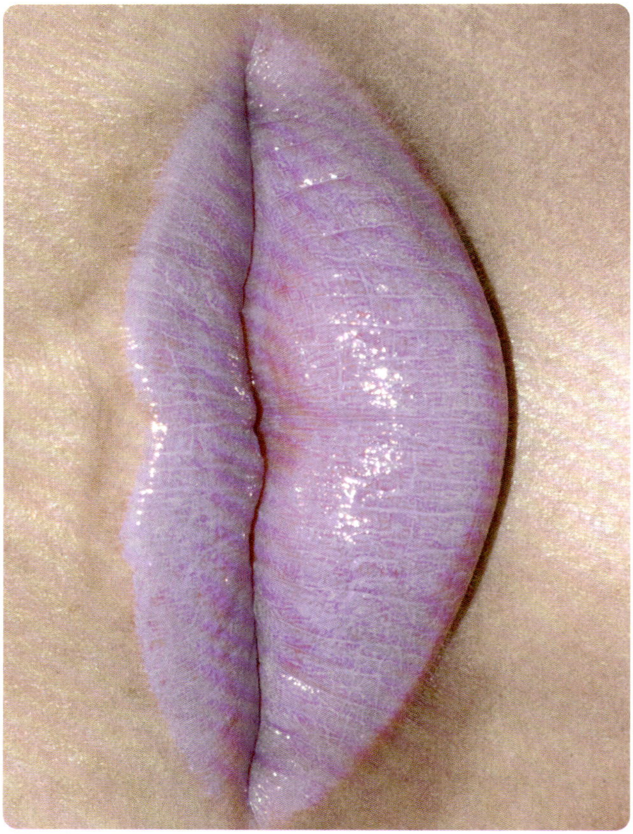
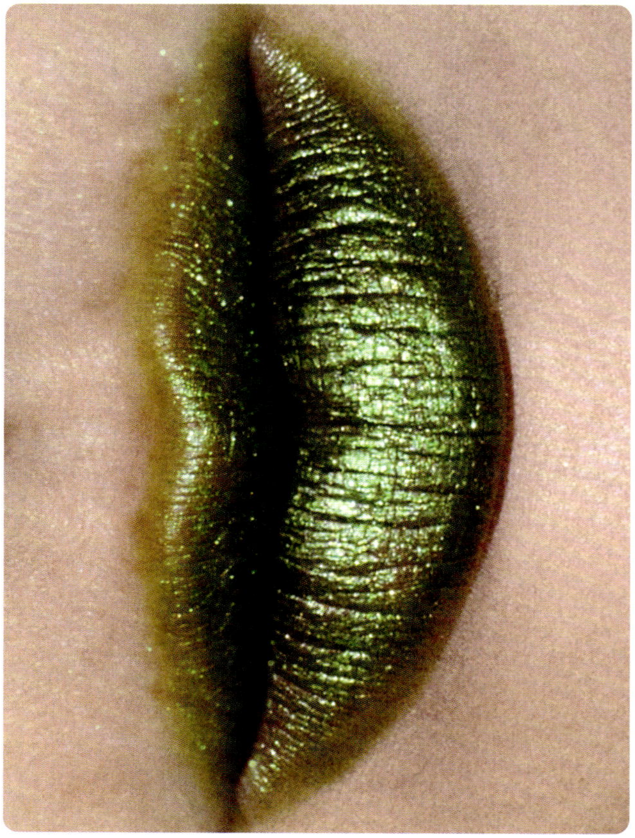
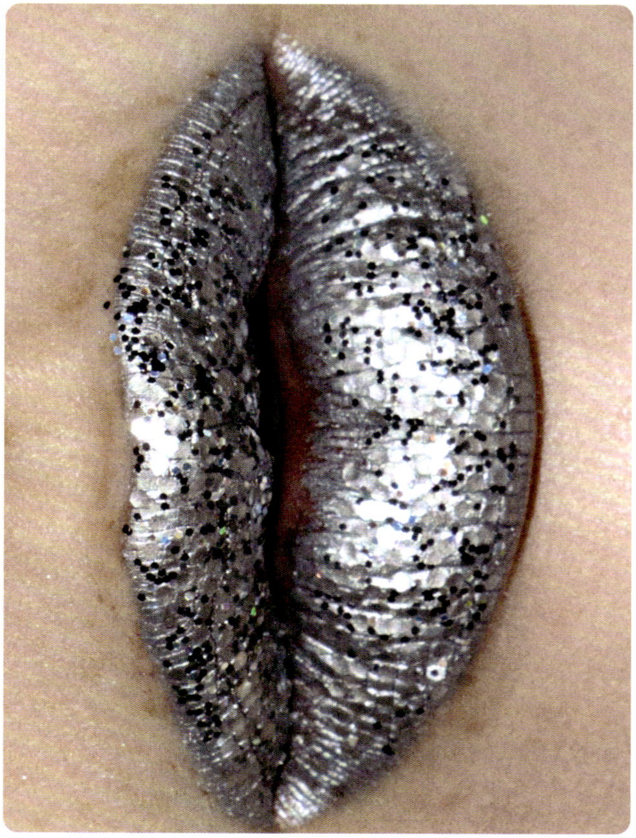

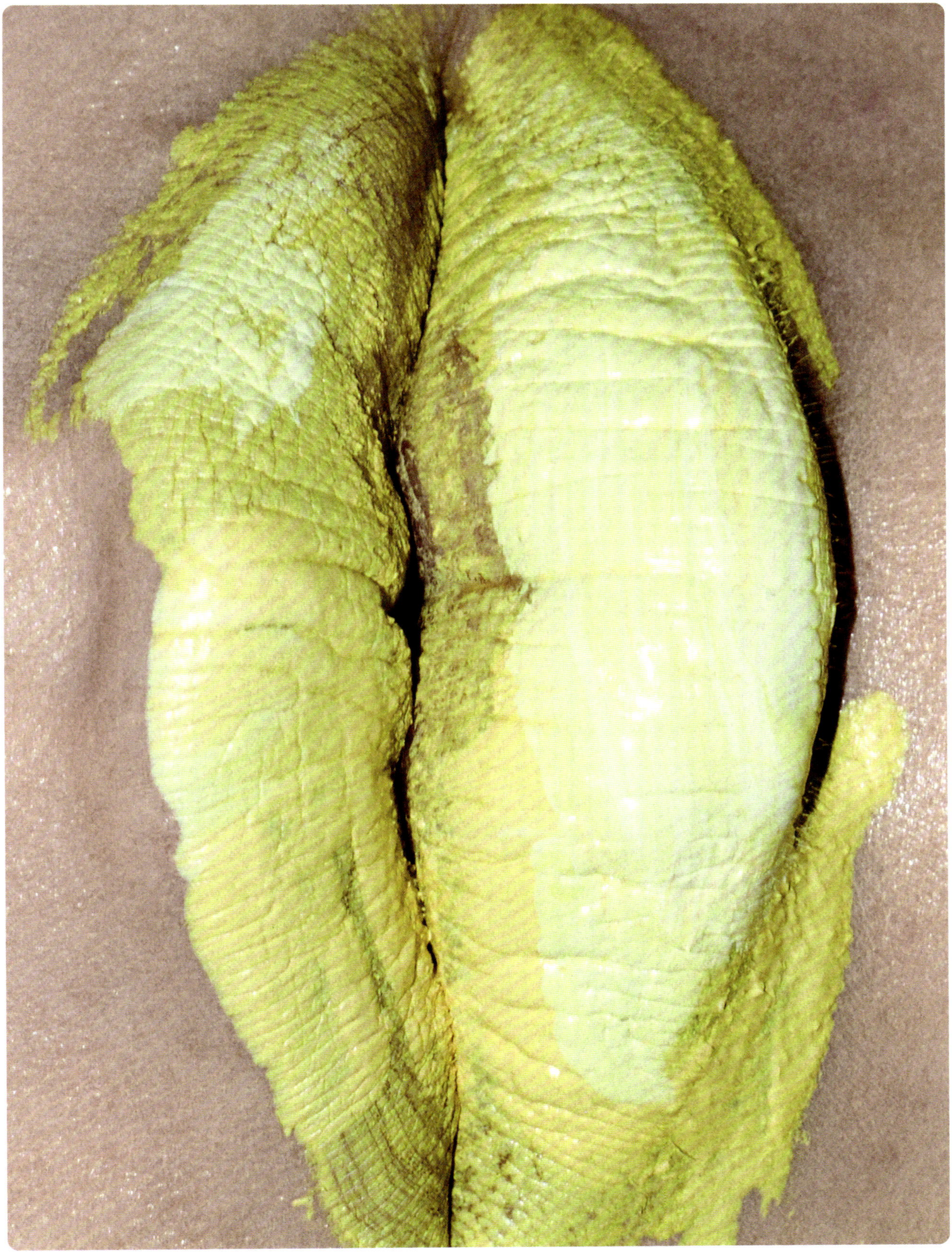

KIMCHI CHIC BEAUTY
Marshmallow Butter Lippie (shade Cafe au Lait). I am a nude lip girl through and through. I actually discovered this product on TikTok Shop and fell *in love*. I used to use concealer after lining my lips because I couldn't find a lipstick that was nude enough for me. This one is the perfect matte nude with a touch of pink. It always makes it in my bag on a night out with me, hehe.

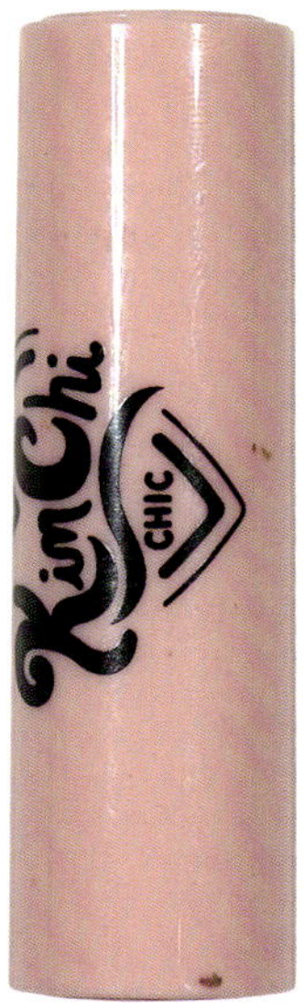

LANCÔME
Juicy Tubes Lip Gloss (shade Marshmallow Electro [Sparkle]). This lip gloss takes me back to the 2000s, hehe. This will elevate any look and bring it to the next level of glam. They smell delicious and come in many fun shades to play around with!

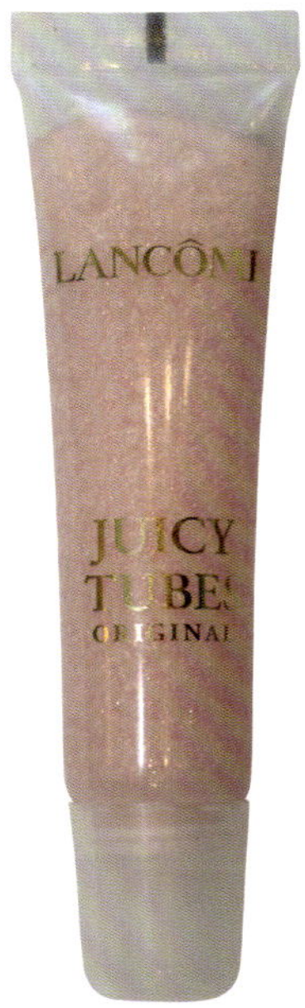

OLE HENRIKSEN
Pout Preserve Peptide Lip Treatment (shade Citrus Sunshine). My go-to alllll the way! I have been using this ever since it launched. It honestly became a staple in my everyday life. I use it when I wake up, throughout the day, and when I go to bed. I even use it on top of my lip liner for a super juicy lip. The formula is so long-lasting, and I love how well it layers and doesn't strip my lip liner off.

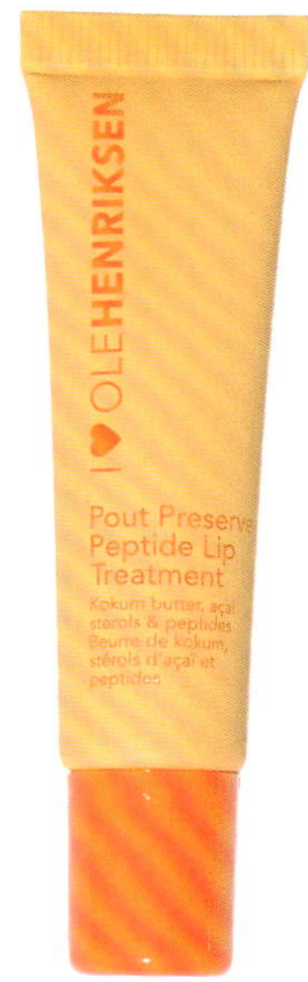

NÉCESSAIRE
The Lip Balm. I'm a lip balm girl through and through. I hate having dry lips, so I take this step very seriously. I love this lip balm because it has a cooling metal tip that provides the best application! It's also minty, so it gives the lips a nice plump!

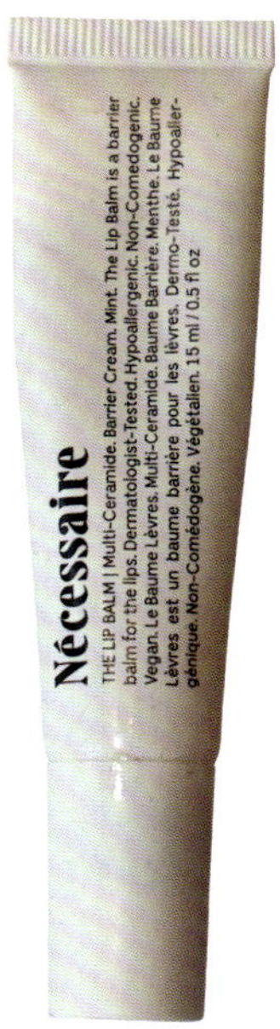

DIOR ADDICT
Lip Glow Butter in Glazed Lavender (shade Glazed Lavender). Yummmm, these are the juiciest, nonsticky lip butters. The charm is such a cute edition (I'm a big packaging girl). Who doesn't want their lip gloss to have charms on it??!!

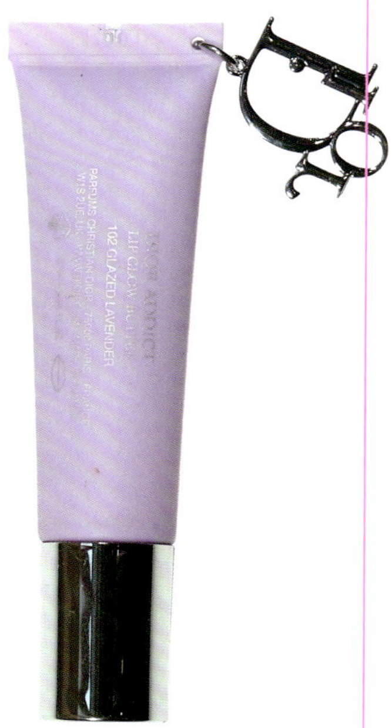

BENEFIT COSMETICS
24-Hour Brow Setter Gel. My skinny little 90s brows love this product. It's not flaky, and it doesn't make your eyebrows feel crusty and hard. The applicator is amazing for brushing, snatching, and lifting. A must-have in my makeup bag for sure.

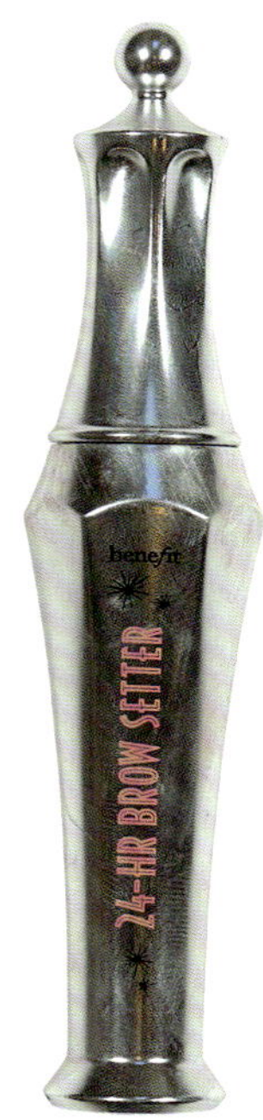

L'ORÉAL
Extensionist Mascara. This mascara has been a fave of mine for a while. It's extra-special because L'Oréal bedazzled it for me... how glam! My lashes look like I've just gotten a fresh lash lift after using this. PRO TIP: For an extra level of volume, use a lash curler beforehand.

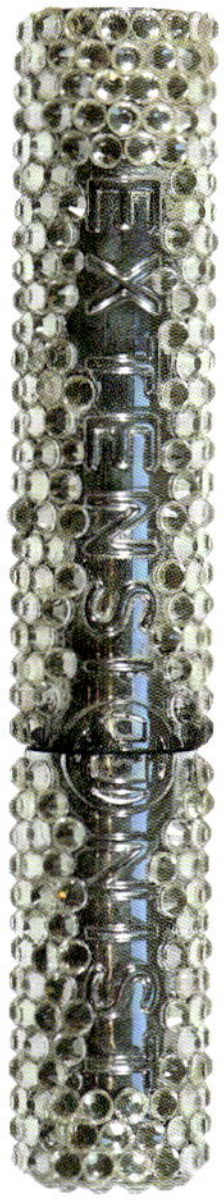

CHARLOTTE TILBURY
Exagger-eyes Mascara. Wow, wow, wow! If I could give an award for mascara packaging, this one would be the winner. It is so luxurious and feels like something out of a princess's makeup bag. The formula is great and doesn't bleed under your eyes. It lasts all day and gives a great lift!

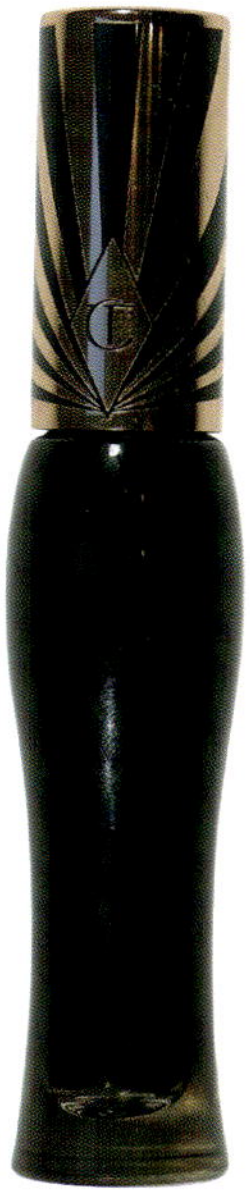

DIORSHOW
Overvolume Extreme Volume Mascara. If you want extreme volume for your lashes, reach for this baby.

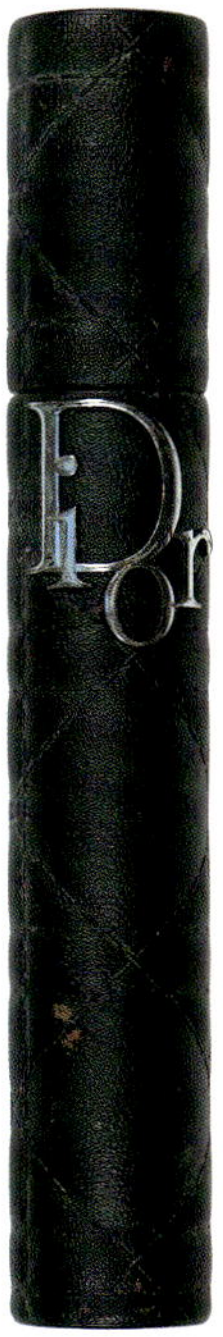

PAW PAW BLENDING SPONGE
This is another thing I cannot do my makeup without. A Paw Paw is the ultimate beauty sponge, and you can get a big pack on Amazon. They are the bounciest, softest beauty sponges out there. PRO TIP: Soak it under the faucet and ring out all the water before using it.

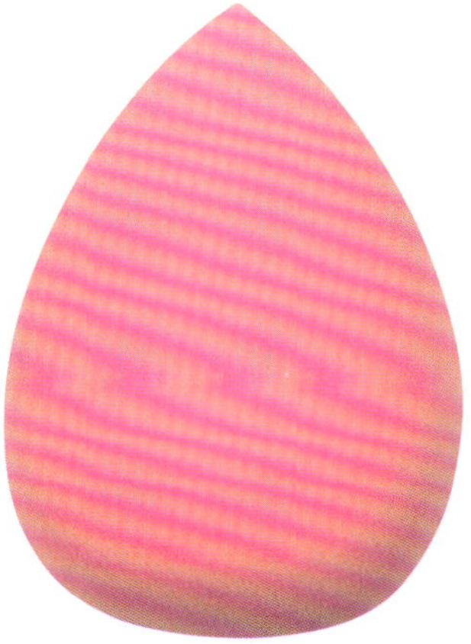

POWDER PUFF
I can't do any makeup look without a powder puff. If you're using a brush to set your face with powder, switch to this and watch how soft your skin is going to look. It's a game-changer. PRO TIP: Dip into loose powder, then dab it onto the backs of your hands before pressing it into your skin. You'll get a more airbrush finish.

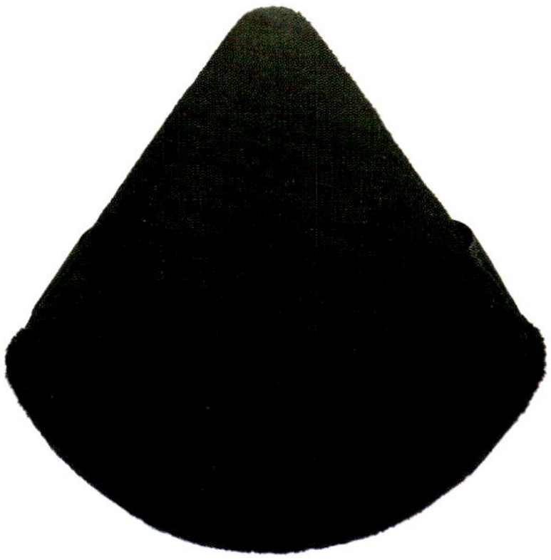

SHARPENERS
Sharpeners are little makeup trinkets that follow me everywhere. I have one lying around in every purse. It's a tool I can't live without. If you want that snatched look... your pencil liners need to be nice and sharp.

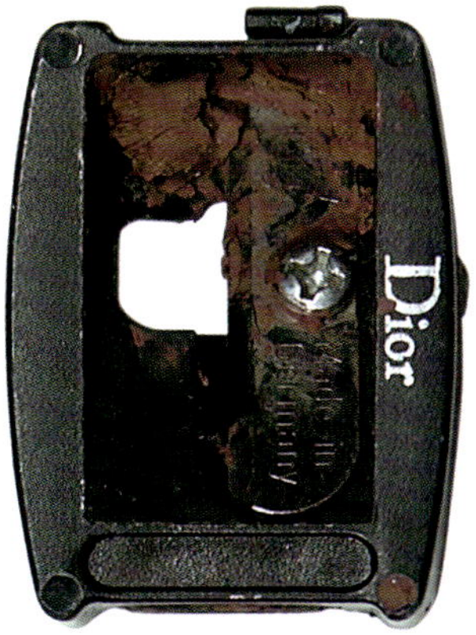

LASHES, LASHES, LASHES!

Lashes are a great accessory. They can totally complete a look and take it up a notch if you want a little more of a glam moment! Some of my favorites are from KISS Lashes, Kylie Cosmetics, and Lilly Lashes. PRO TIP: Ardell Duo Lash Adhesive is the best lash glue out there!

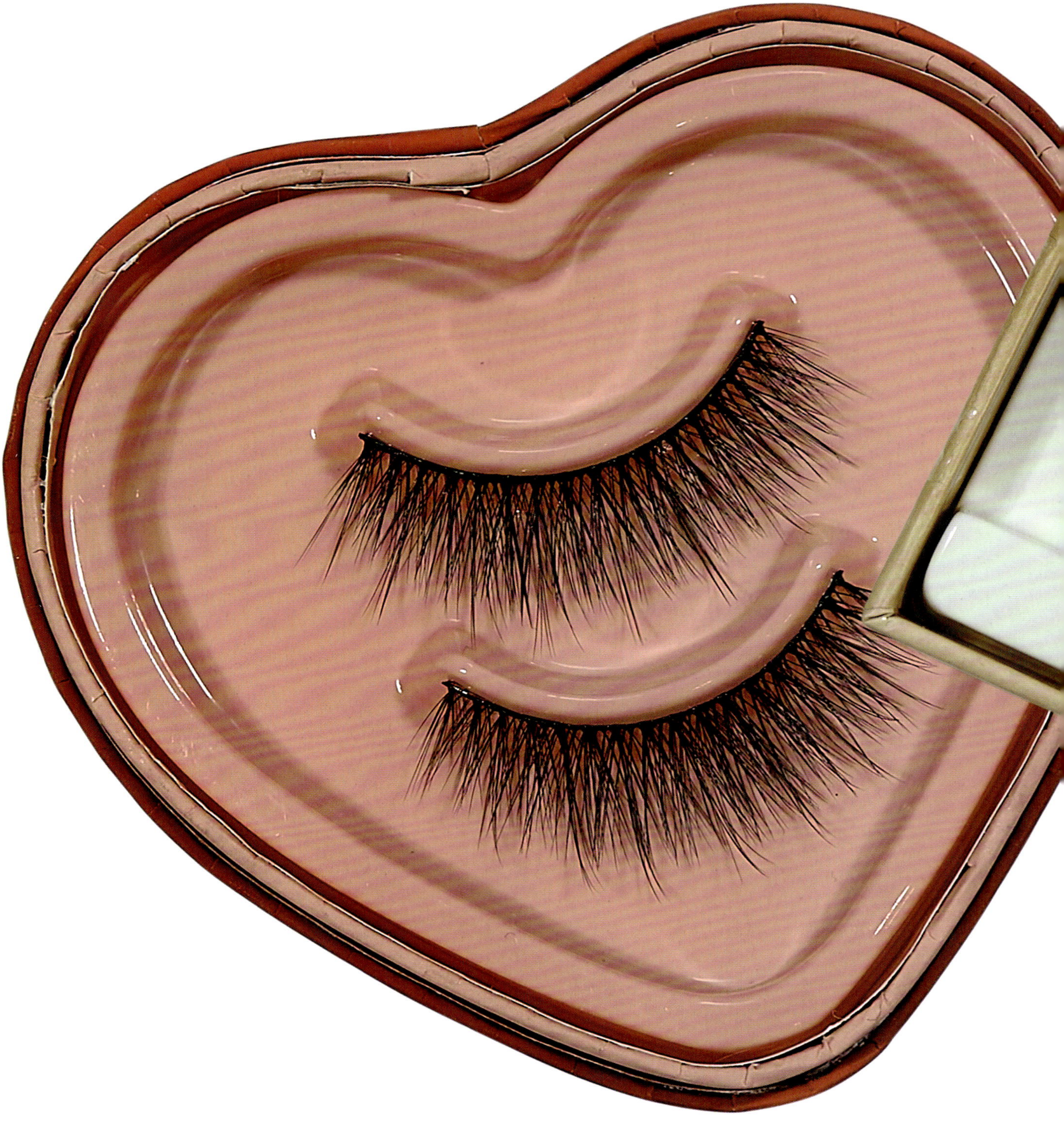

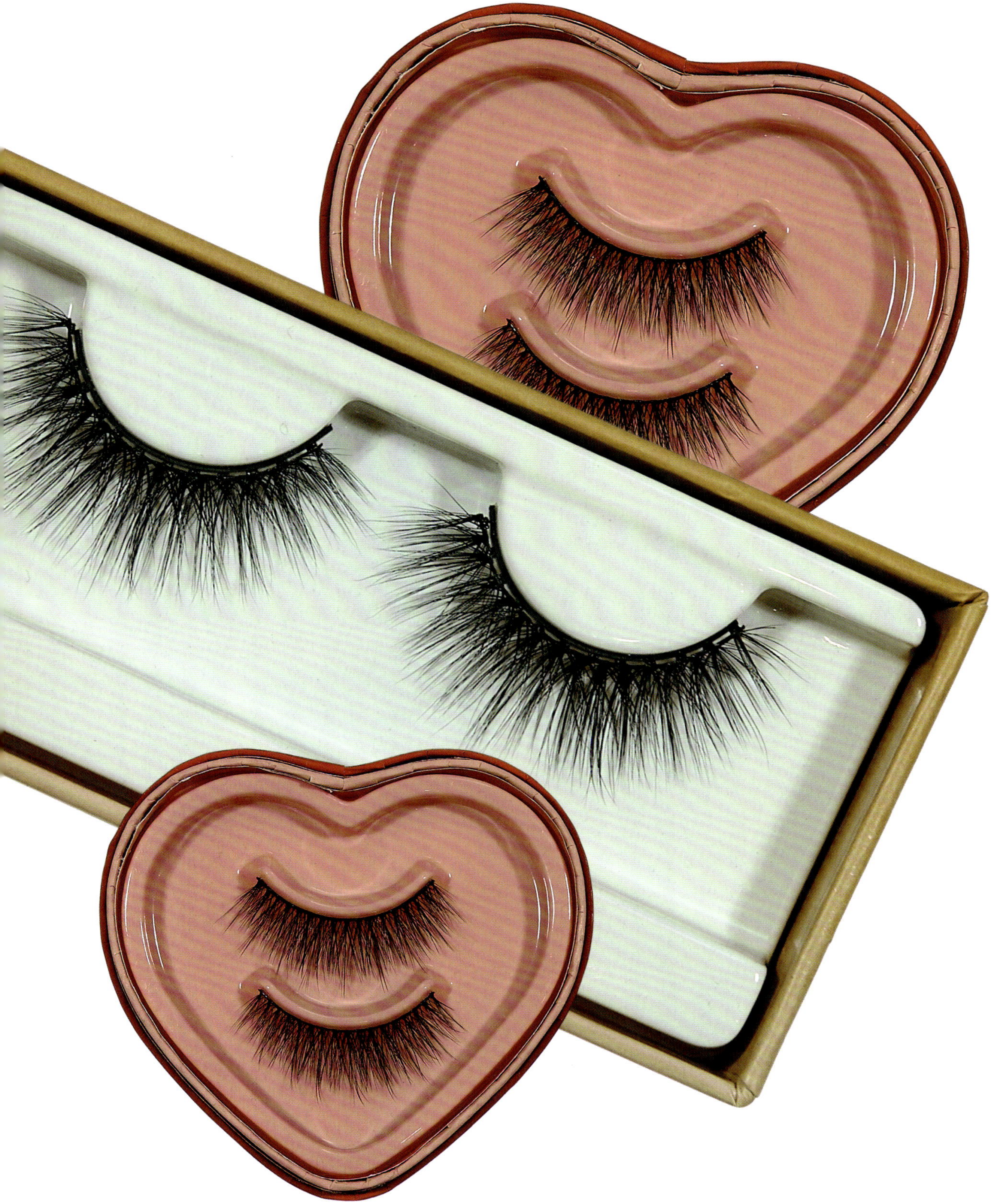

E.L.F. PR BOX
I save all of my PR boxes to remind me of all the amazing opportunities. I've been lucky enough to have collaborated with some of my dream brands. This was the PR box for my "face of" campaign with e.l.f., launching their O Face lipsticks!

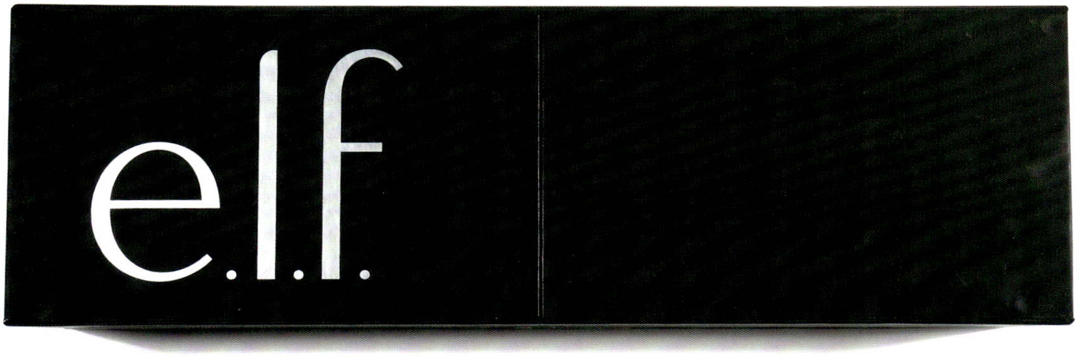

KISS PR BOX
KISS Lashes are one of my favorite false-eyelash brands, so it was an absolute dream to work with them on my very own collection. This was the PR box that included the collection inside!

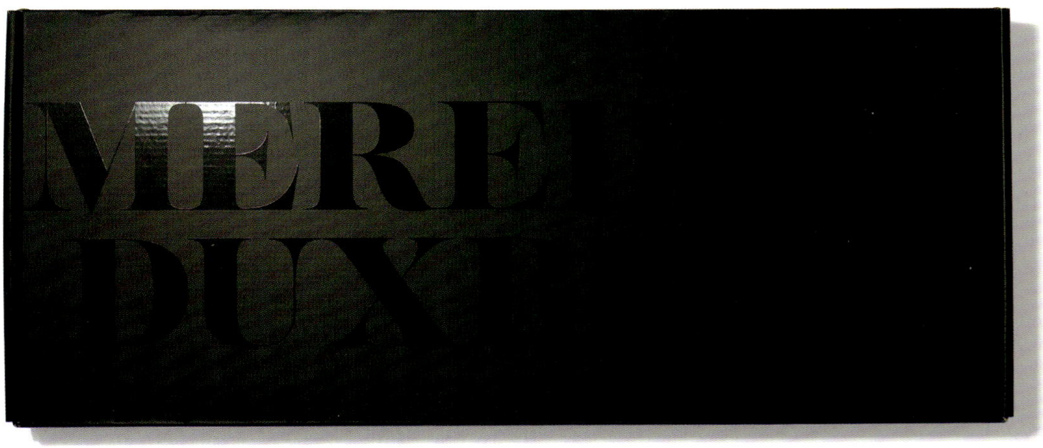

MORPHE X MEREDITH DUXBURY PR BOX
This is the PR box of my collection with Morphe Cosmetics. I spent so much time on this project, and it really showed my love for color and glam. This photo was shot on a rooftop pool in New York City—how iconic!

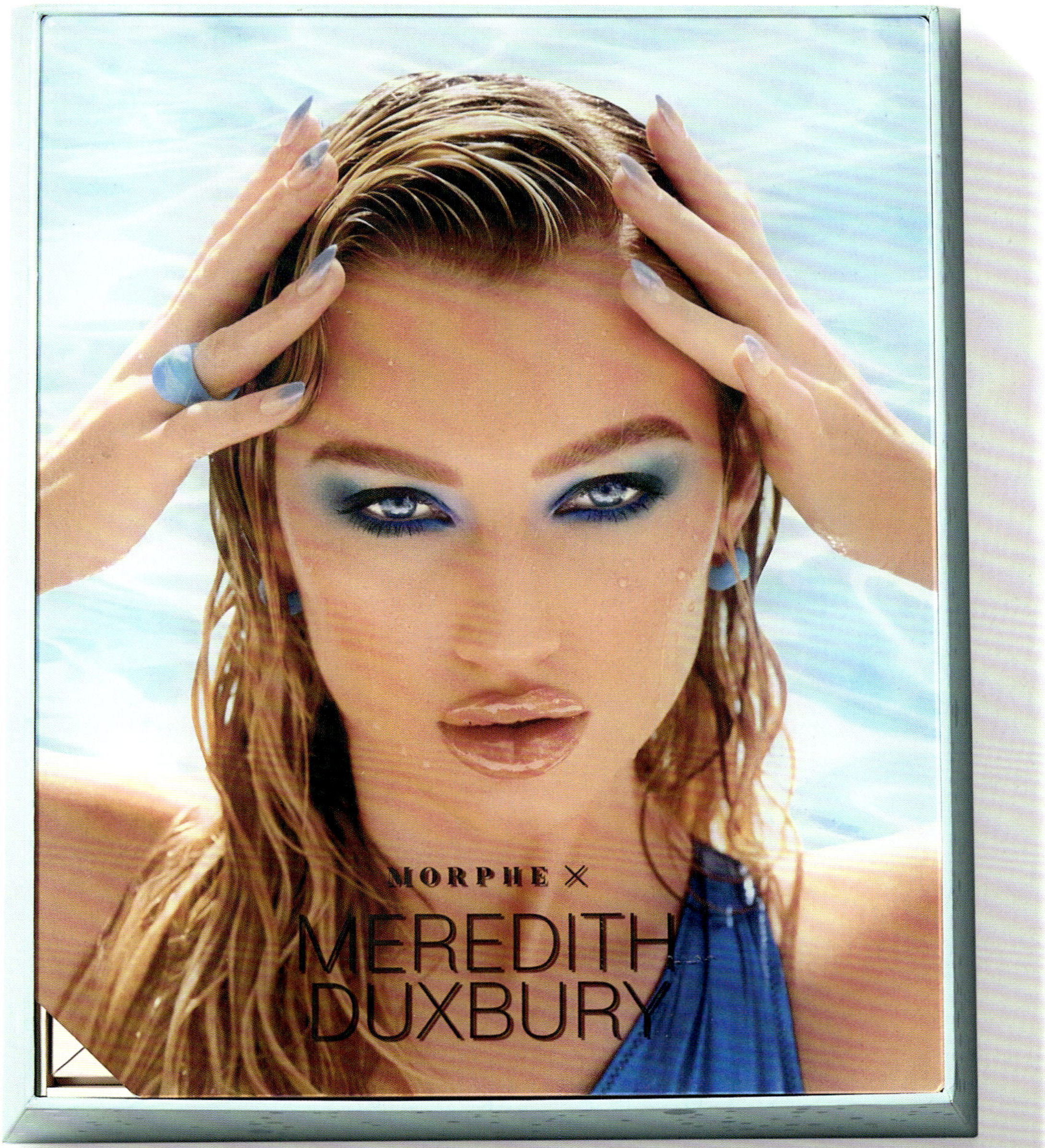

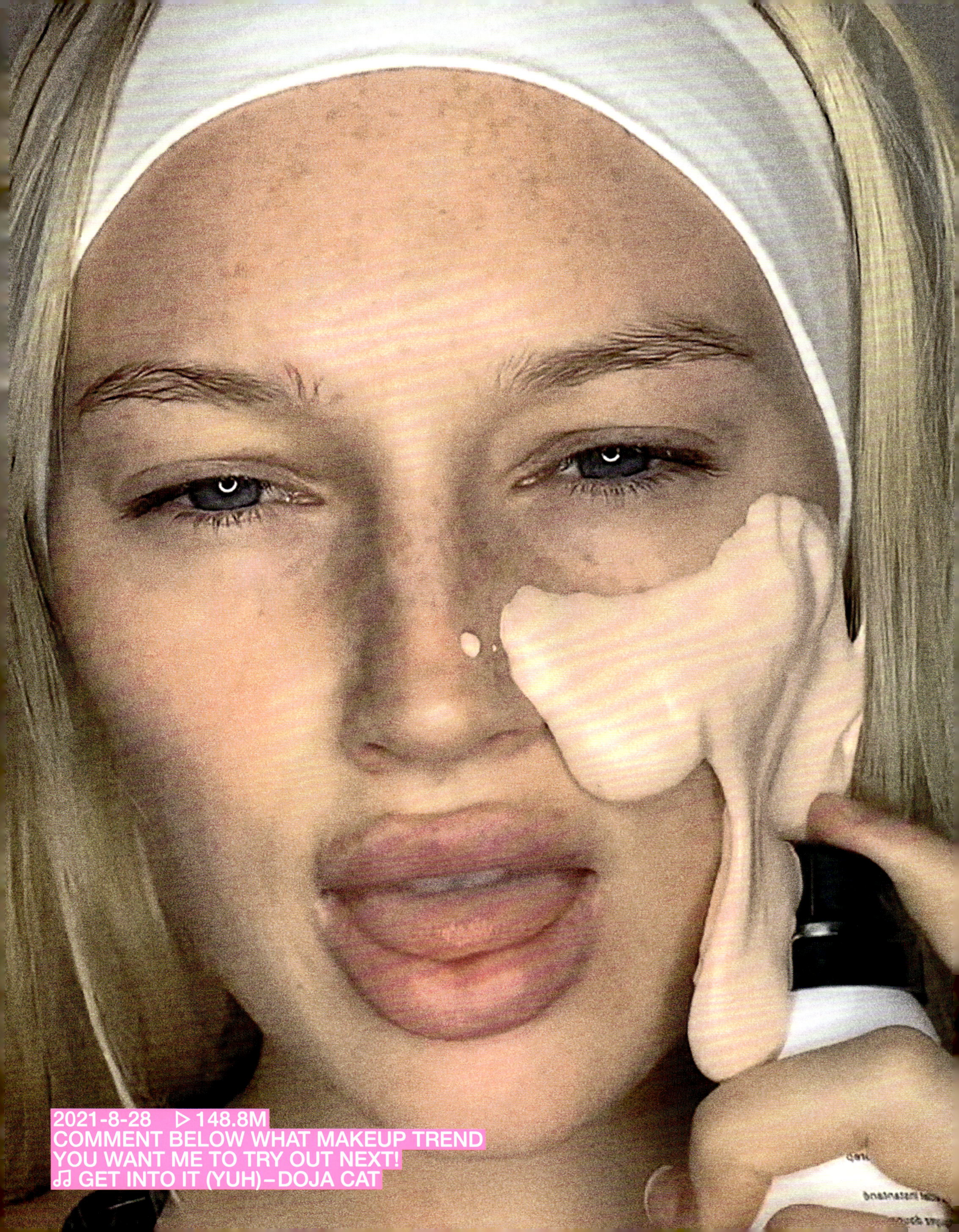
2021-8-28 ▷ 148.8M
COMMENT BELOW WHAT MAKEUP TREND
YOU WANT ME TO TRY OUT NEXT!
♫ GET INTO IT (YUH)–DOJA CAT

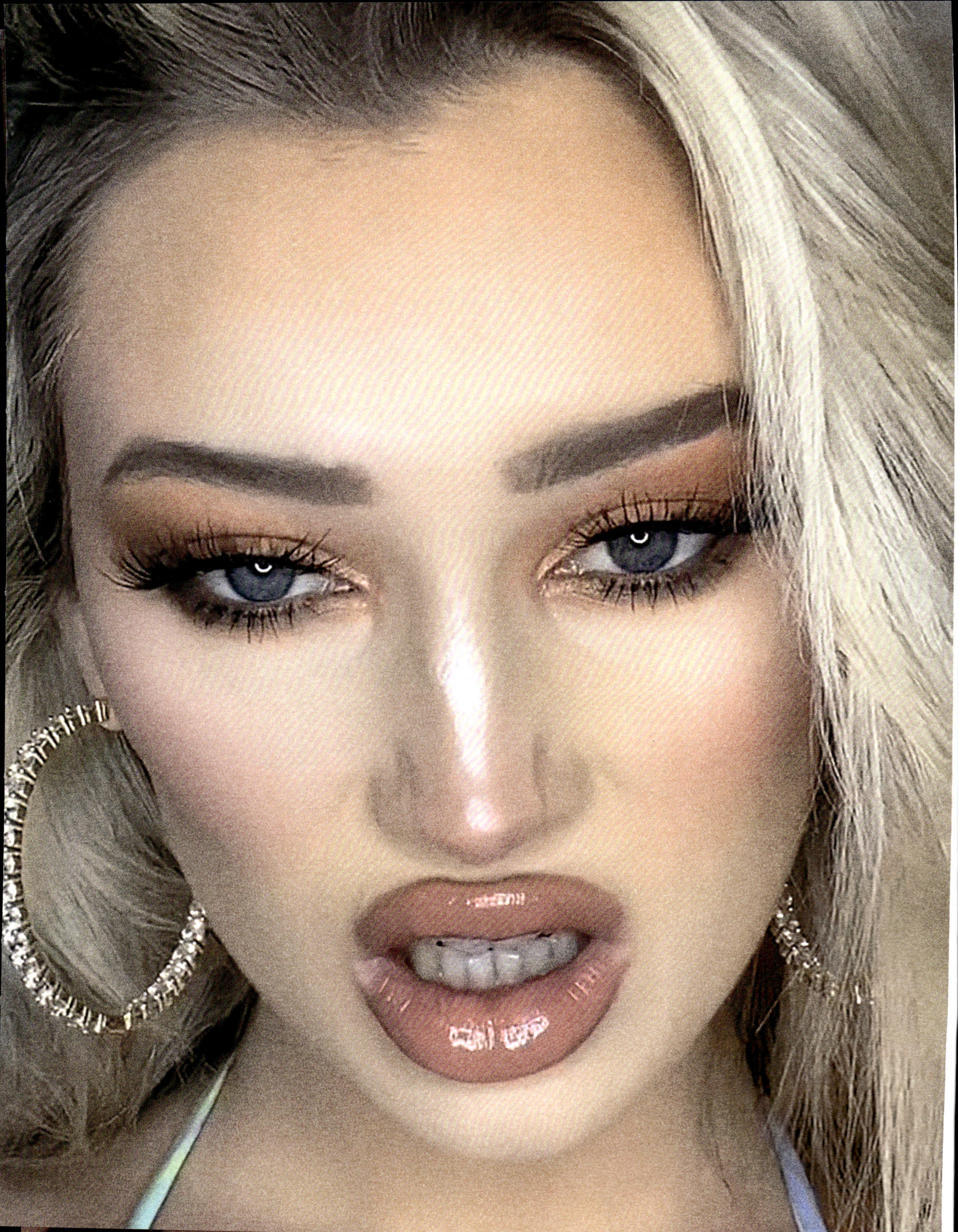

YOUTUBE 1 MILLION GOLD PLAQUE CREATOR AWARD
In an industry where everything is digital and online, it's really nice to have something tangible to show off your accomplishments and work. YouTube sent me this plaque for reaching 1 million subscribers. Shout-out to my YouTube fam, I love you guys beyond!!!

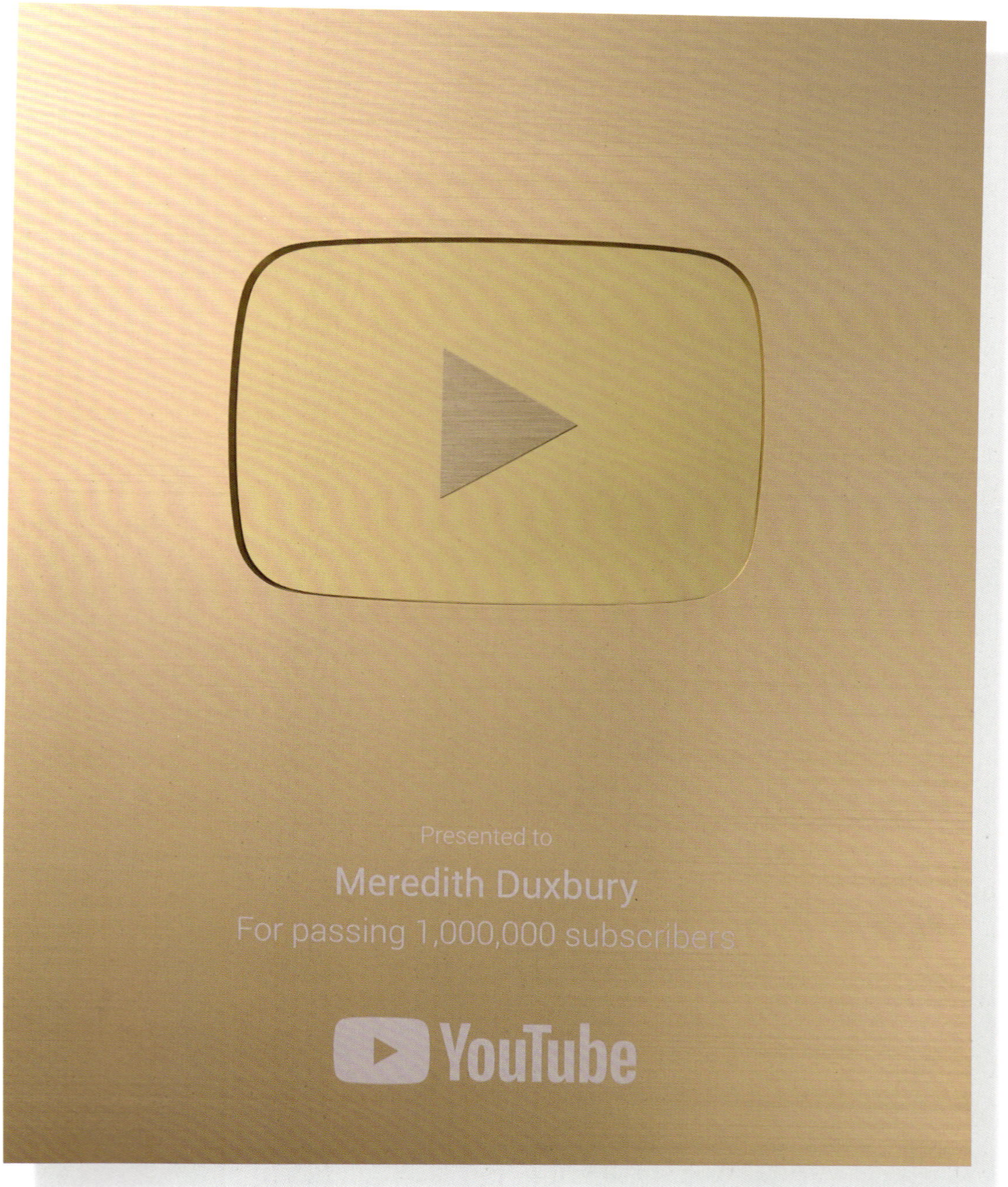
Presented to
Meredith Duxbury
For passing 1,000,000 subscribers
YouTube

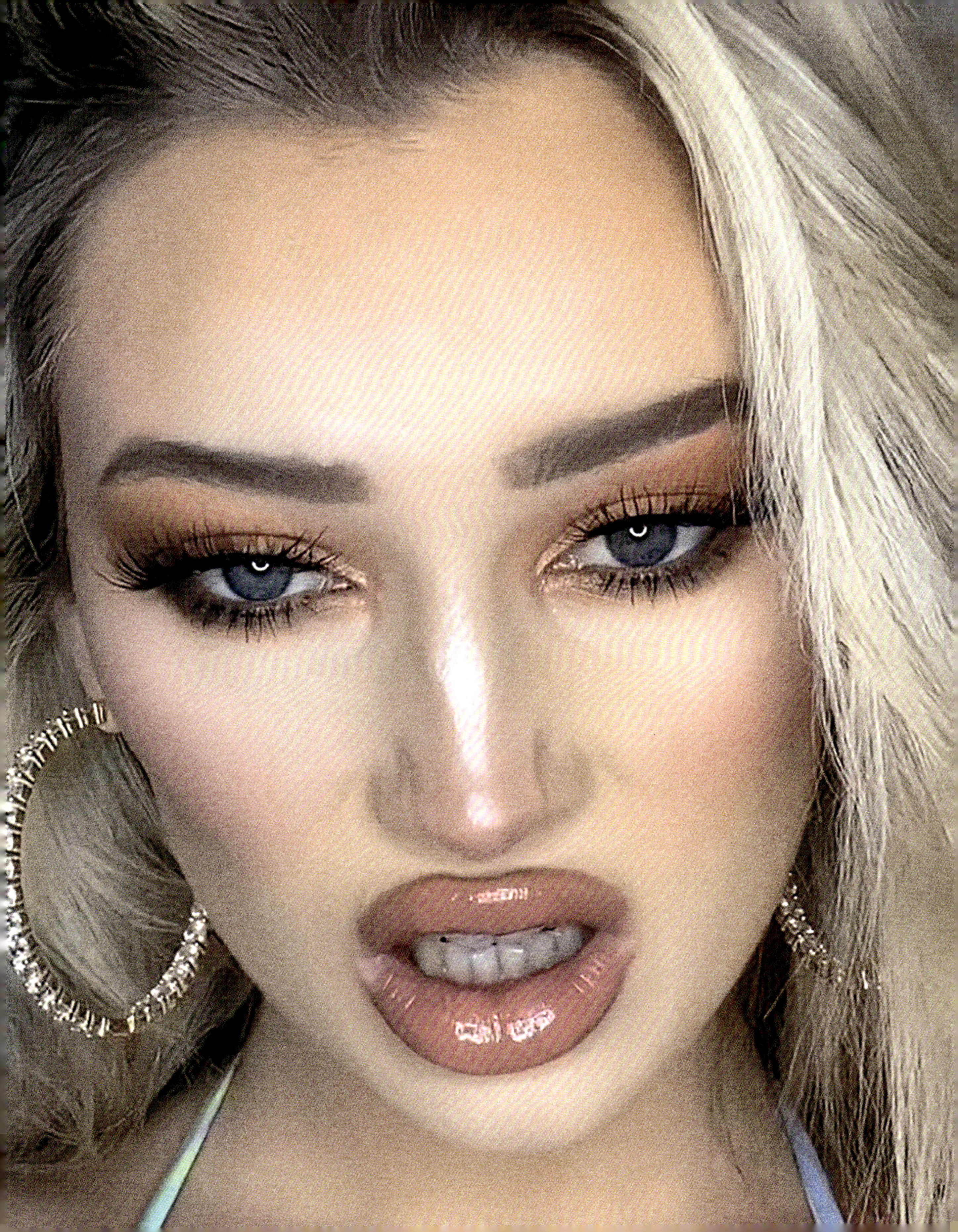

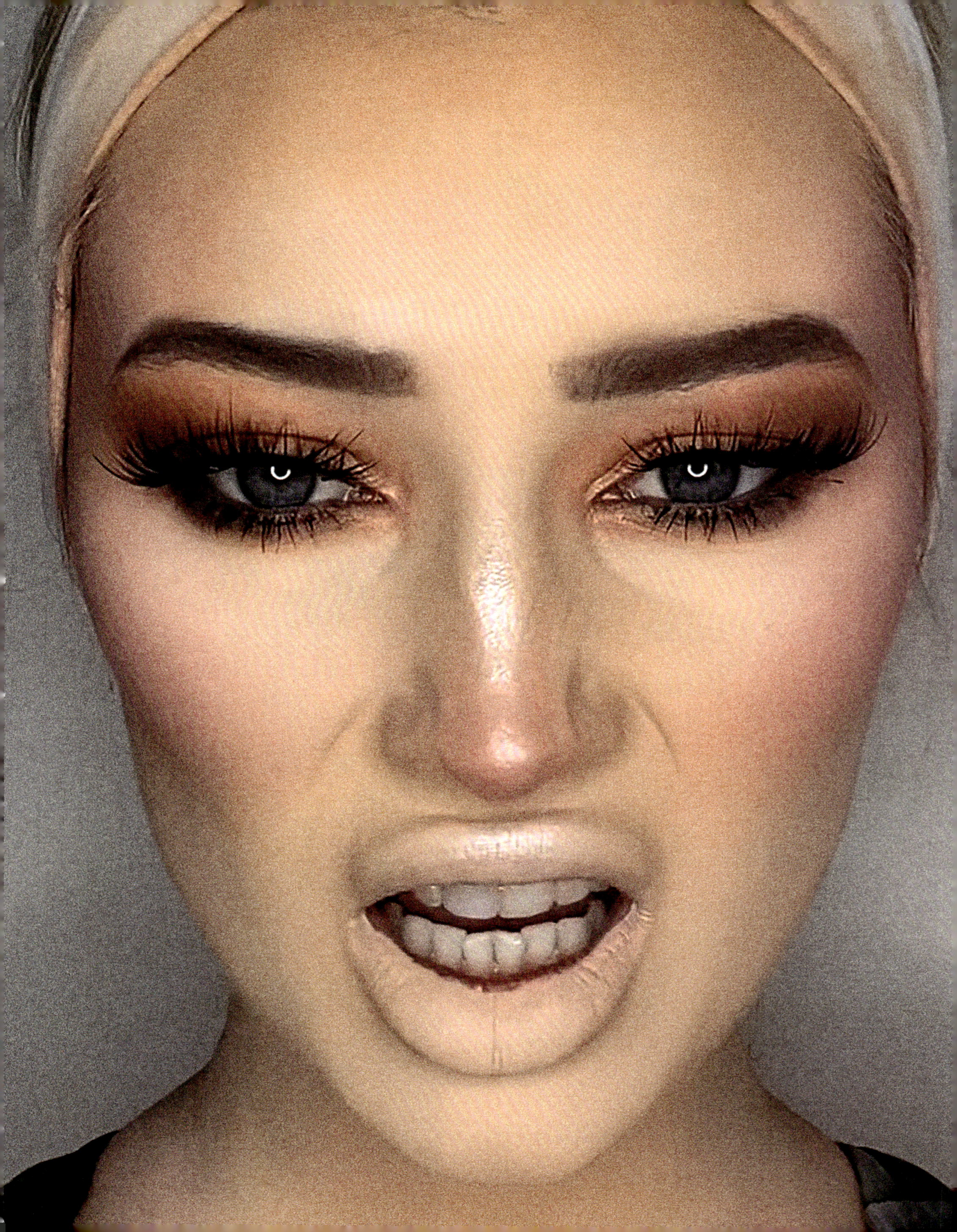

YOUTUBE 1 MILLION GOLD PLAQUE CREATOR AWARD
In an industry where everything is digital and online, it's really nice to have something tangible to show off your accomplishments and work. YouTube sent me this plaque for reaching 1 million subscribers. Shout-out to my YouTube fam, I love you guys beyond!!!

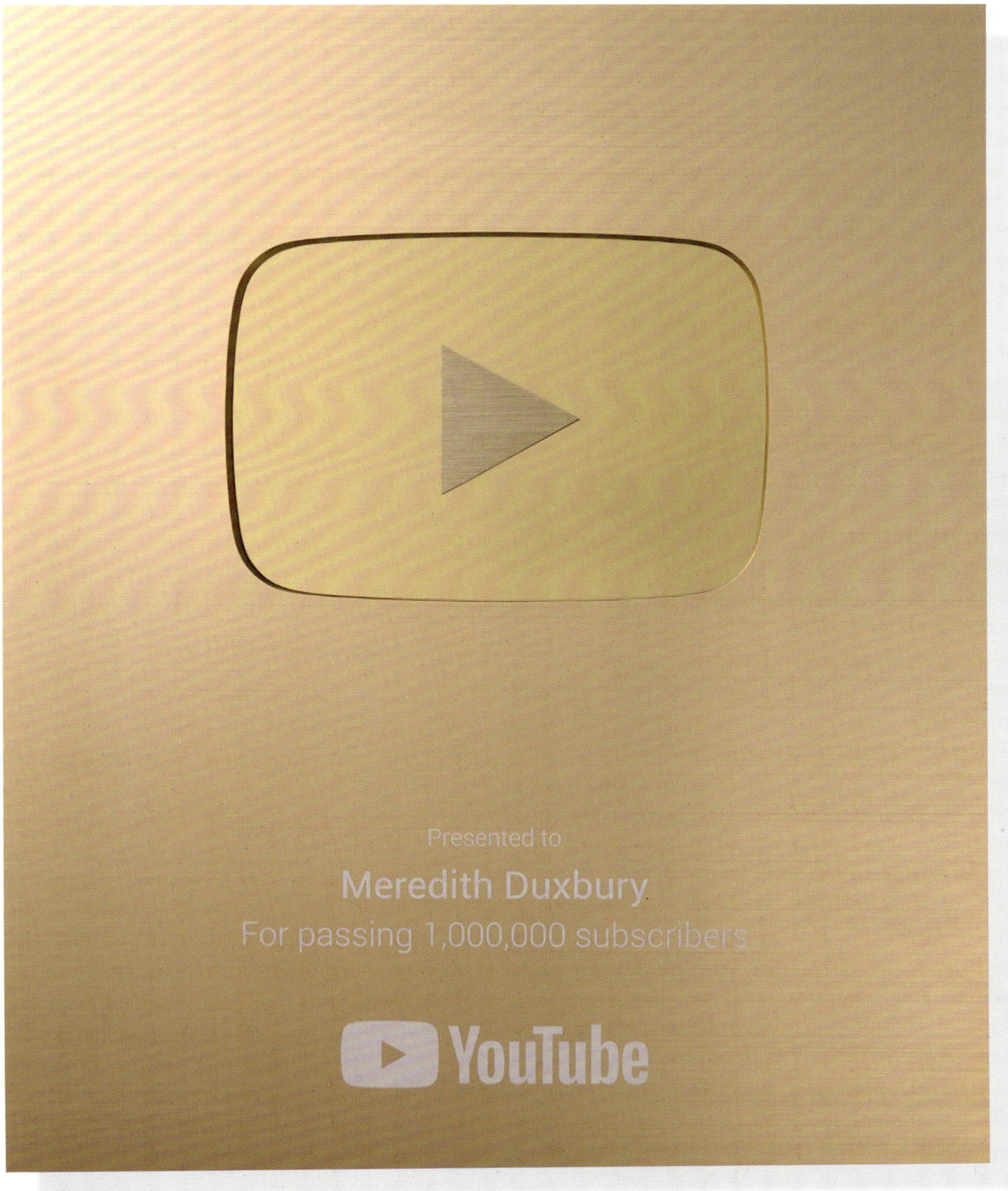
Presented to
Meredith Duxbury
For passing 1,000,000 subscribers
YouTube

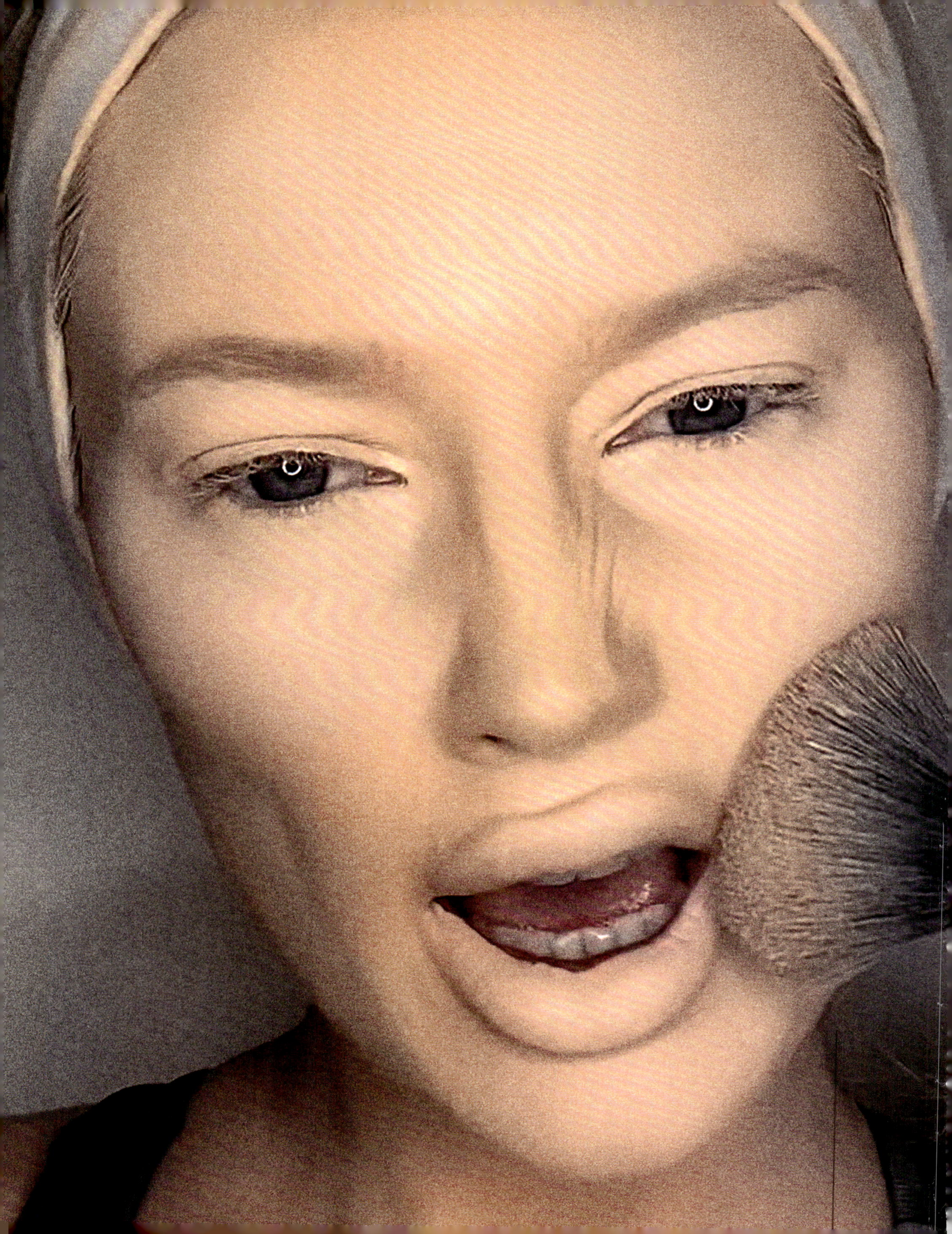

MORPHE X MEREDITH DUXBURY
35-Pan Artistry Palette. This is one of my favorite palettes I've ever owned, not only because I created it from scratch with Morphe, but because it has everything in one: it's so versatile, it has shimmers, mattes, neutrals, and fun pops of color! I always reach for this when I want to feel inspired.

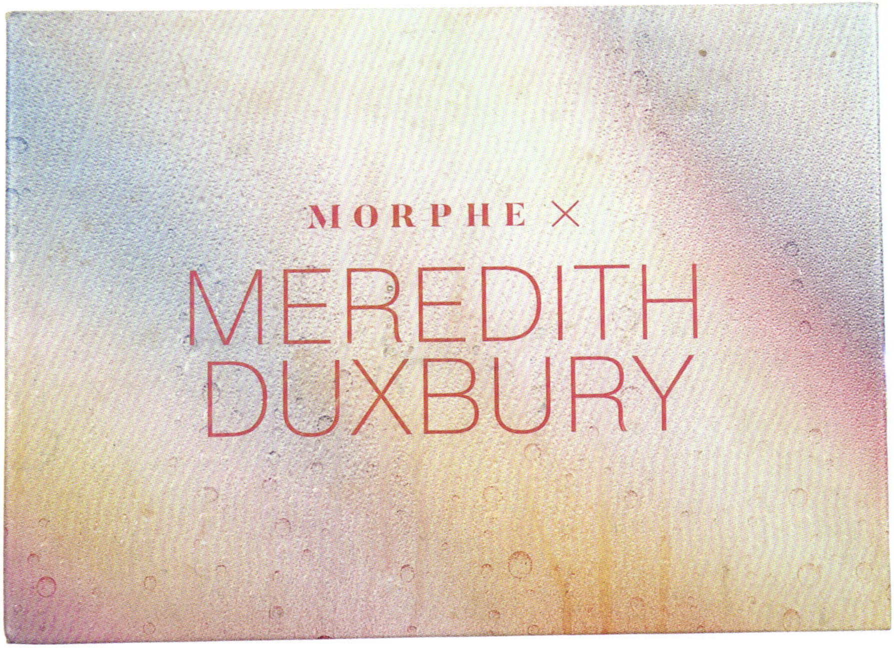

KISS X MEREDITH DUXBURY
I've been such a fan of KISS lashes for so long, so when they came to me to do a collaboration, I was beyond excited to create some of my favorite styles with them! These are for when I want to glam it up and feel like *that* girl....

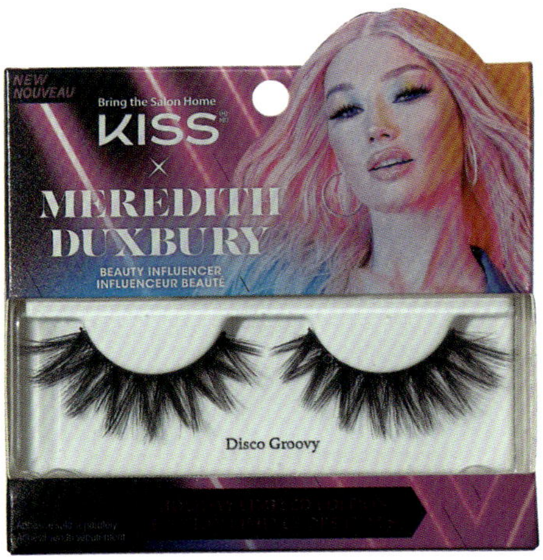

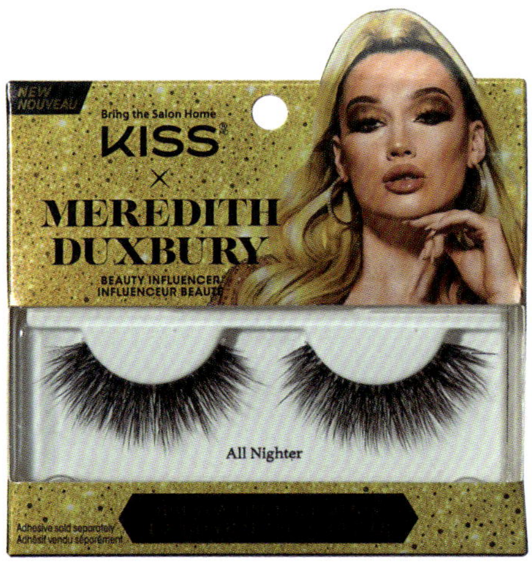

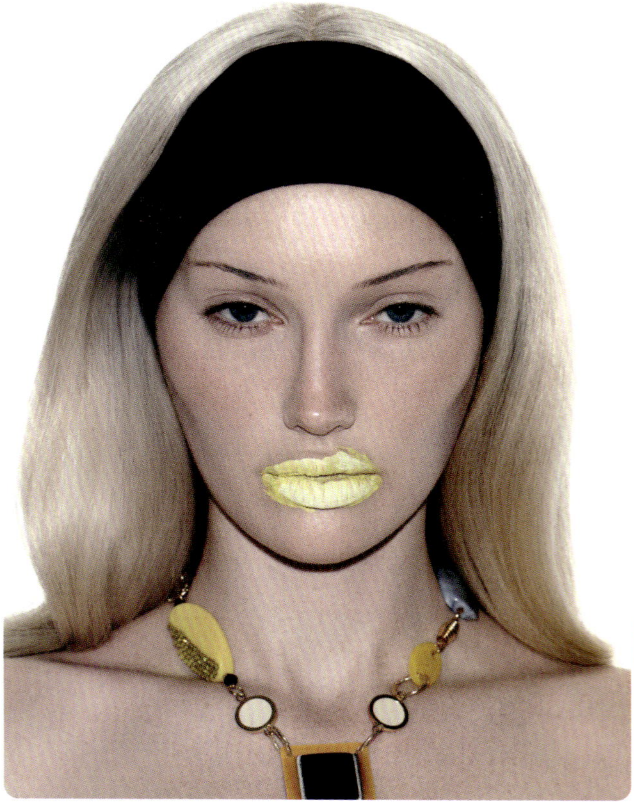

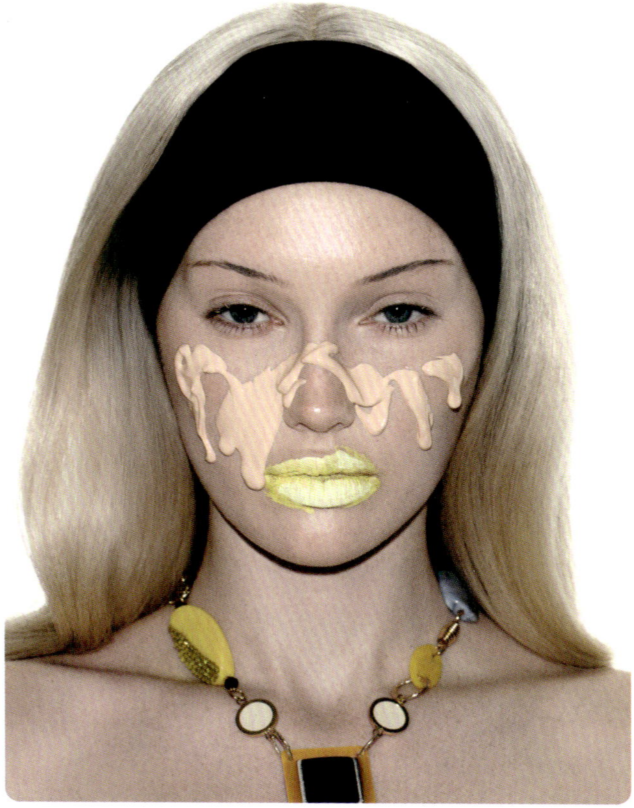

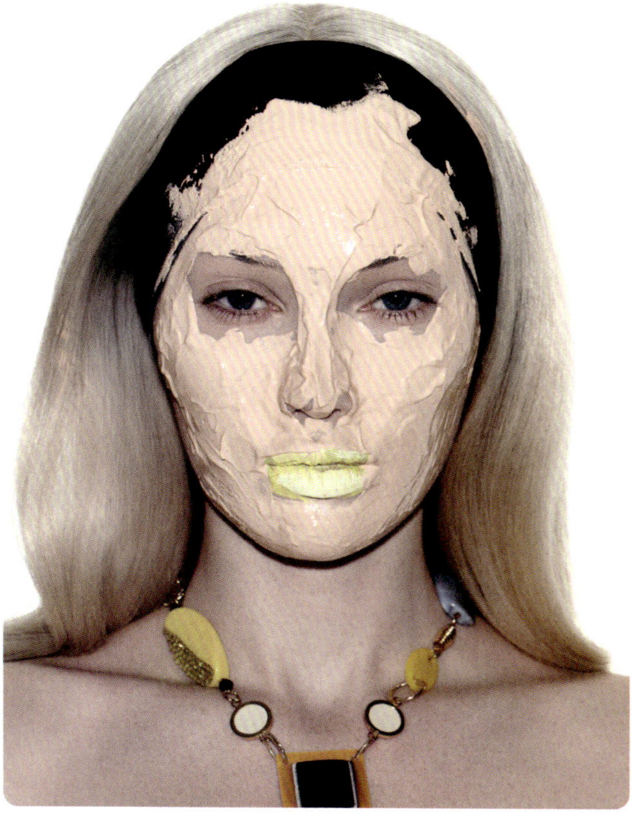

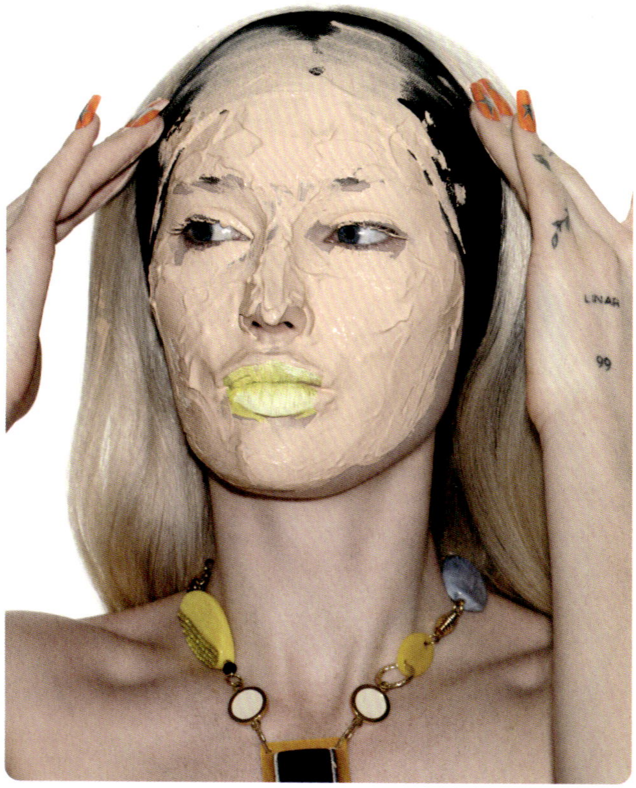

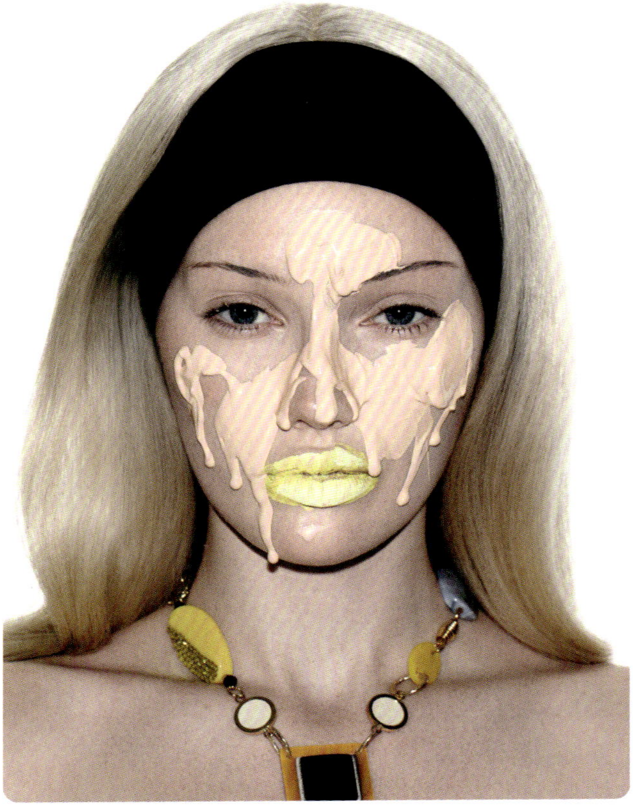

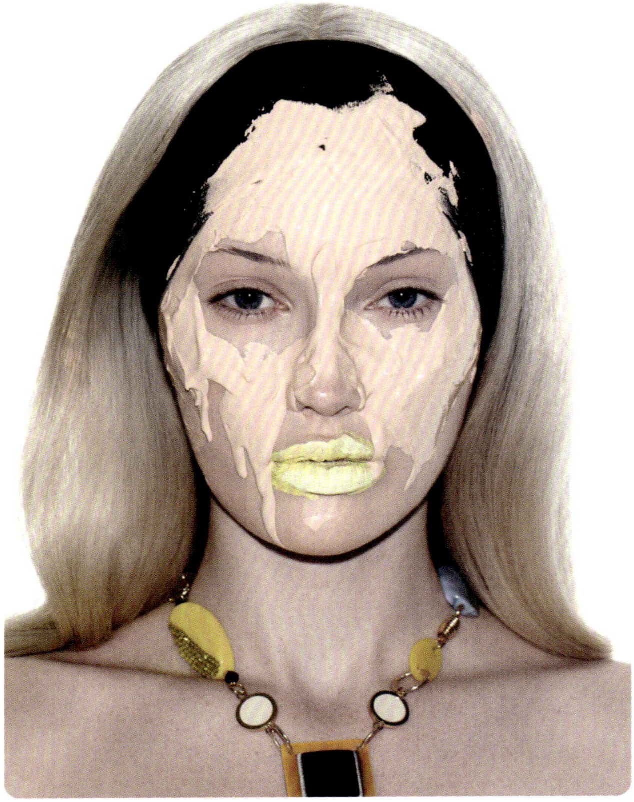

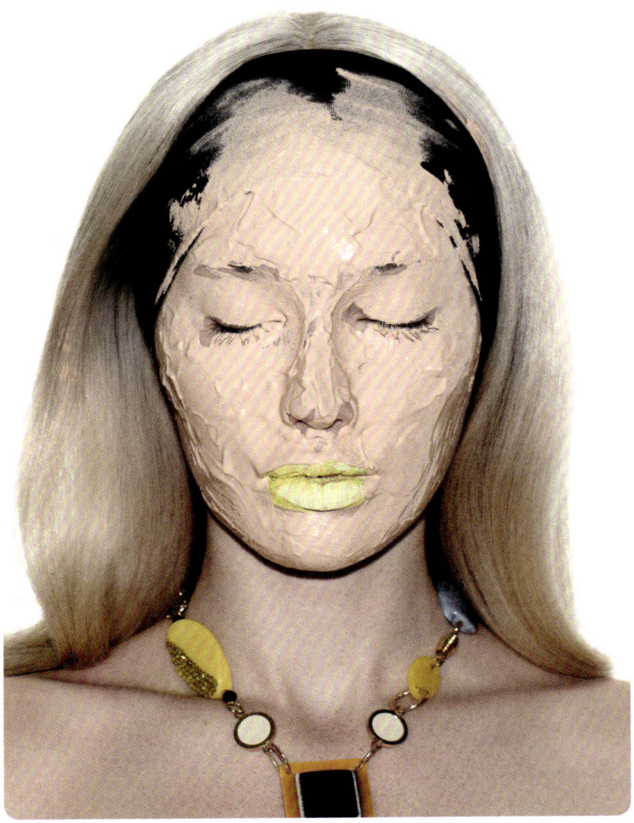

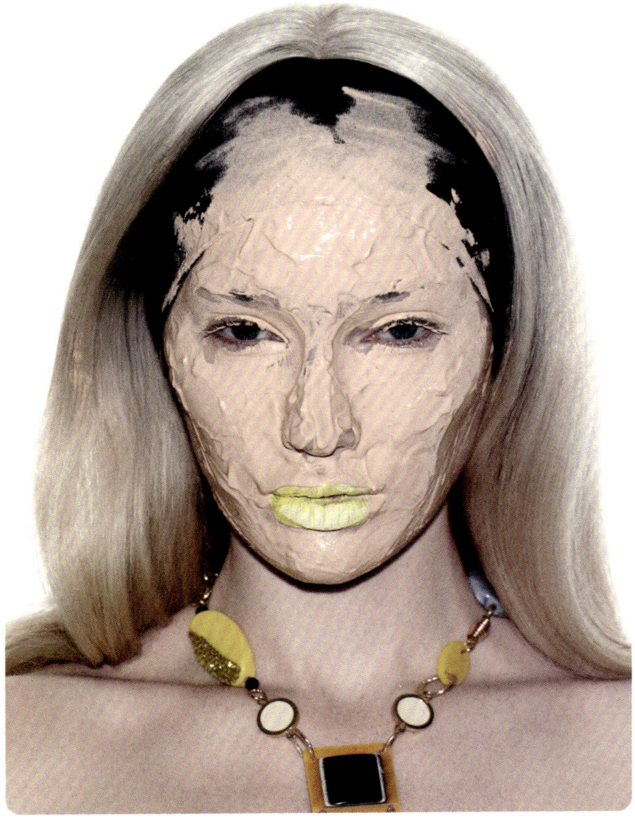

"EMBRACE MESSY GIRL MAKEUP, IT DOESN'T NEED TO BE PERFECT"

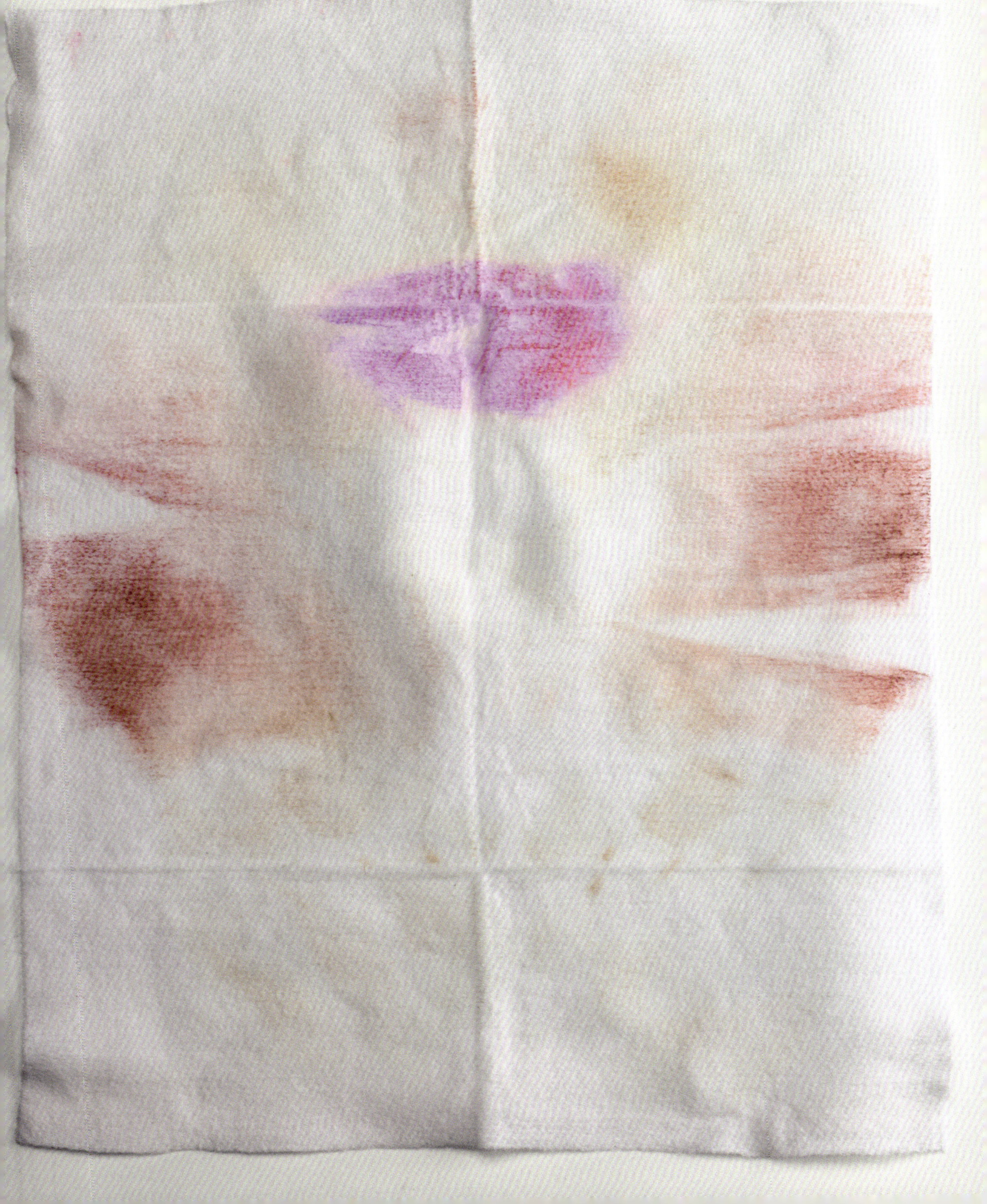

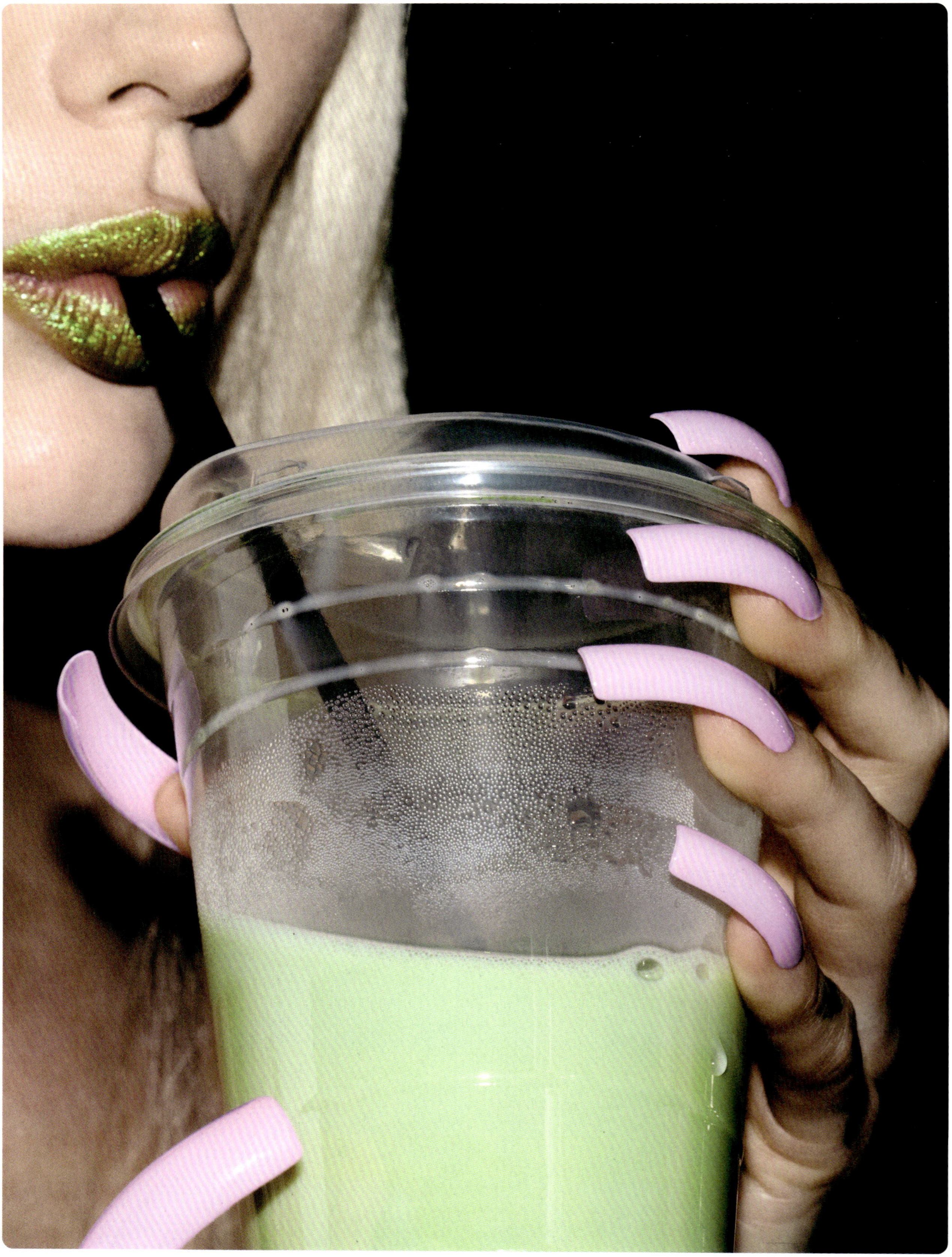

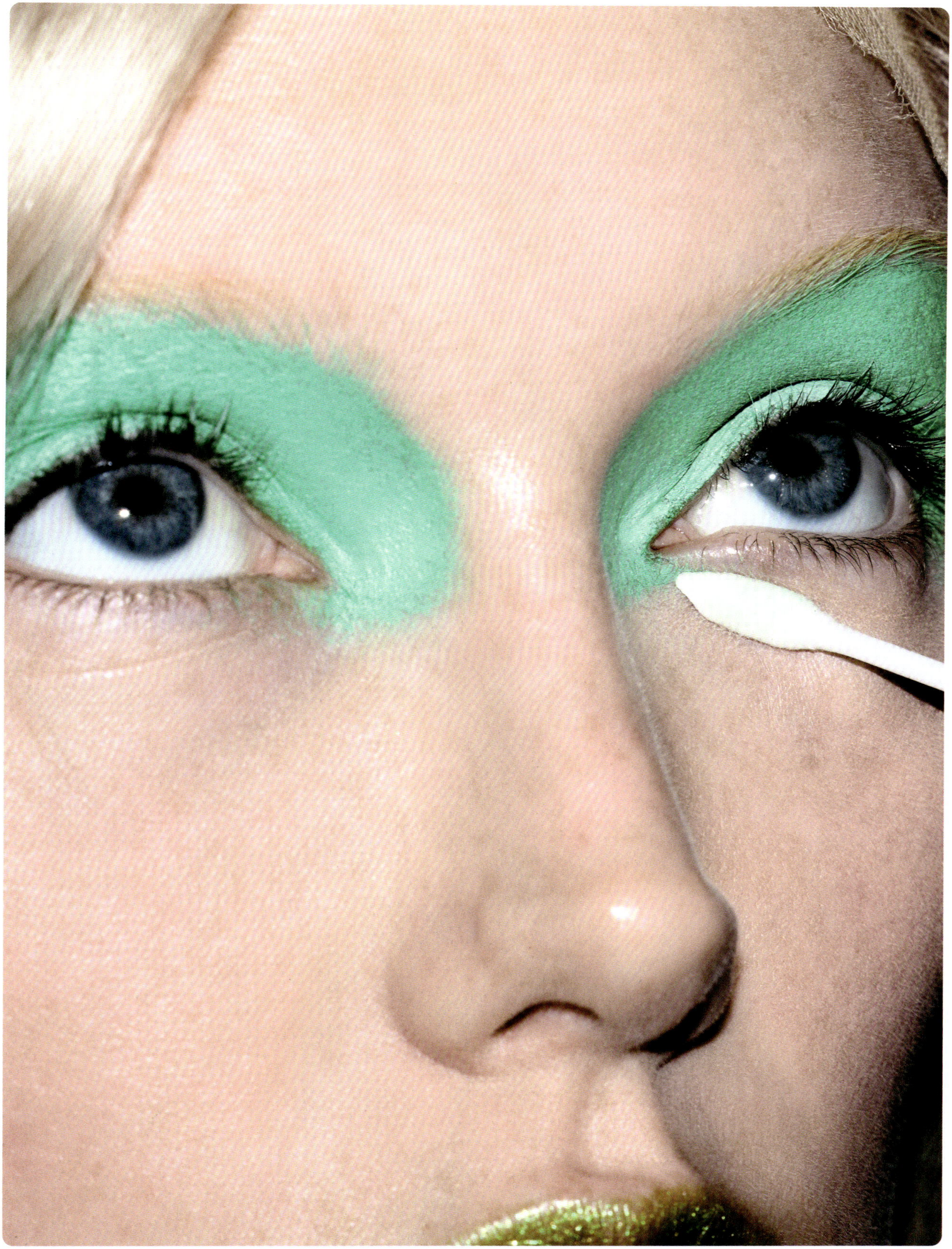

Q Okay, let's talk about the specifics of building a look. You've told me that when you sit down, you sometimes look at a palette or just what is around you. Are there any specific eras, artists, or aesthetics that you actually really love and grab onto?

A Right now, I would say retro—like the sixties—is very inspiring to me because it's colorful and kind of funky and different. Sixties looks offer me a way to express my messiness in a way that people can relate to.

I'm also really inspired by Julia Fox—the way she dresses up and does her makeup when she goes to events and shows is so fun. She is always pushing boundaries and taking risks. Whenever I see something she does, I'm inspired to go out there and do a really fun, quirky look and not give a f*** what people think.

Q You've got to meet and work with a lot of amazing makeup artists and brands. What is one that has stood out to you?

A Charlotte Tilbury is definitely one of my biggest mentors and someone I admire deeply. Not only has she built an incredible brand, but I also love everything she stands for in beauty and how she dares women to dream big. She really has the warmest soul, and we've had some amazing experiences together.

Q TikTok is known for its challenges, so I want to know what the craziest one you've done?

A The craziest challenge I've done is doing my makeup with kitchen utensils—it was very challenging, hahaha. When I finished, I didn't know what to do with all the utensils. I was like, "Am I supposed to shove them in my dishwasher????"

Q Tell me about some of the utensils that you used.

A I used a spatula, fork, knife, and spoon. I think I may have used tongs, too. I just used the weirdest things. I never imagined that I would ever do my makeup with food, but I did freckles with a piece of broccoli, which was very interesting. I once covered my whole face with 1,000 dots of foundation and rubbed it all in.

Q Was that also a TikTok challenge?

A Yeah, but again: free will.

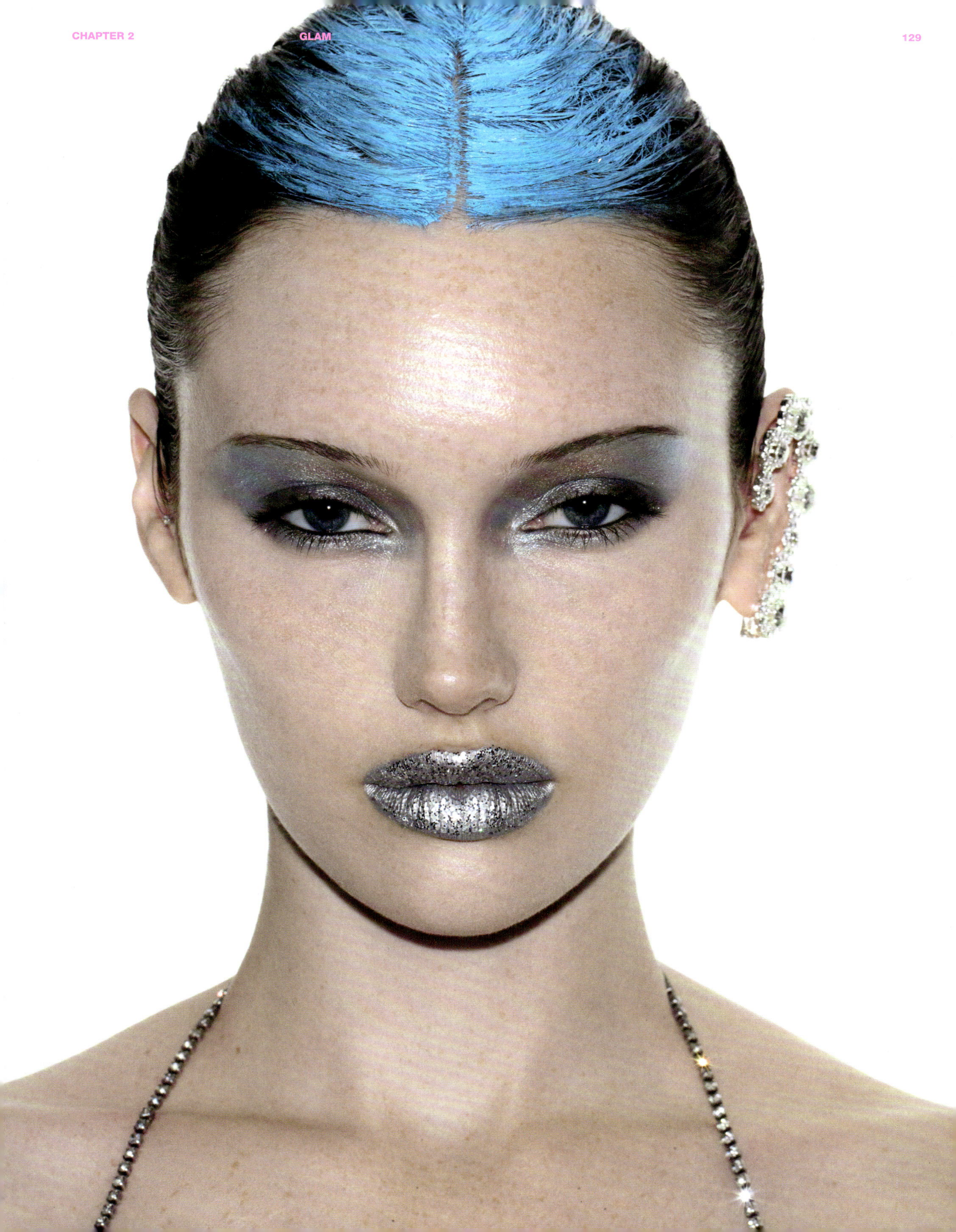

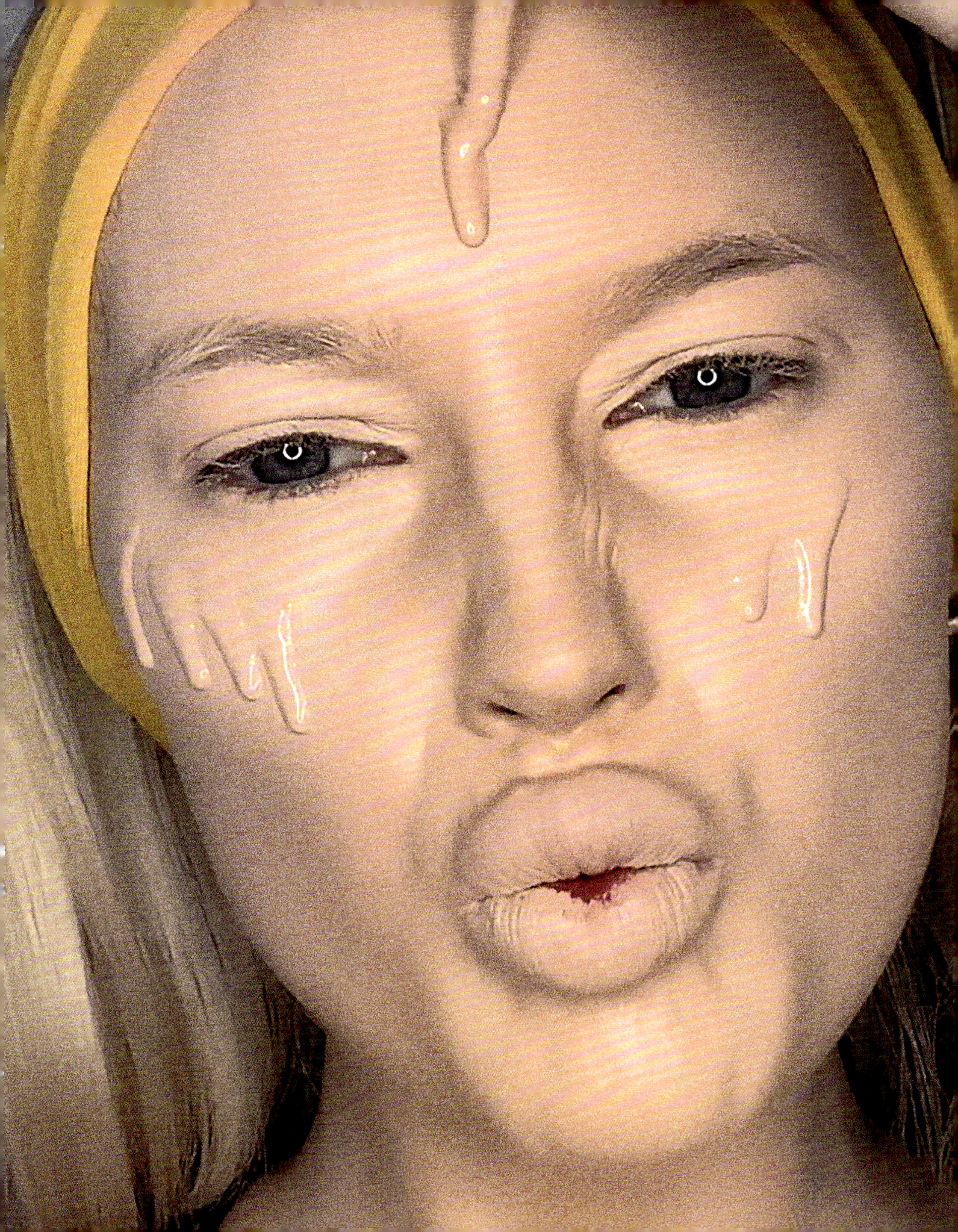

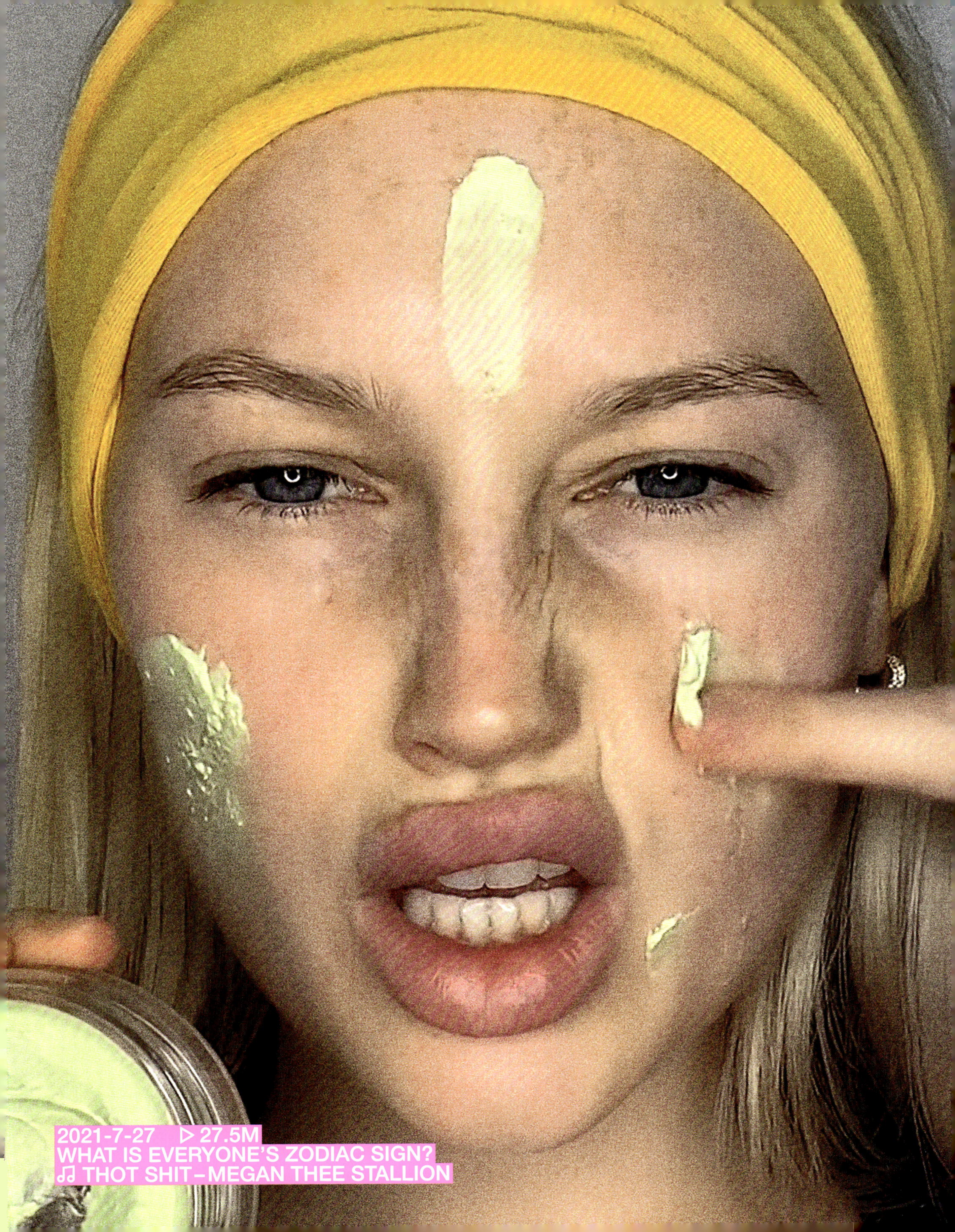

2021-7-27 ▷ 27.5M
WHAT IS EVERYONE’S ZODIAC SIGN?
♫ THOT SHIT–MEGAN THEE STALLION

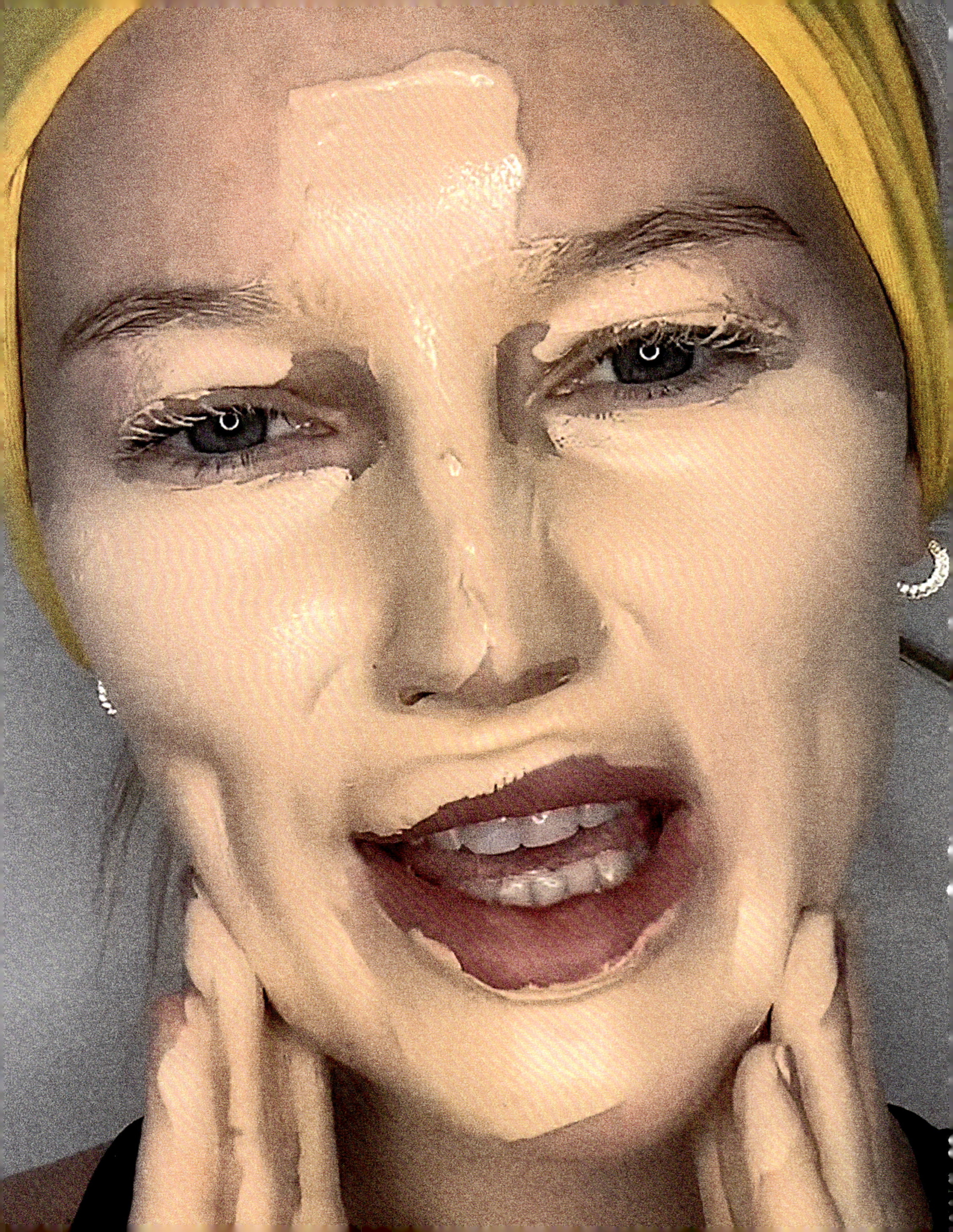

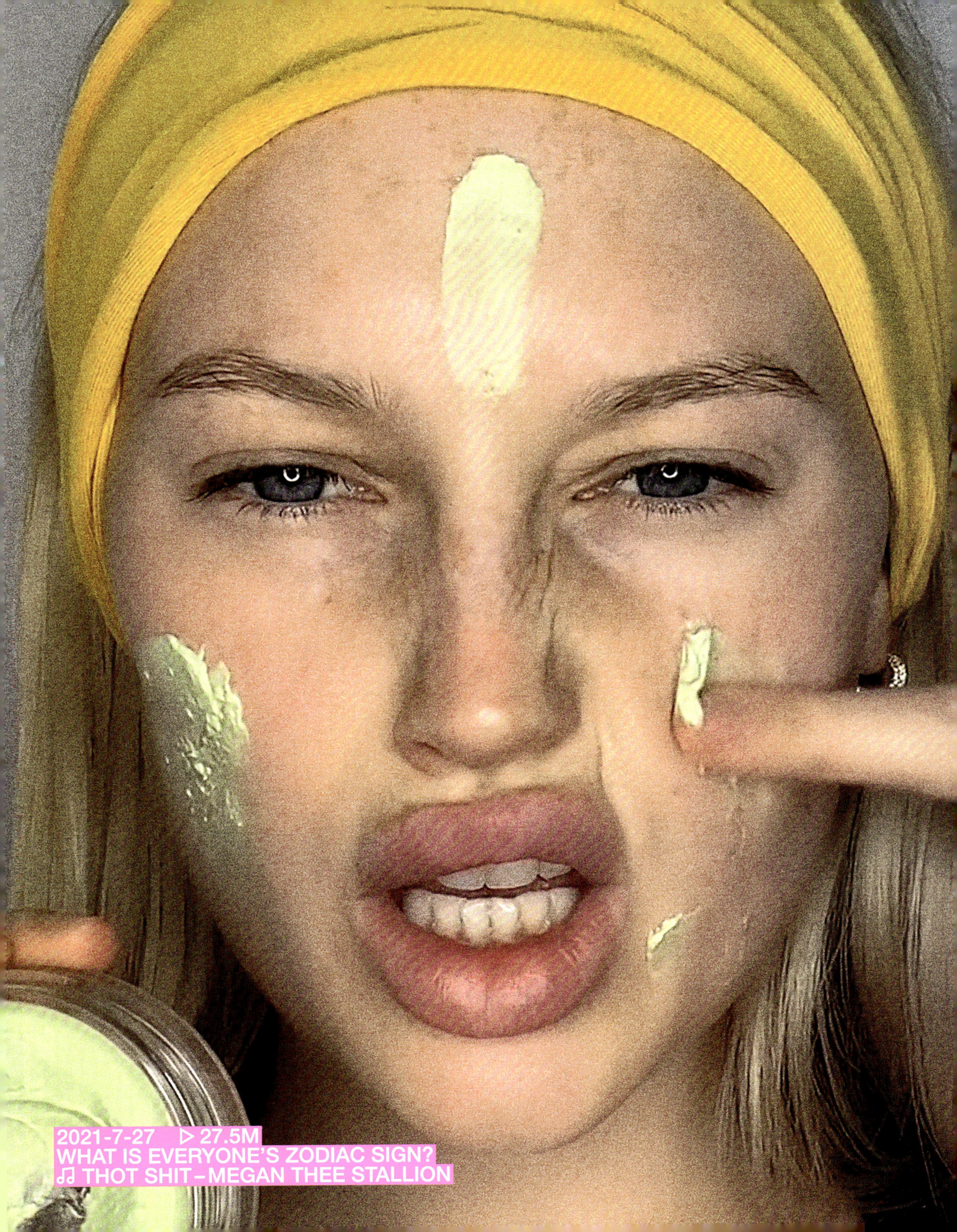
2021-7-27 ▷ 27.5M
WHAT IS EVERYONE'S ZODIAC SIGN?
♫ THOT SHIT–MEGAN THEE STALLION

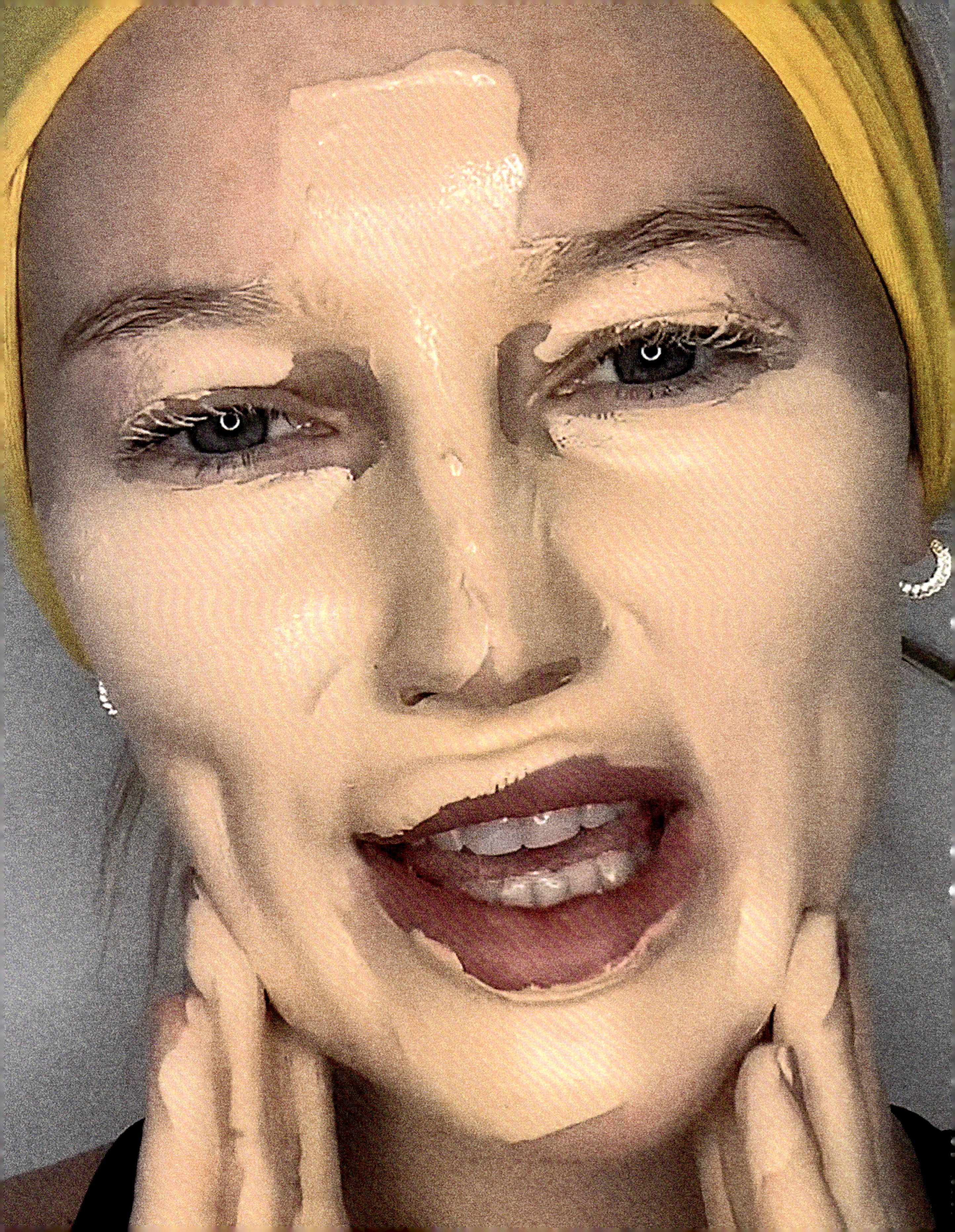

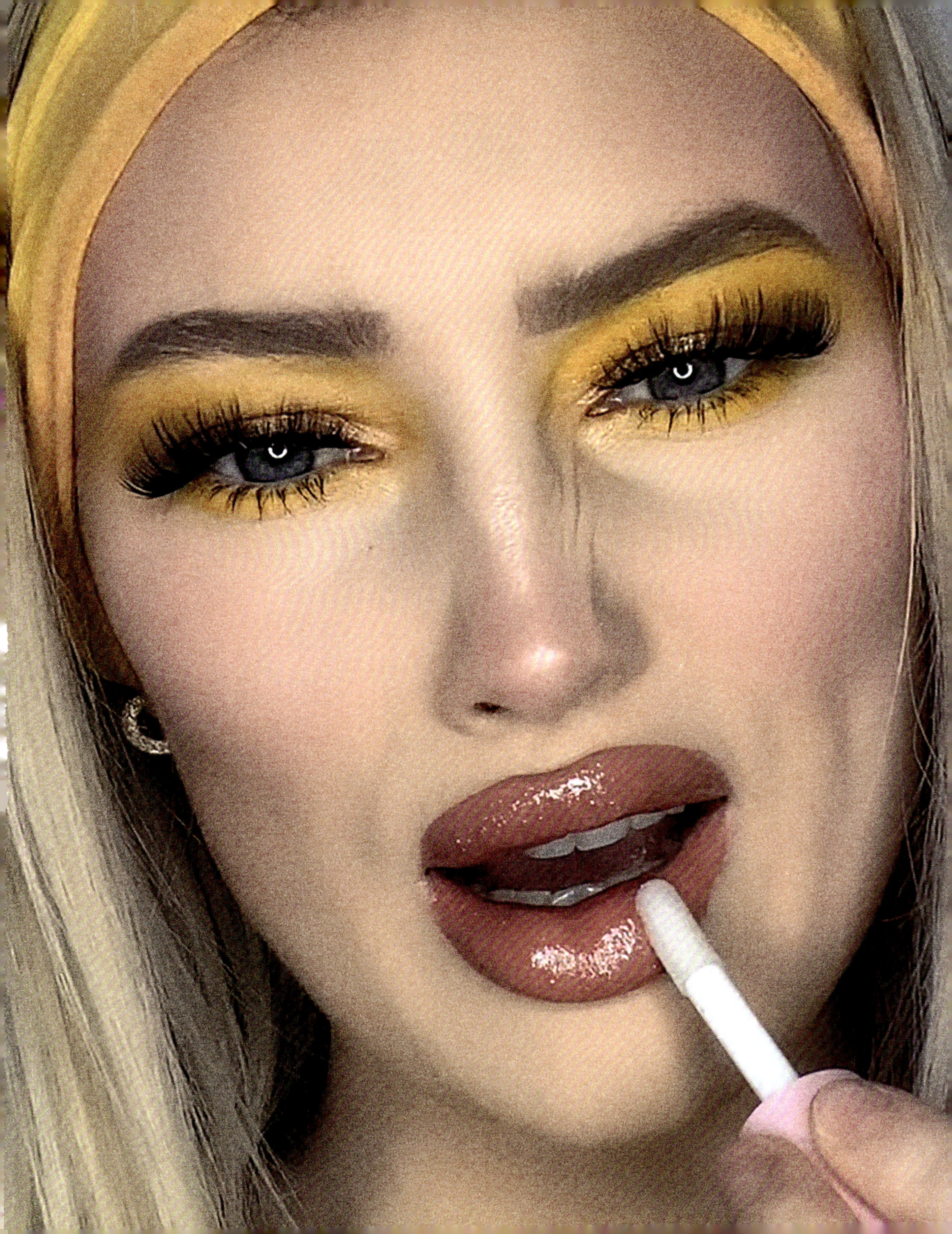

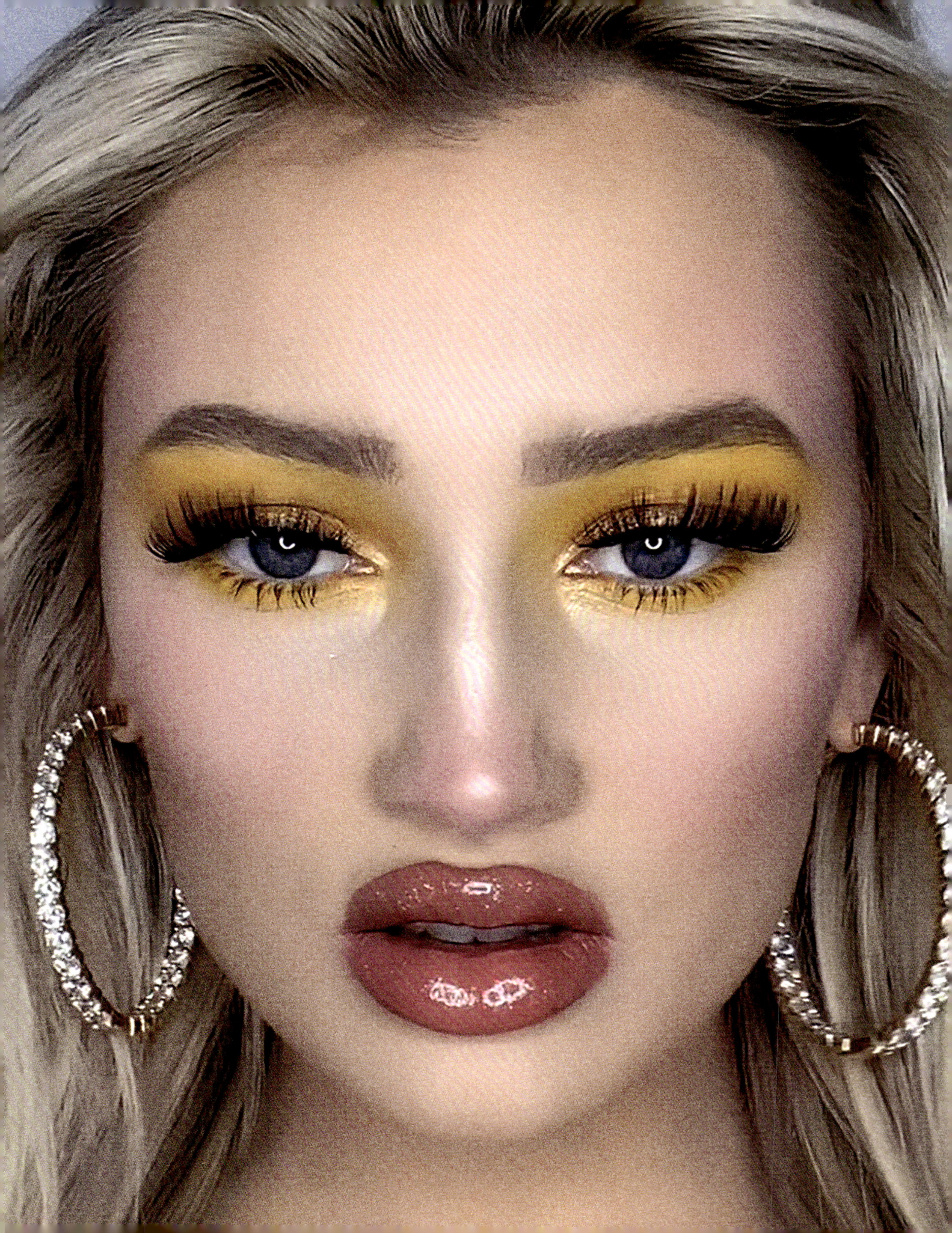

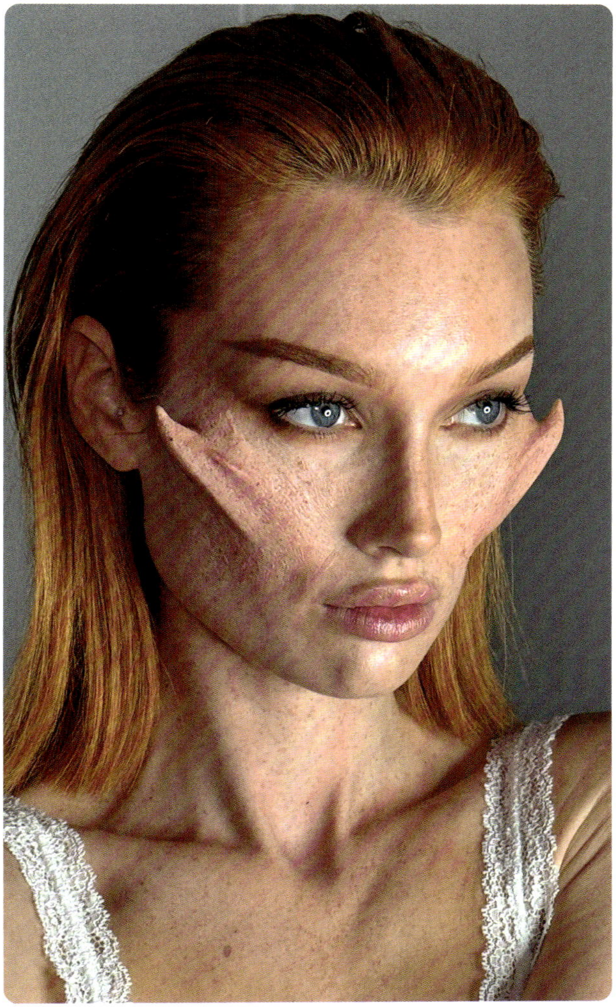

TOP: I worked with another makeup artist who specializes in special effects makeup and experimented with these prosthetics. The glam process is so different when using these because the skin can't have anything on it that would cause them to slide off. It definitely changes how you would usually do your makeup! BELOW: A look I did for Halloween that took me around four hours to complete. I cut up white lace and glued each piece to my face, matching them perfectly so they fit seamlessly together. After that, I created a makeup look on top of the lace to create a doll-like character. So cute!

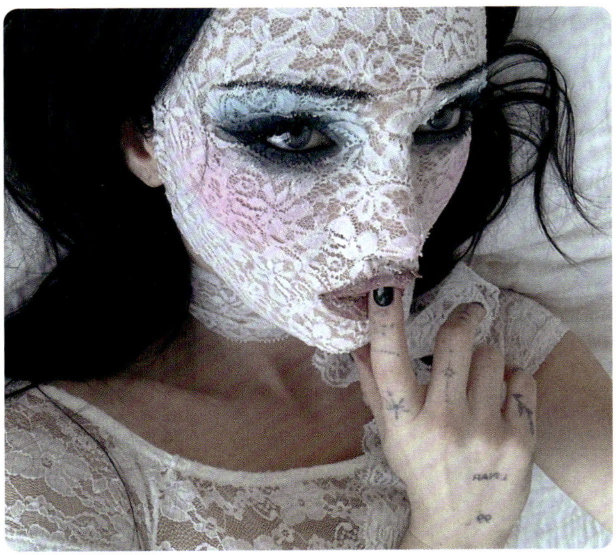

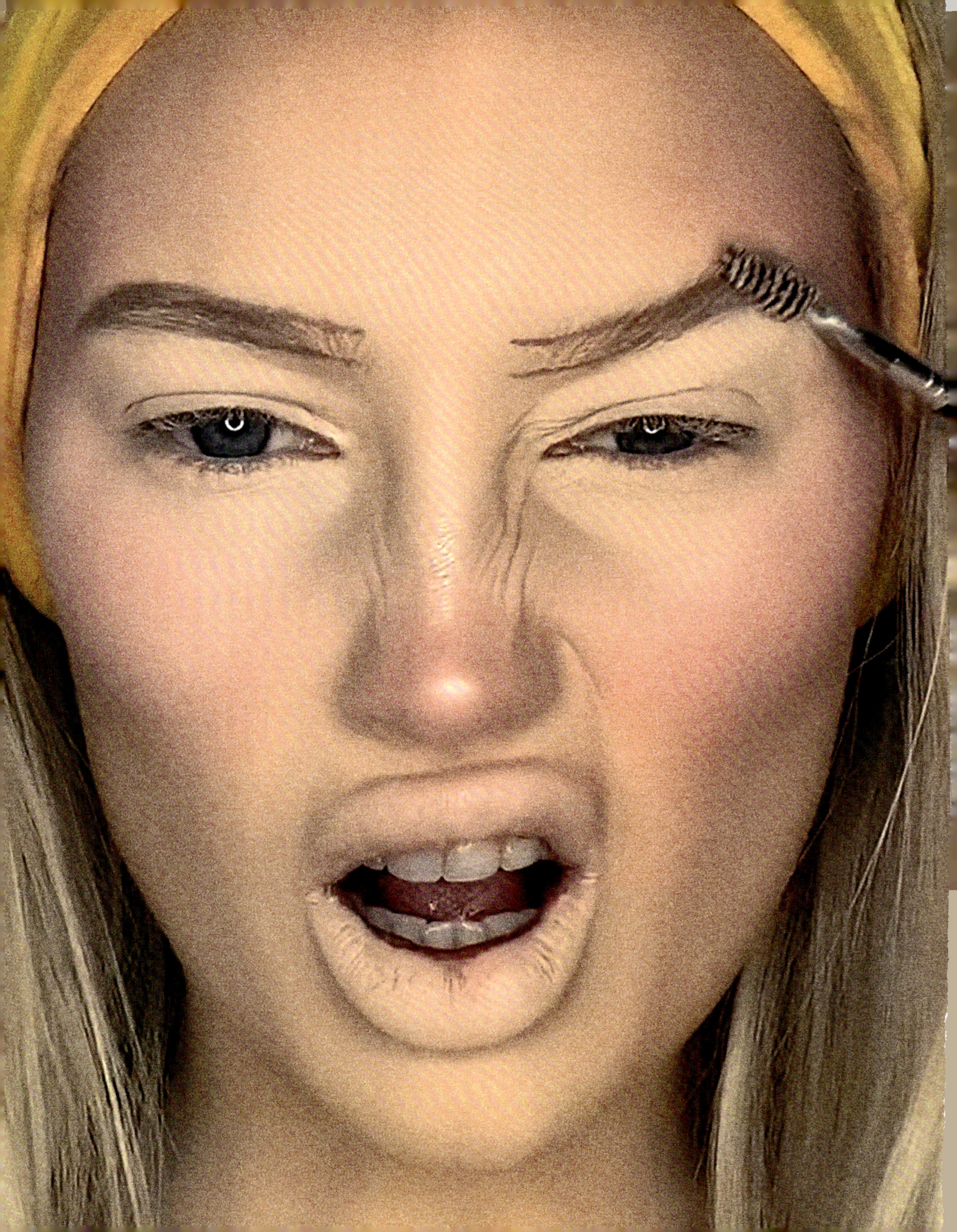

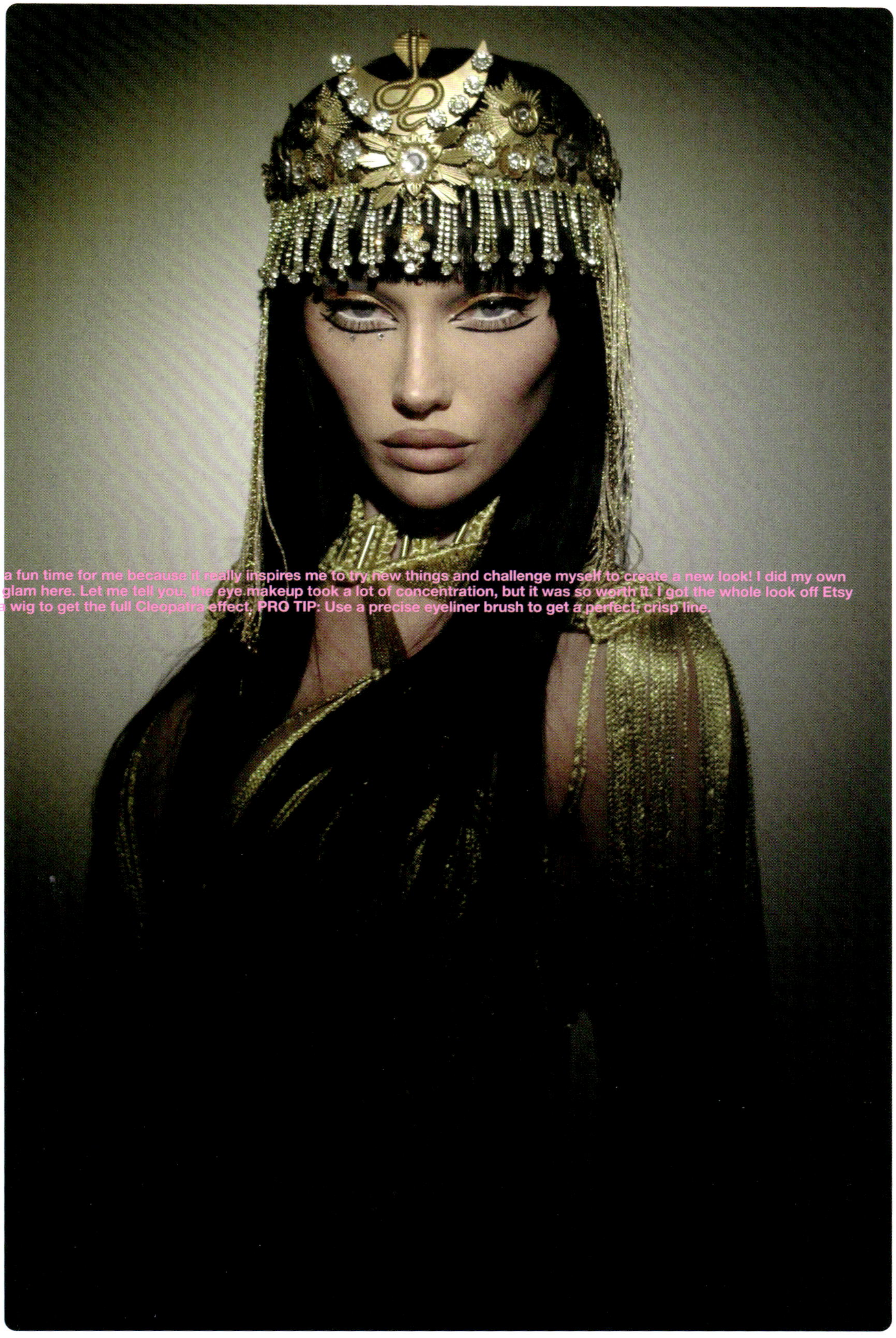

Halloween is such a fun time for me because it really inspires me to try new things and challenge myself to create a new look! I did my own take on Cleopatra glam here. Let me tell you, the eye makeup took a lot of concentration, but it was so worth it. I got the whole look off Etsy and paired it with a wig to get the full Cleopatra effect. PRO TIP: Use a precise eyeliner brush to get a perfect, crisp line.

Q Now that you work with glam teams, how do you effectively communicate your vision while letting other people who tend to have their signature looks reinterpret what you're going to look like?

A It's so important to be straight up and talk over your vision before you start getting into glam, because there are so many times when people will sit there for an hour or two hours and then end up hating their look because they have a signature way that they like to do their lip or eye.

It's essential to express to your glam team what you like in advance of sitting down. You need to say, "Hey, I like my part super-centered," or "I like my hair slicked straight back, middle part." Or "I like my cupid's bow to be super-sculpted out" or "I like my blush placed higher on my cheekbones." Your glam team will appreciate it so much—they can still bring their creative input and talent to take your ideas and create a masterpiece that you like.

Q Is that a skill? It must take time, though. The first couple of times that you sat in a glam armchair, was there ever a moment when you were like, "Oh, my God, I don't like how I look!"

A For sure! It takes time to learn how to collaborate well with others within what you're comfortable with—sometimes we are scared to speak our minds. You have to endure a few mess-ups and a few glam looks you might not like in order to understand how to do it right the next time. But knowing how you like your makeup to look and expressing it is important.

Q I want to talk a little bit about hair. At one point, you said, "Cut your hair! You only live once!" Do you still live by that?

A Yeah, I still live by that! You should take risks, make those decisions, and have fun with them. Because for me, life is all about learning through mistakes. I'm not saying cutting my hair was ever a mistake, but you don't know if you like something until you try it.

Q What is the boldest hair decision you've made on a whim?

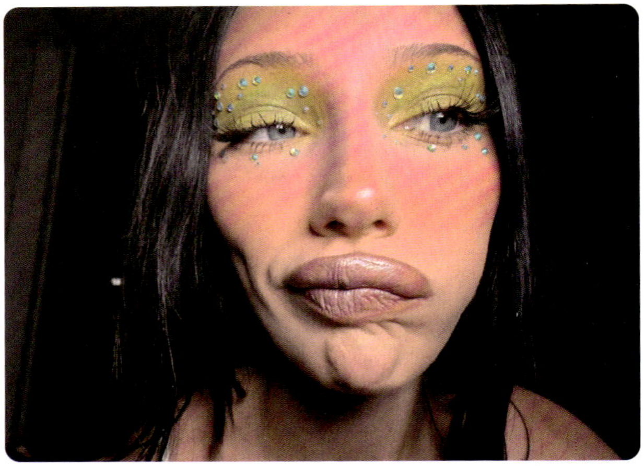

TOP: This was my take on the Zara Larsson tour makeup that was trending on TikTok! PRO TIP: Gems are such a fun way to play up an eye-makeup look! CENTER: This lip liner and I have a special bond... the Charlotte Tilbury Lip Cheat Lip Liner in Iconic Nude, the perfect cool-toned nude lippie.

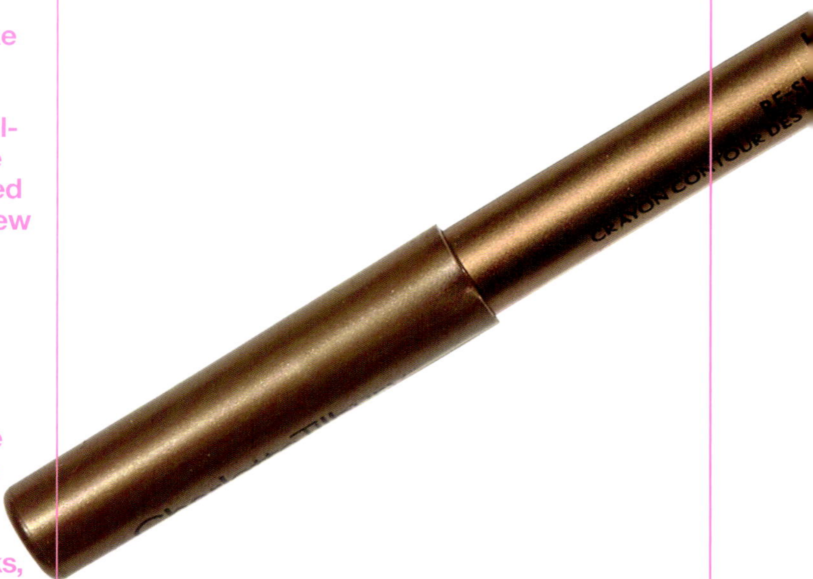

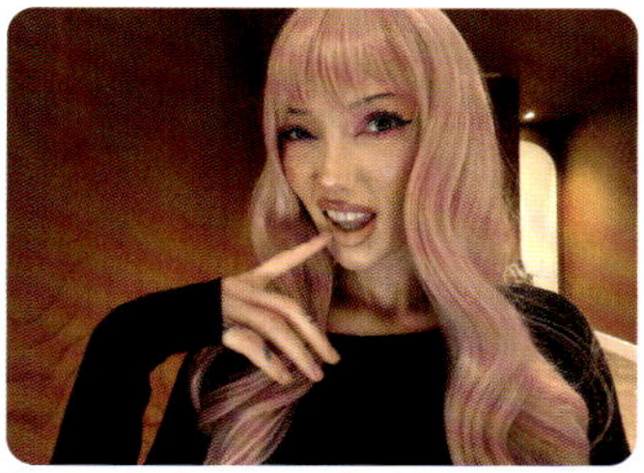

I love playing around with wigs whenever I want to switch up my style, but without fully committing to a new look!

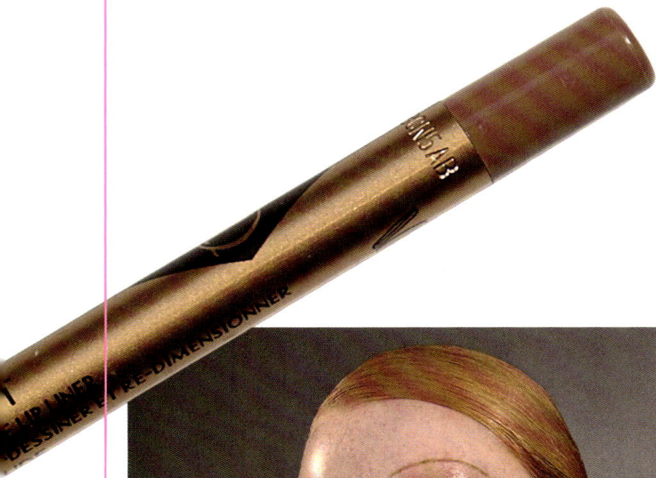

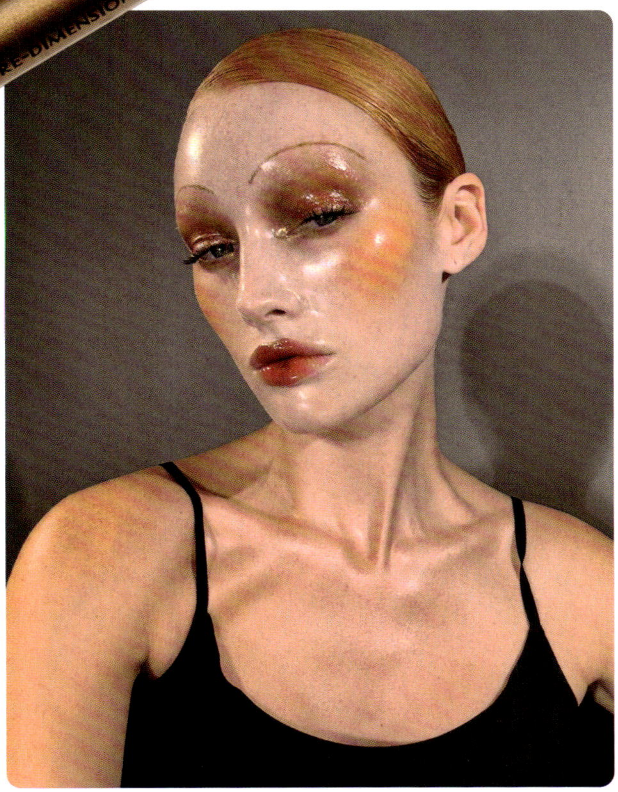

Pat McGrath has been such an inspiration to me. She has been an amazing mentor throughout my whole journey in the beauty industry. She pushes limits like no other and truly has the most creative mind. This was her iconic glasslike skin makeup look that she created for the Maison Margiela Couture Spring/Summer 2024 show, which I was lucky enough to have her recreate it on me. I had to stay still for hours during the application process to make sure nothing creased. Let's just say my ADHD didn't make this easy.

A Dyeing it red and cutting it into a bob from long, blonde hair.

Q What inspired you to do that? Were you just sitting there and thinking red could be cool?

A I'm very impulsive and spontaneous. I love switching up my look. My team had suggested it to me, and red just sounded like a fun idea!

Q Did it pay off?

A For sure! I feel like in fashion and modeling, it definitely helped me make my stance and kind of let it be known I'm here. I want to do runway, and I can be a chameleon and embrace different looks across these industries.

Q Have you ever cried after a haircut?

A Who hasn't, tbh.

Q And did you cry in the chair or when you got home?

A I cried when I got home. I was definitely having a mini panic attack, and then I had to run out of there and pretend like I liked the haircut. But I've learned to speak up; it can feel embarrassing, but it's your hair, and hair holds a lot of weight in people's confidence.

Q If you had to dye your hair right now, what color would it be?

A Baby blue or baby pink. I just love looking in the mirror and seeing different versions of myself. With makeup, it's so easy for me to do that, and that's why I love putting on wigs too. If I actually went through and dyed my hair baby blue, I would get the biggest adrenaline rush.

Q Tell me about your hair color era. You have had several hair colors. How would you define each one?

A So blonde hair was the foundation of Barbie-girl Meredith, who was just doing her thing and being glam to the max. And then red hair was more my modeling-fashion intro era. It was also my single-girl era.

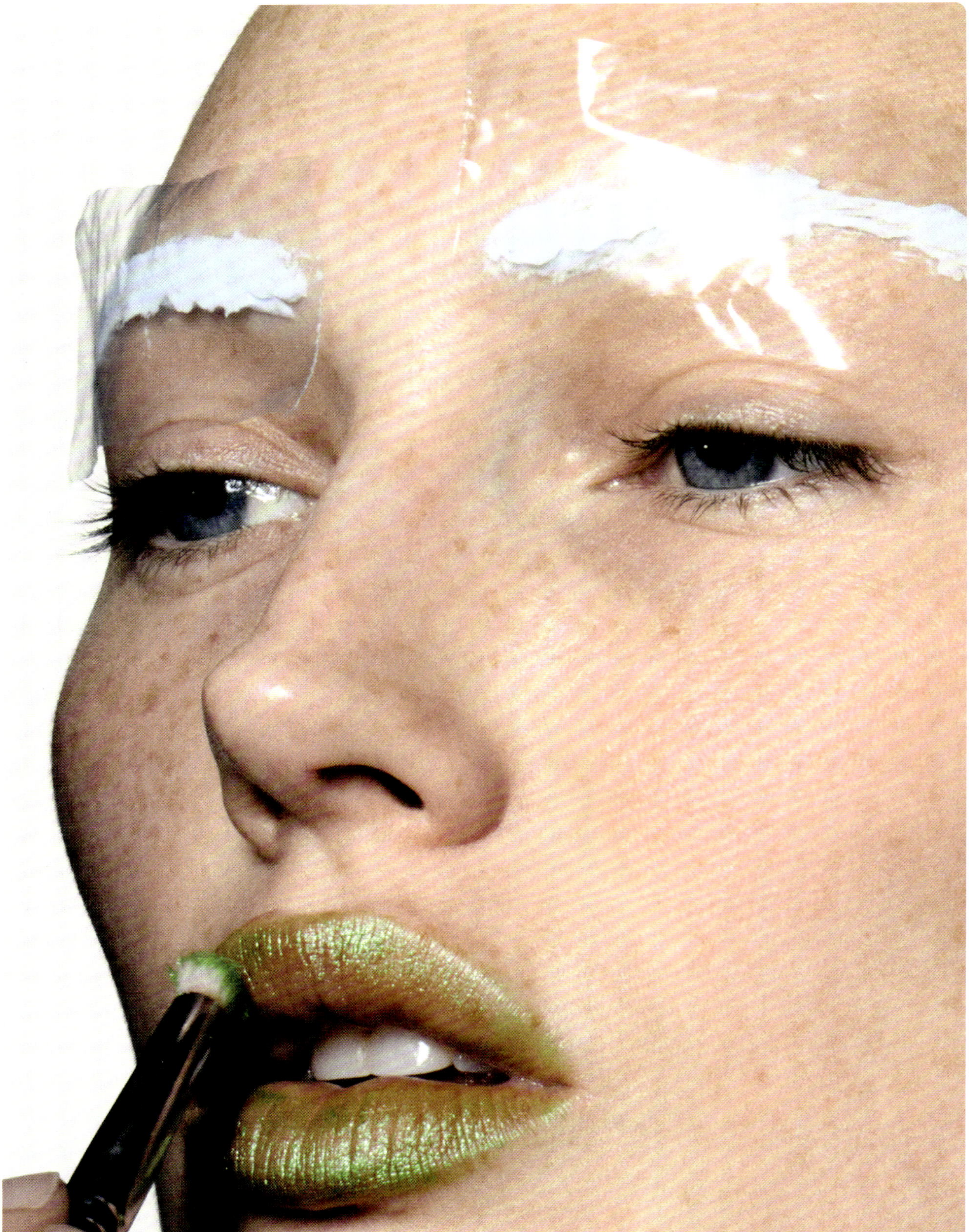

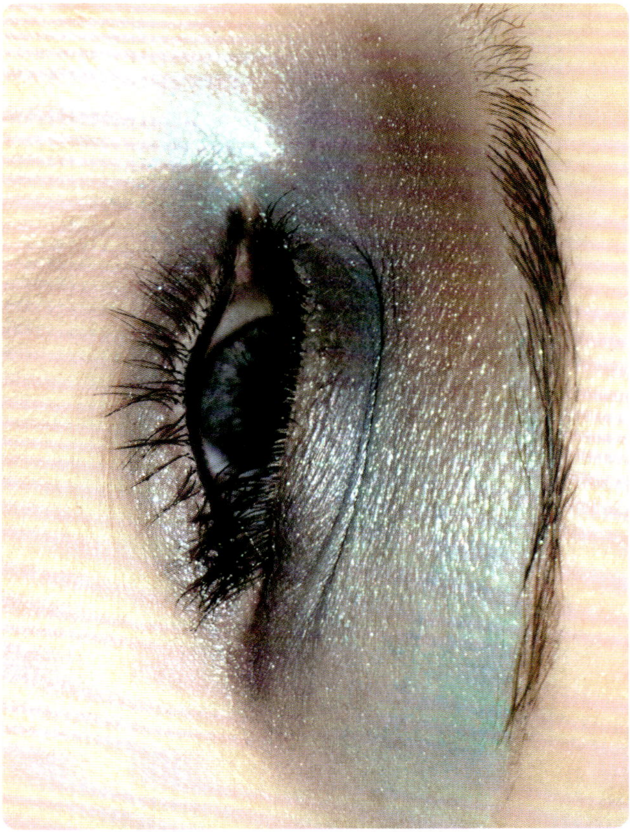

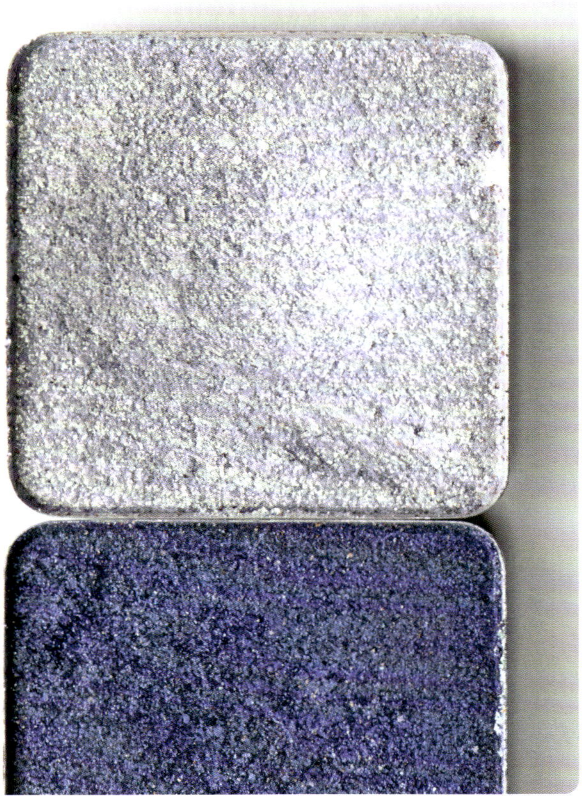

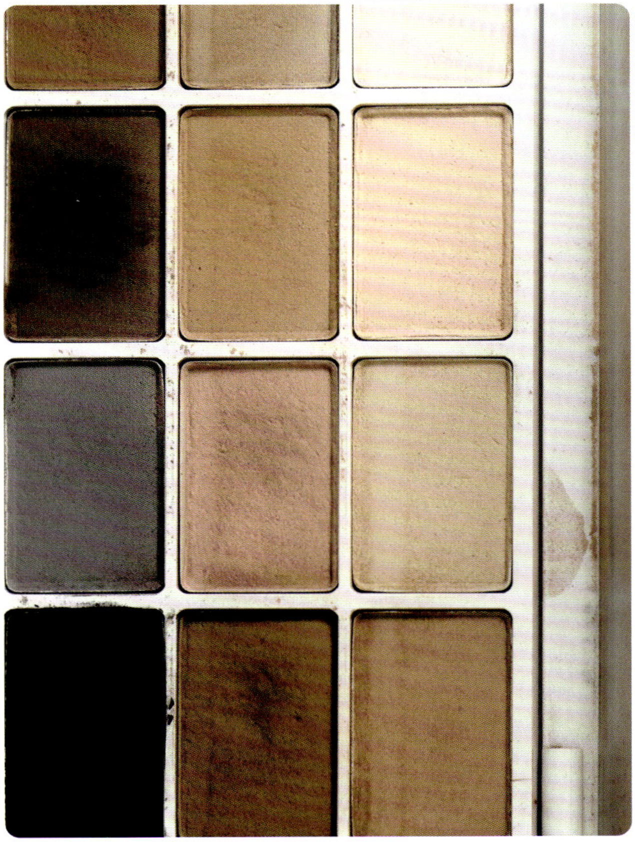

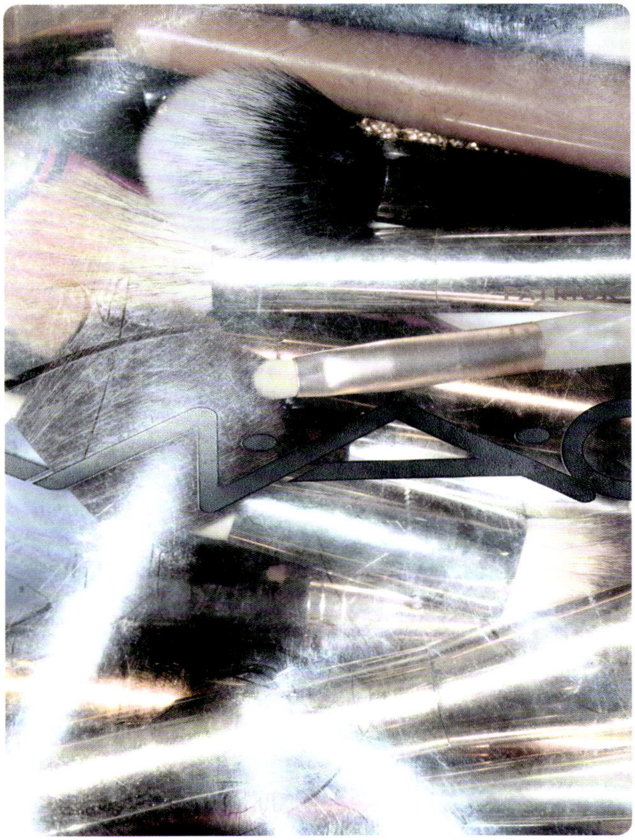

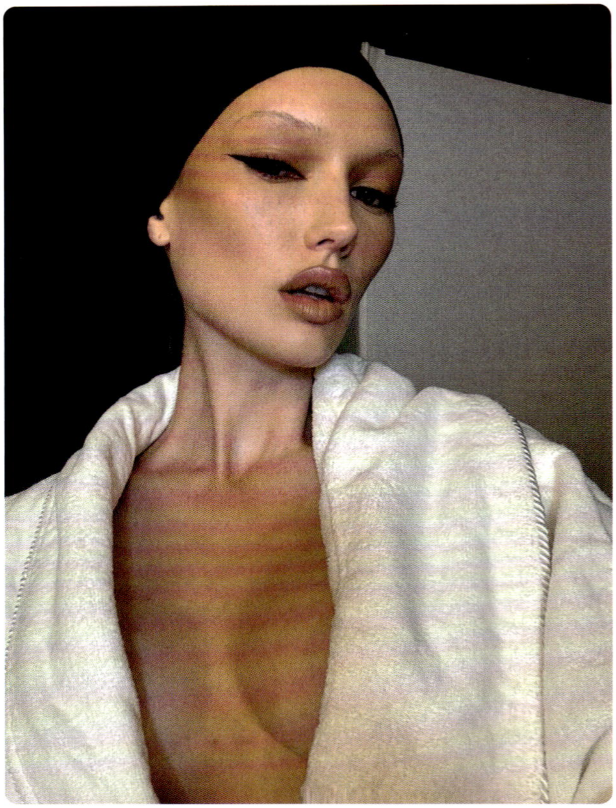

I love a glam backstage selfie. It's fun to look back at these moments and see how much I've accomplished.

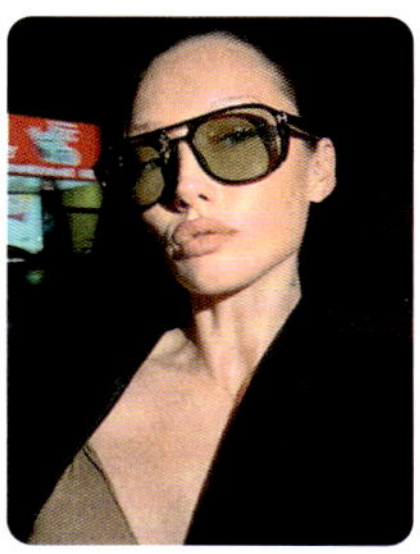

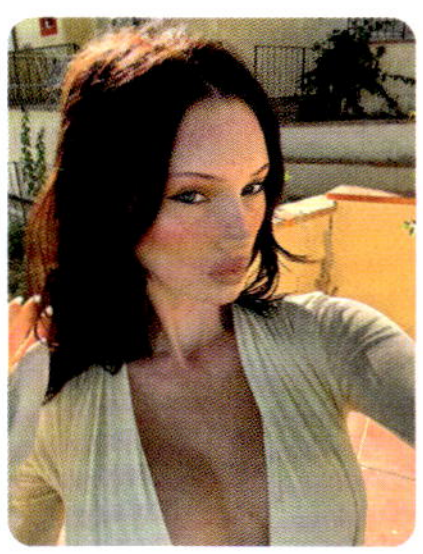

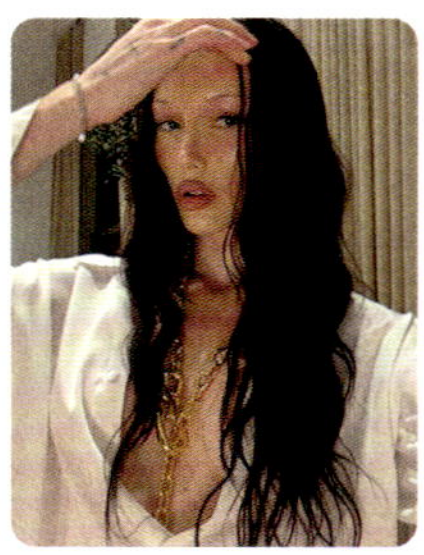

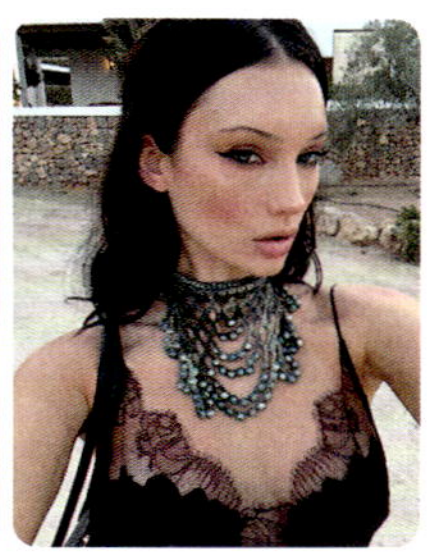

A few of my fave selfies, taken when I felt my prettiest and loved my glam! Some are natural; others are more bold! Always take a selfie before walking out the door. It's nice to be able to bring yourself back to a moment when you felt your best!

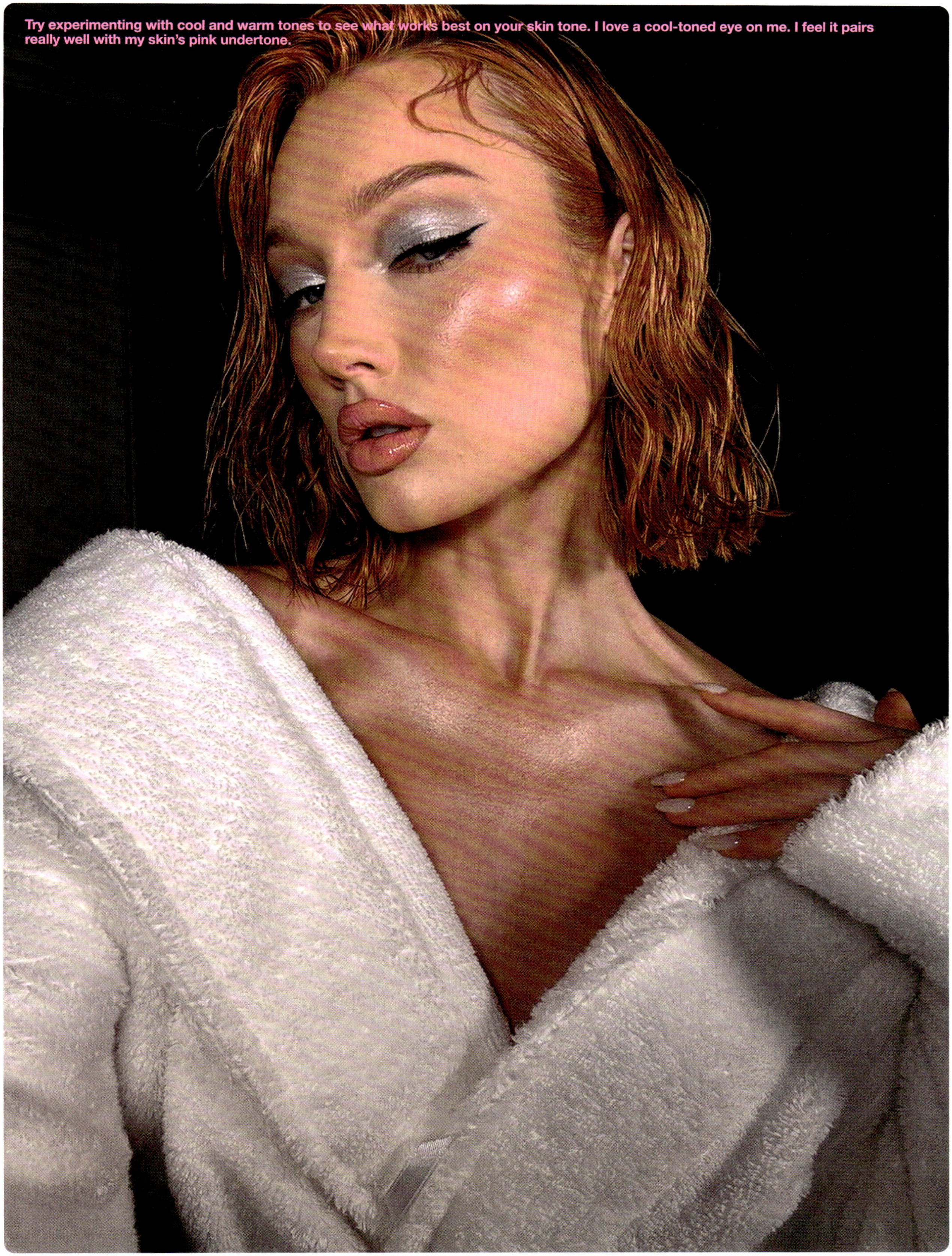

Try experimenting with cool and warm tones to see what works best on your skin tone. I love a cool-toned eye on me. I feel it pairs really well with my skin's pink undertone.

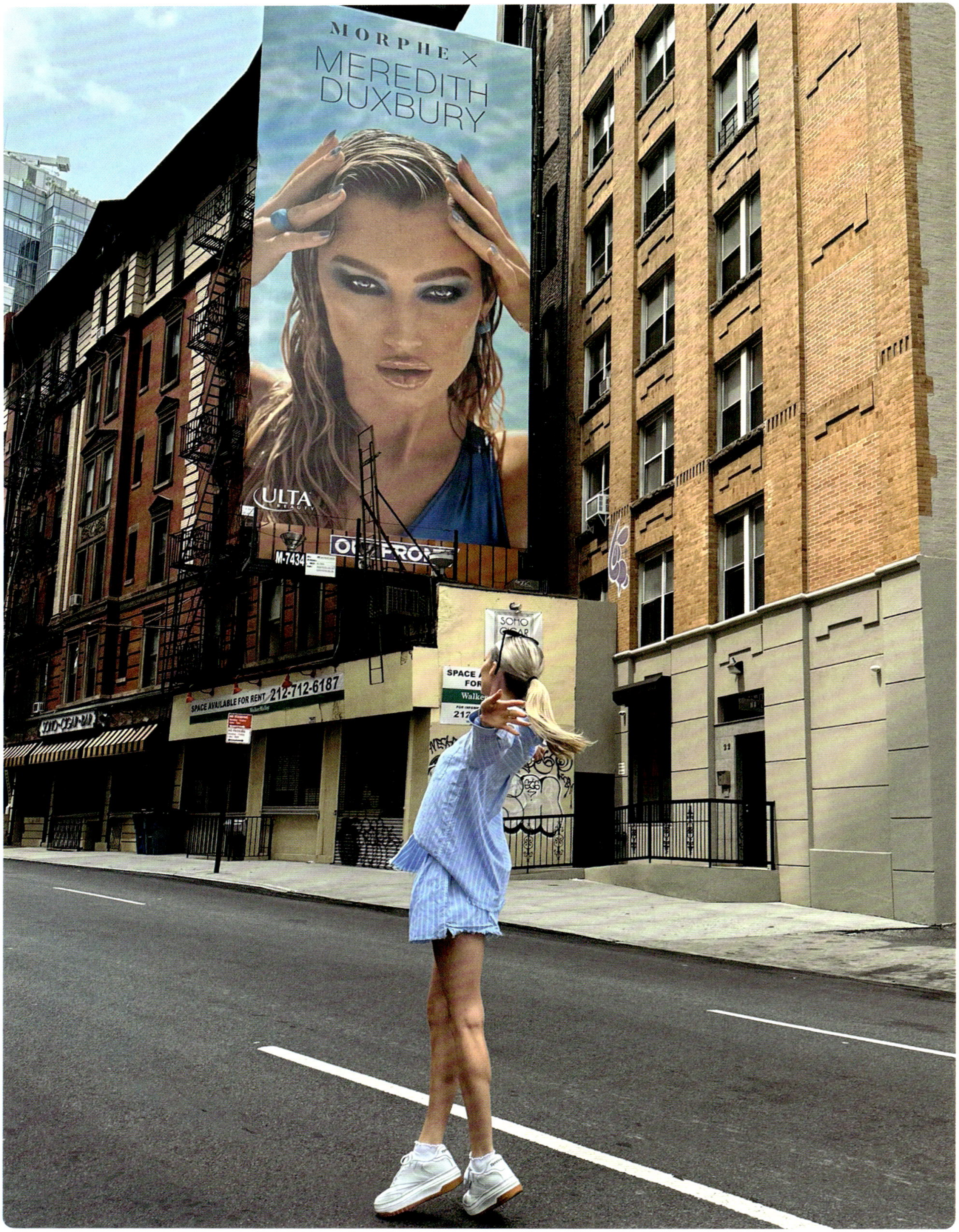

Wow! I remember the first time I saw this, I had tears in my eyes. I walk by this billboard in SoHo all the time with my dogs, so to see my face...fathom!

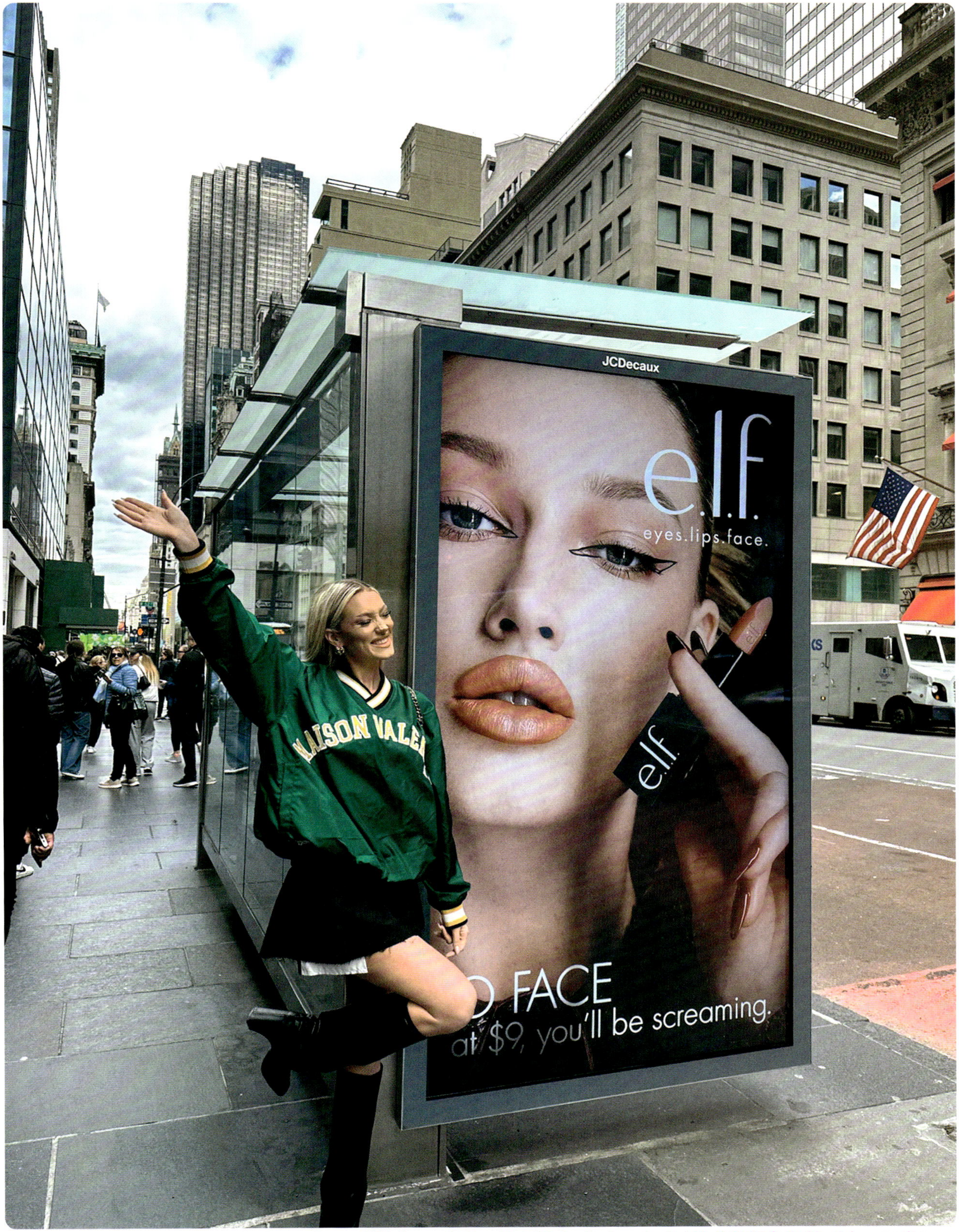

This was such a pinch-me moment, having my face on Fifth Avenue in New York City for the launch of e.l.f.'s O FACE Satin Lipstick campaign. Thank you, e.l.f., for making the little girl in me's dreams come true!

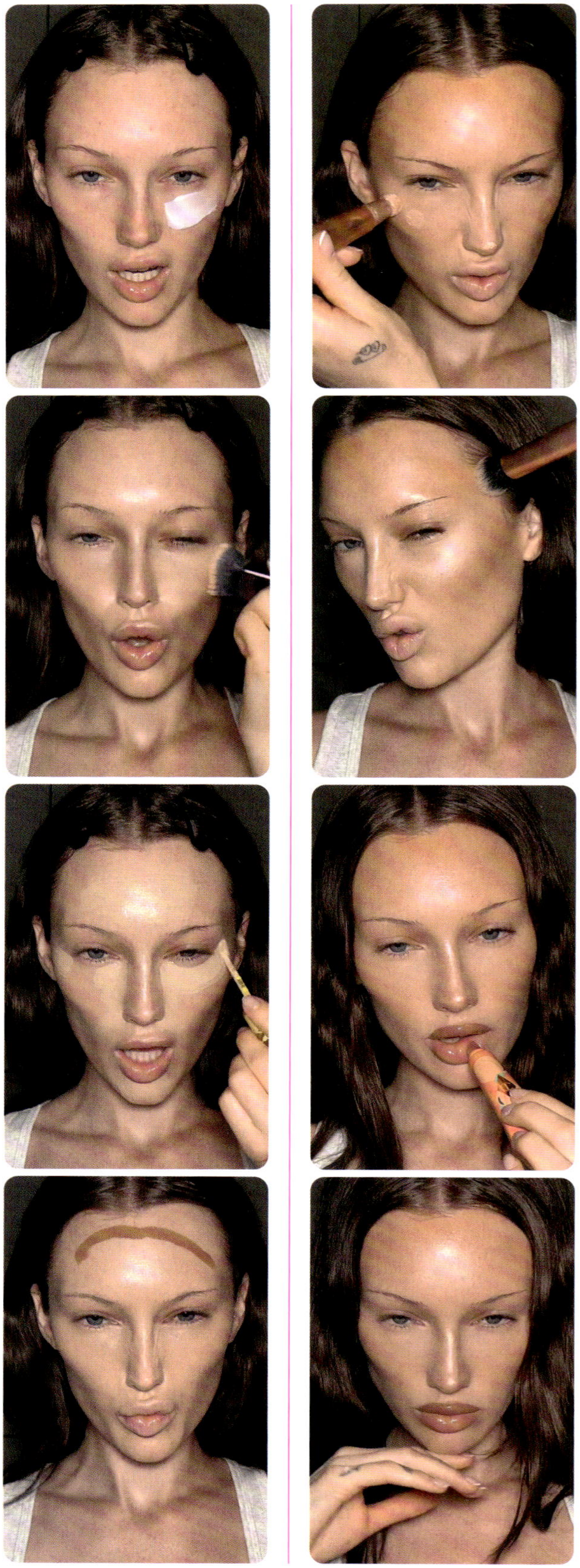

She was thriving, and she was that b****. Now, my black hair is my dark, feminine era. She's a little rebellious, she knows how to have fun, and she's really building on everything she has ever worked toward and wanted.

Q Tell me about your glam nonnegotiable. What is something that instantly makes you feel like you? You told me earlier that you love a nude lip, but is there more to it?

A I would say an overlined lip. Any shoot I'm on, if the lip is not overlined, I'm like, "We have to bring that up a notch."

I would also say a really sexy eye is a nonnegotiable. During the day, I will go more casual, but when I'm going out, my nonnegotiable is that the eye needs to bring my alter ego out. It needs to bring the drama.

Q Your eyeliner looks really good right now.

A Why, thank you! It's so funny because when I do my liner, I don't breathe. I don't like anyone being in the room while I do it. And no one can talk to me.

Q What is one beauty rule that you think we can throw out? What rule should we retire?

A We need to retire the idea that makeup needs to be done a certain way. Makeup can be done however you want to do it.

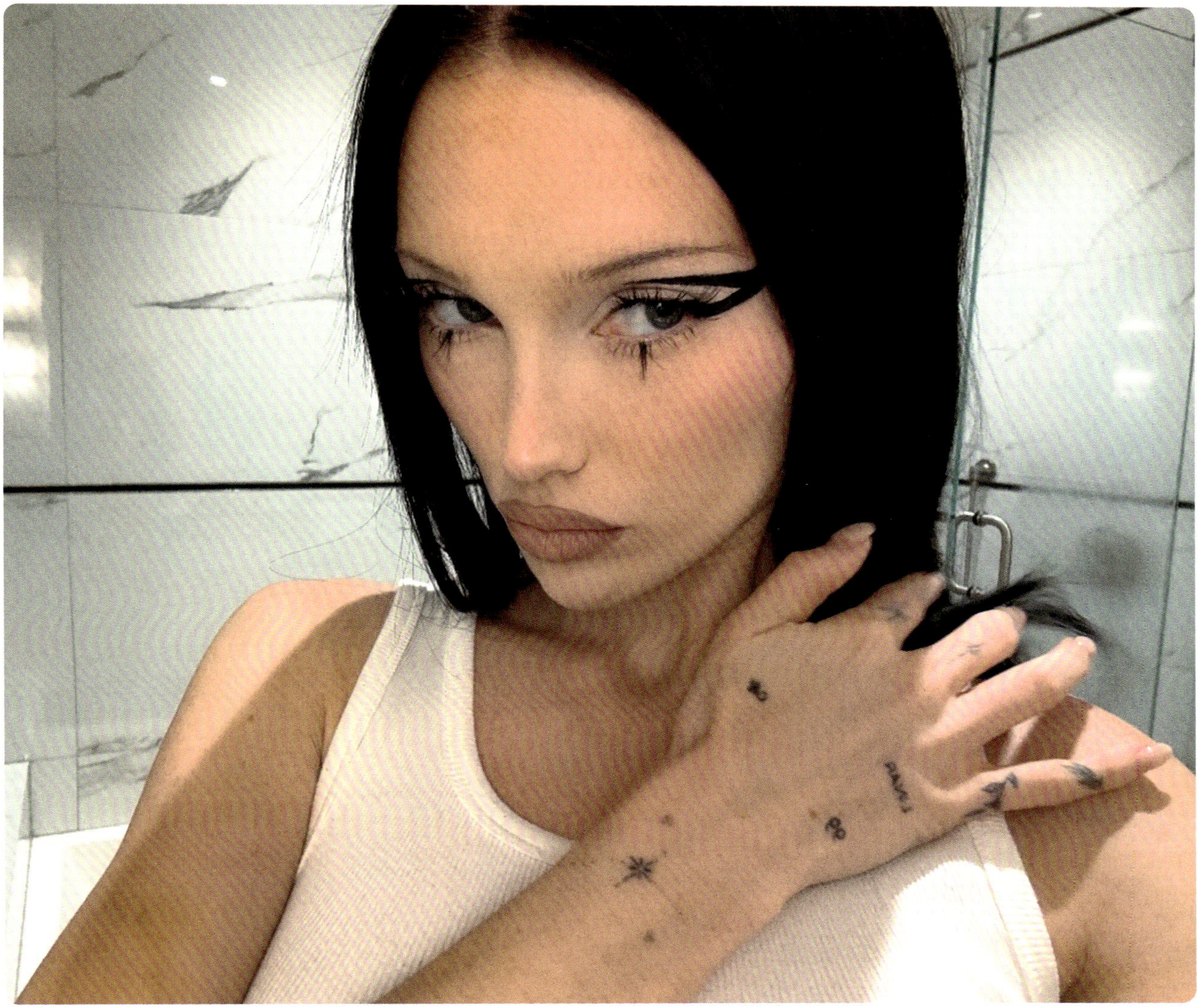

The lashes and liner added all of the drama! Don't be afraid to use a lash in an unconventional way!

GLAM-TREND ROULETTE

Q Let's play glam-trend roulette. Okay, what is one trend you never want to see again?
A The no-makeup makeup.

Q Honestly, what is one trend that you are thrilled has survived?
A My foundation technique. I mean, come on…it's iconic.

Q What is one trend that you are manifesting now?
A Skinny brows. I love them. People are saying that I'm going to regret that in thirty years when I have no brows. But eyebrows grow back. I have to shave them twice a week. I'm like, "Guys, this is maintenance!"

Q I am curious about your mood when you first saw yourself with skinny brows.
A Oh, I became more of a bad b****, more snatched!

Q Is it like after a breakup, and you feel like you have to chop off your hair?
A Honestly, yes. Out with the old, in with the new!

GLAM RAPID FIRE

Q You can only use one palette for the rest of your life. What's the color story?
A Oh, it would be a cool, toned, smoky, gray-blue palette with some shimmers.

Q Gorgeous. What is one product you would want to be buried with, just in case there is glam in the afterlife?
A Charlotte Tilbury Iconic Nude Lip Liner.

Q If aliens landed and asked you to teach them makeup, what would you show them first? Are you giving them skinny brows?
A Hell, yeah. I feel like aliens might not have brows. They might need some sort of foundation because I feel like their skin may be questionable.

Q Do you have any toxic glam traits?
A Probably. I mean, yeah lol. I don't clean my brushes enough. It's really bad, but I will reuse the same brush. Even when I'm on a two-week trip over the summer or something, my brushes will be so dirty, but I like it when brushes have product in them—I just feel like it blends my makeup in smoother.

Q You can swap makeup bags with one celebrity for a day. Who is it?
A Kim Kardashian.

GLAM F***, MARRY, KILL

Q We are going to play f***, marry, kill. You don't need to explain your answers. Just tell me about these: lip liner, lip gloss, lipstick?
A Marry lip liner, kill lip gloss, and f*** lipstick.

Q Makeup sponges, brushes, hands?
A Marry hands, f*** brushes, and kill sponges.

Q This one's easy: glittery eyes, smoky eyes, natural eyes?
A Kill natural eyes, marry glittery eyes, and f*** smokey eyes.

Q Hair color that never fades, makeup that never cakes, nails that never chip?
A Marry makeup that never cakes, kill nails that never chip, and f*** hair color that never fades.

Q And for our last one, we have a look that gets compliments from: strangers, a makeup artist, your ex?
A Marry the look from the strangers, kill the one from the ex (because who gives a f*** what they think?), and f*** the makeup artist. Yeah.

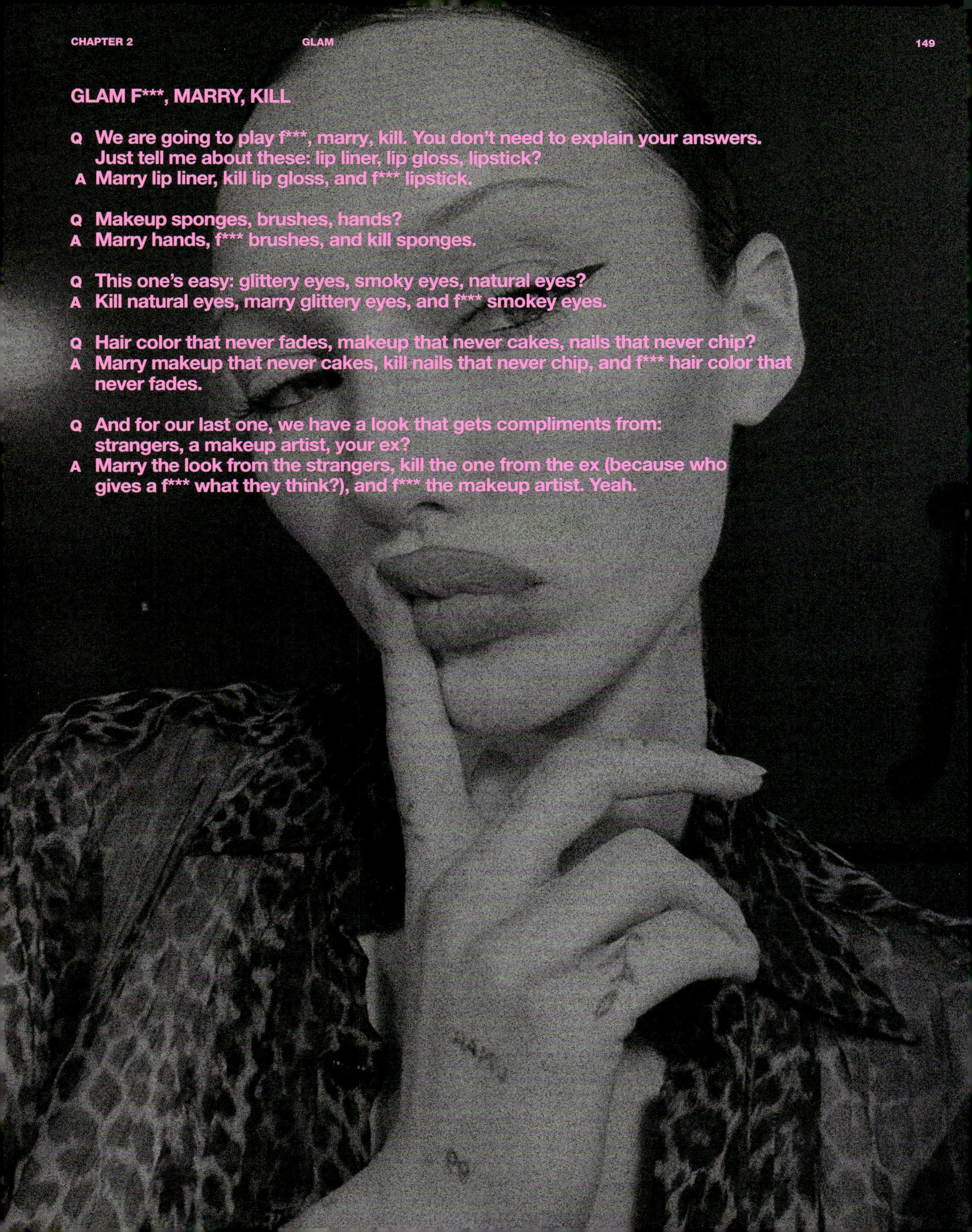

HOW TO: SIREN/CAT EYE

This is my go-to glam for when I want to emulate a sultrier look! It's perfect for a night out when you want a little more drama in the glam, and it gives the eye a really beautiful, lifted, striking effect.

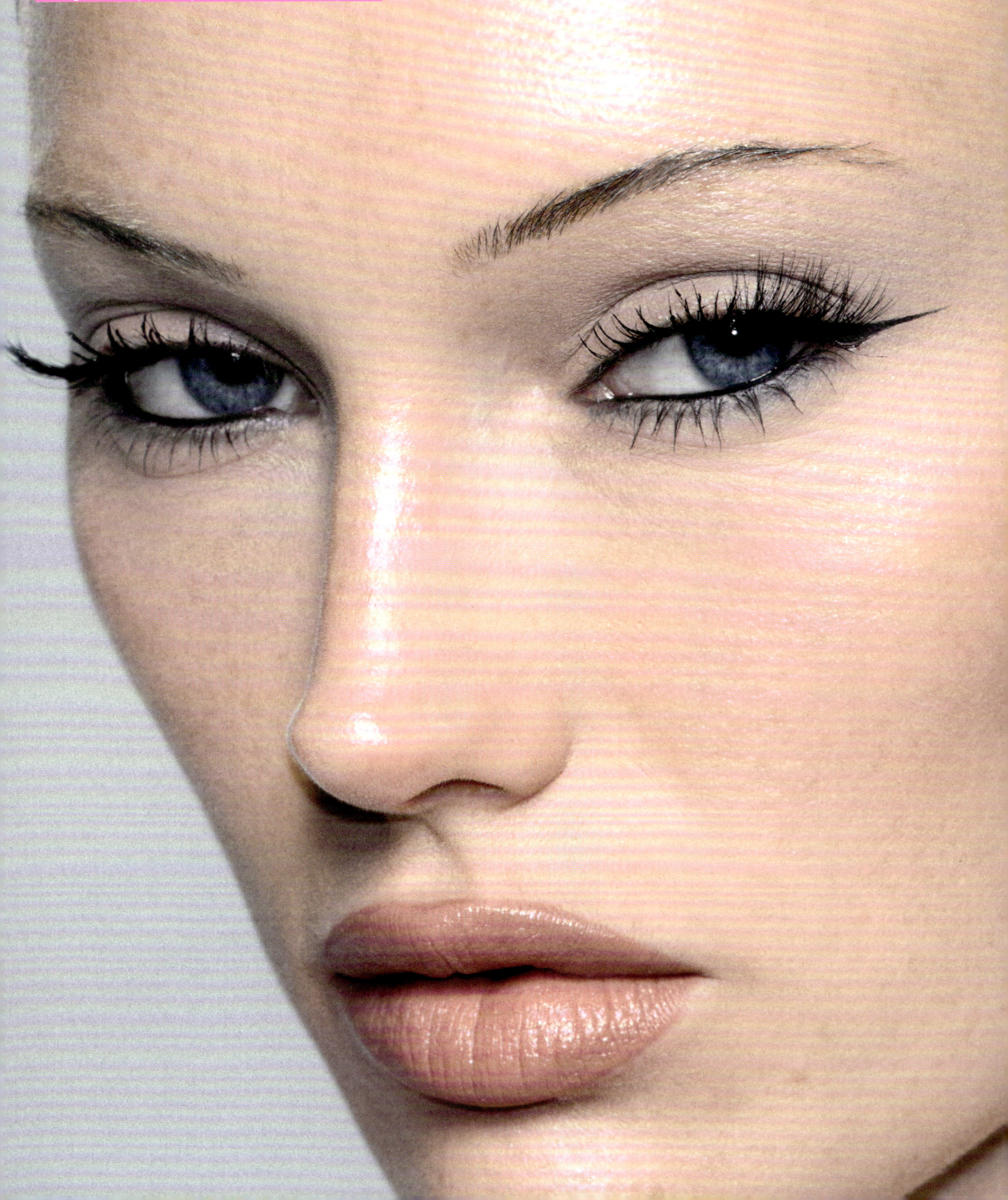

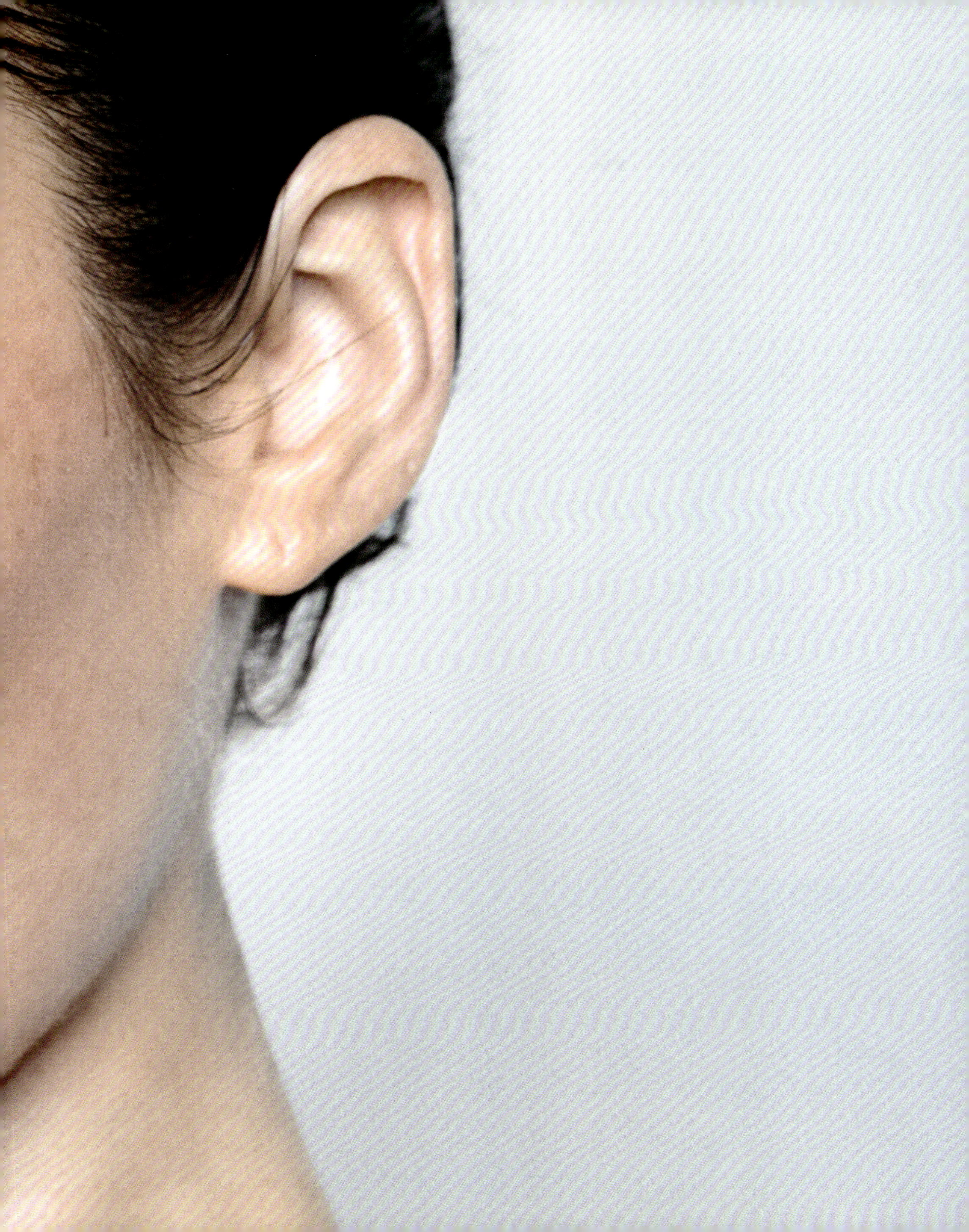

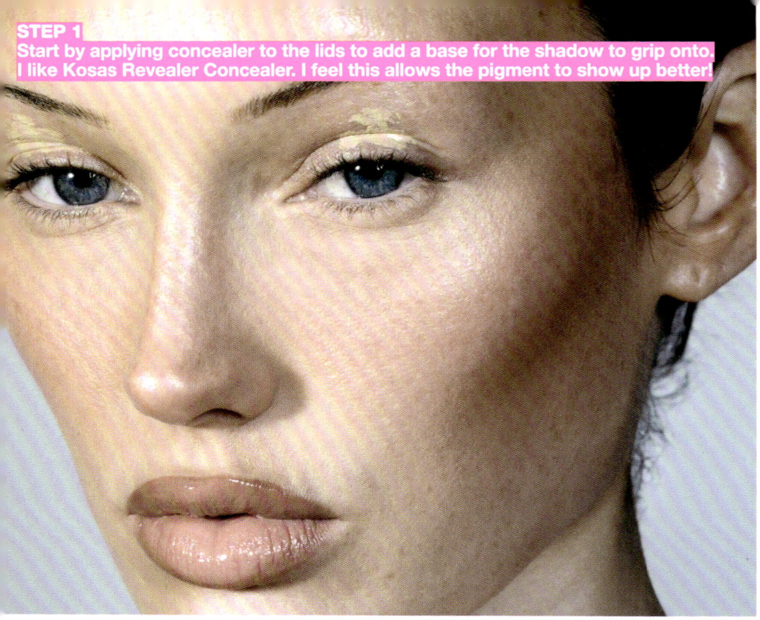

STEP 1
Start by applying concealer to the lids to add a base for the shadow to grip onto. I like Kosas Revealer Concealer. I feel this allows the pigment to show up better!

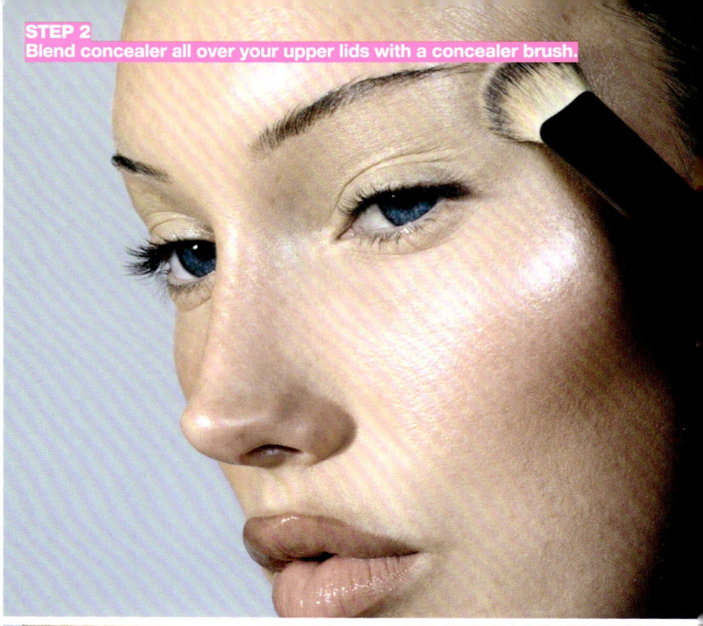

STEP 2
Blend concealer all over your upper lids with a concealer brush.

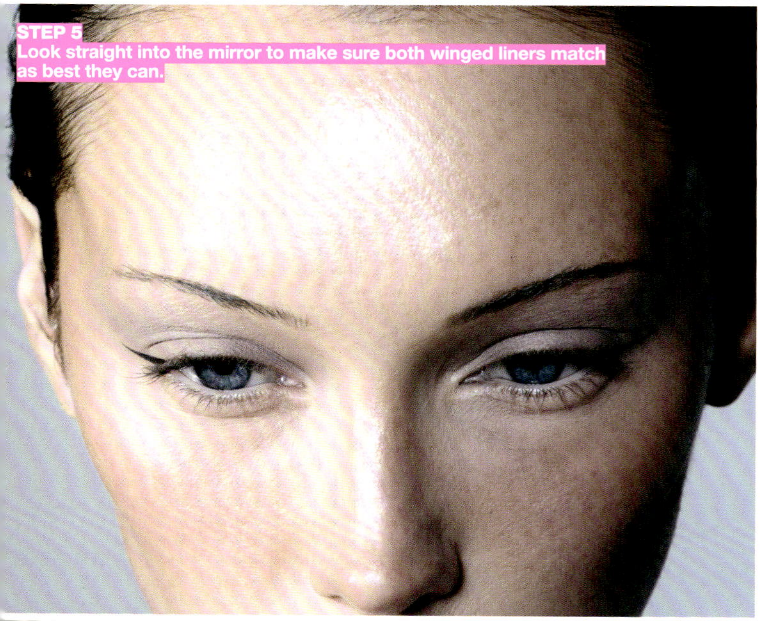

STEP 5
Look straight into the mirror to make sure both winged liners match as best they can.

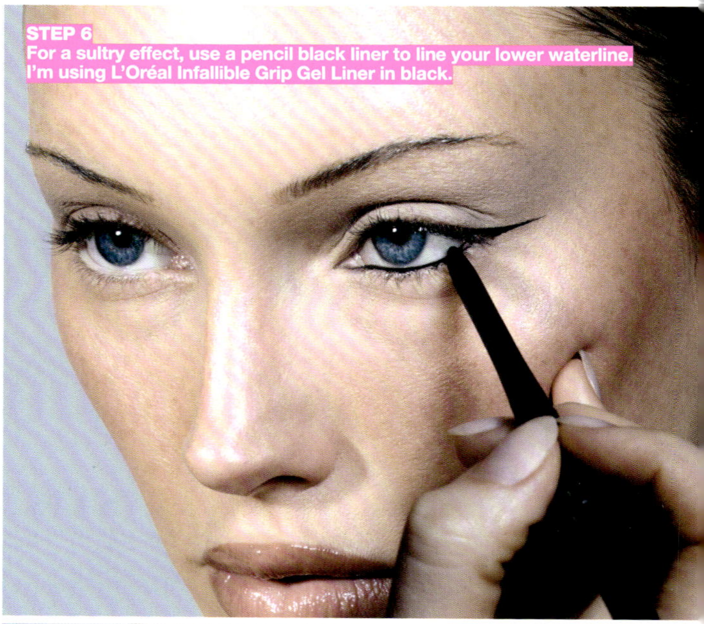

STEP 6
For a sultry effect, use a pencil black liner to line your lower waterline. I'm using L'Oréal Infallible Grip Gel Liner in black.

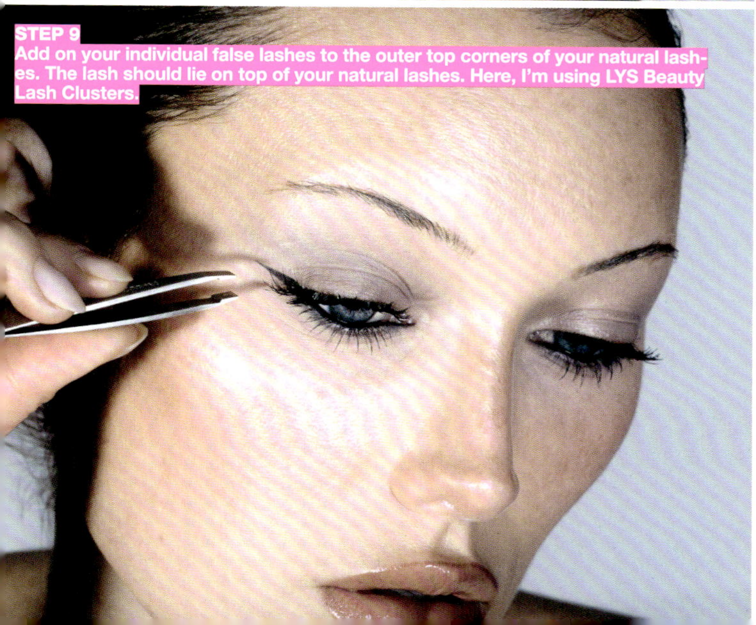

STEP 9
Add on your individual false lashes to the outer top corners of your natural lashes. The lash should lie on top of your natural lashes. Here, I'm using LYS Beauty Lash Clusters.

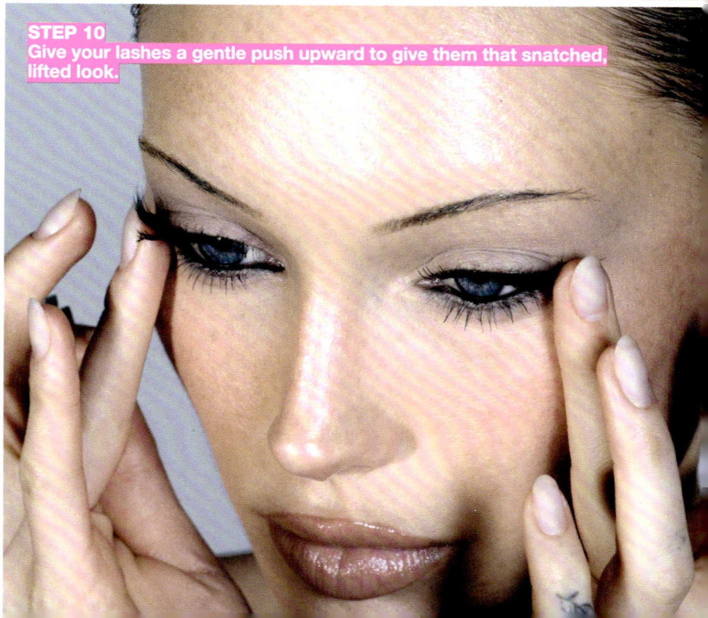

STEP 10
Give your lashes a gentle push upward to give them that snatched, lifted look.

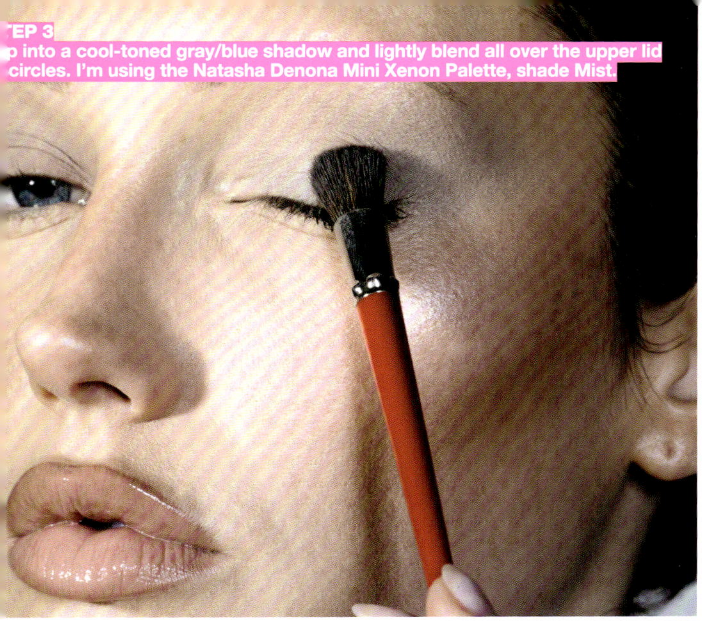

TEP 3
p into a cool-toned gray/blue shadow and lightly blend all over the upper lid circles. I'm using the Natasha Denona Mini Xenon Palette, shade Mist.

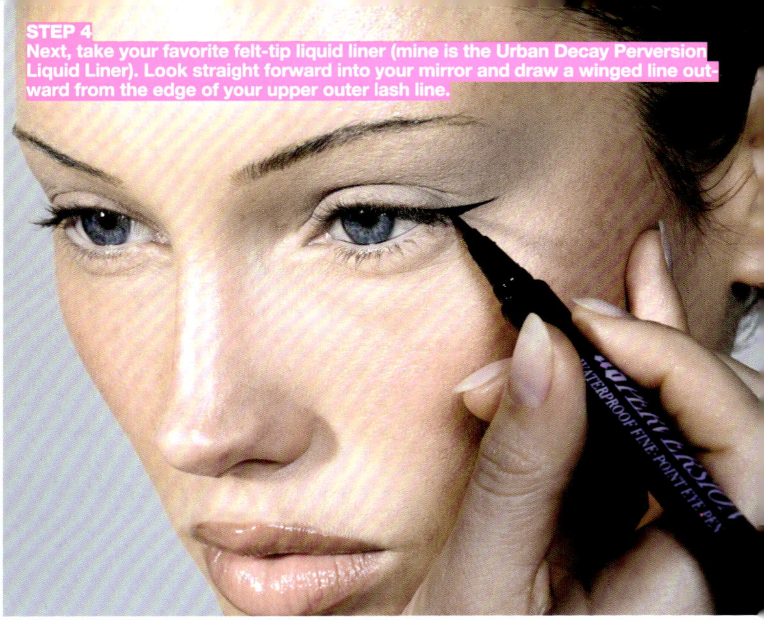

STEP 4
Next, take your favorite felt-tip liquid liner (mine is the Urban Decay Perversion Liquid Liner). Look straight forward into your mirror and draw a winged line outward from the edge of your upper outer lash line.

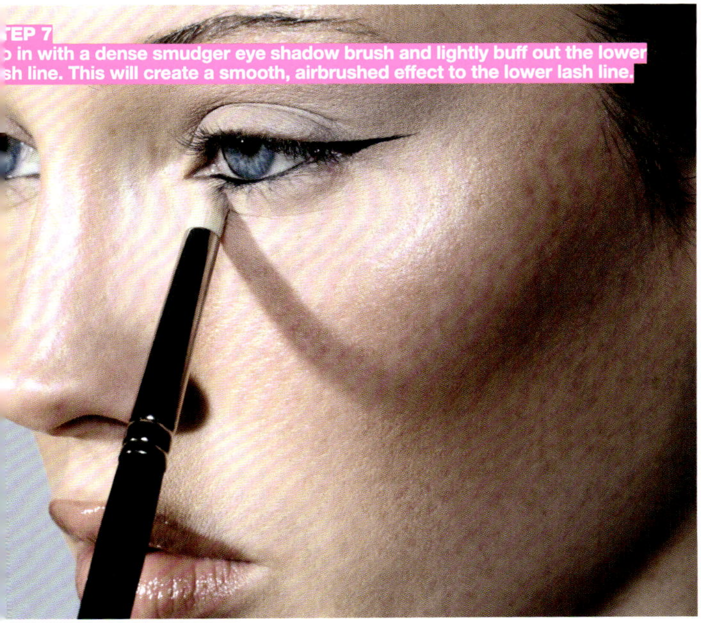

TEP 7
p in with a dense smudger eye shadow brush and lightly buff out the lower sh line. This will create a smooth, airbrushed effect to the lower lash line.

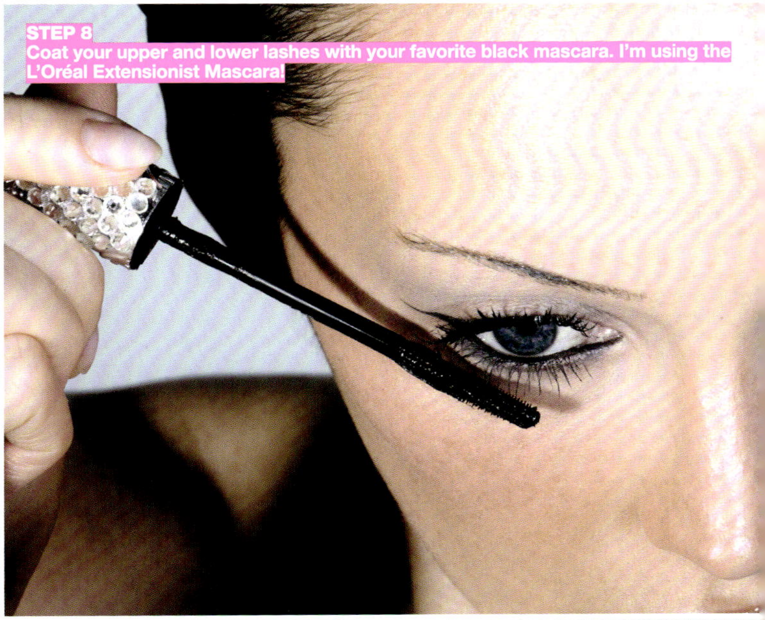

STEP 8
Coat your upper and lower lashes with your favorite black mascara. I'm using the L'Oréal Extensionist Mascara.

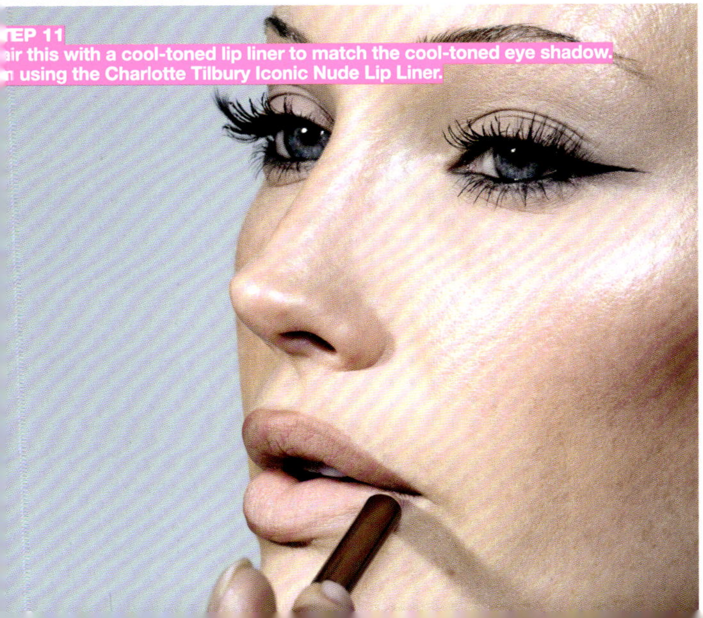

TEP 11
air this with a cool-toned lip liner to match the cool-toned eye shadow.
n using the Charlotte Tilbury Iconic Nude Lip Liner.

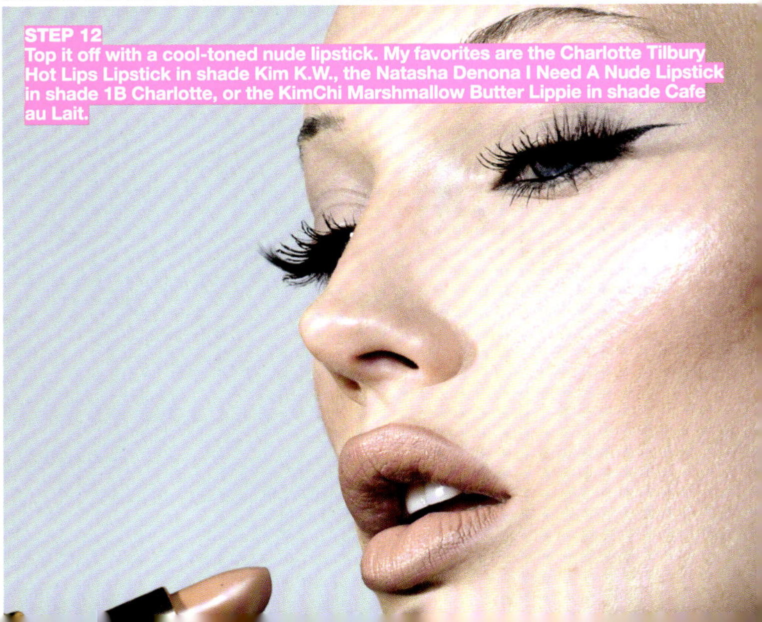

STEP 12
Top it off with a cool-toned nude lipstick. My favorites are the Charlotte Tilbury Hot Lips Lipstick in shade Kim K.W., the Natasha Denona I Need A Nude Lipstick in shade 1B Charlotte, or the KimChi Marshmallow Butter Lippie in shade Cafe au Lait.

HOW TO: GLOWY, NATURAL GLAM

This glam is perfect for days when you want to feel put together but don't have time for a full glam session! It's also perfect for when you want to feel a little lighter and subtle!

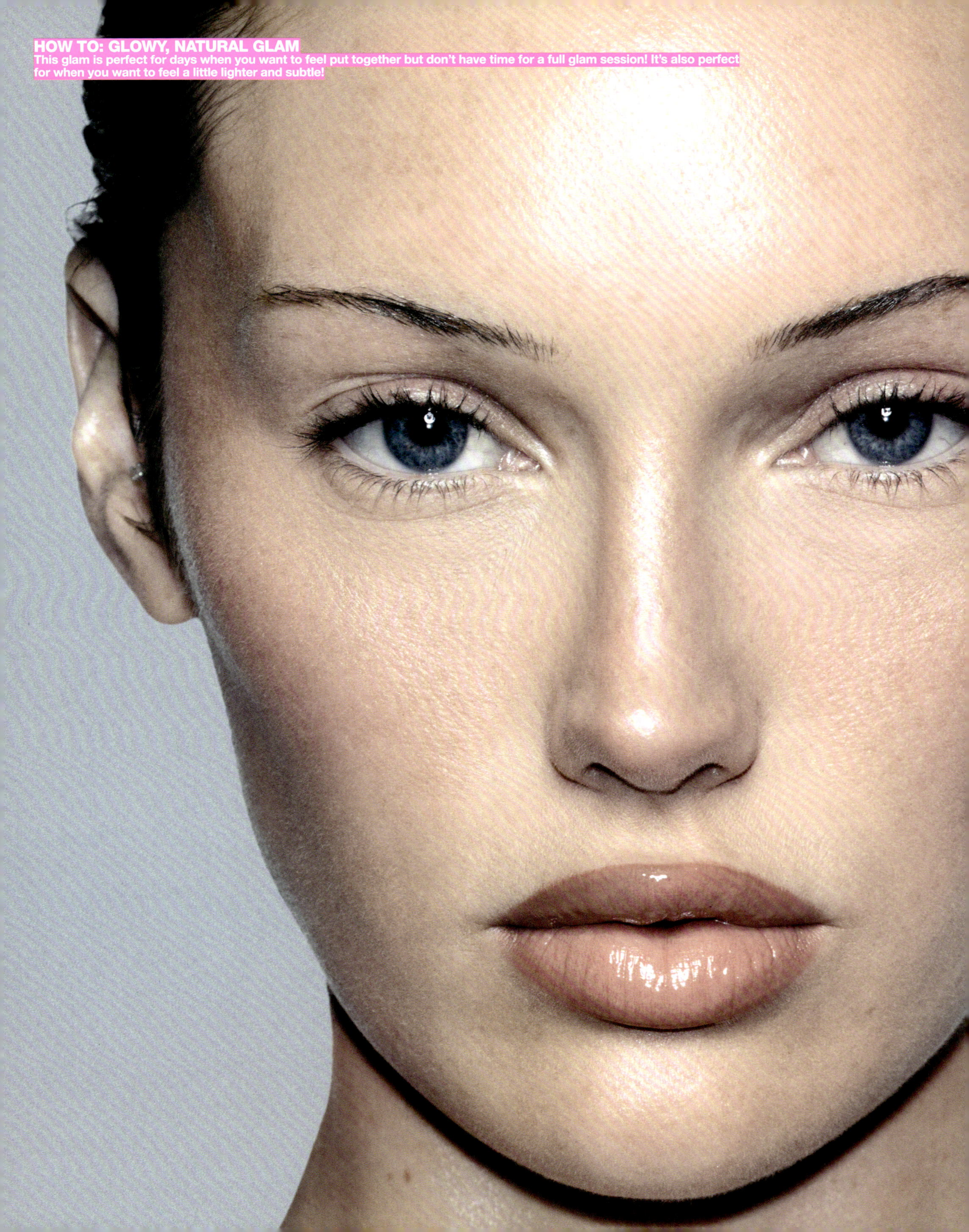

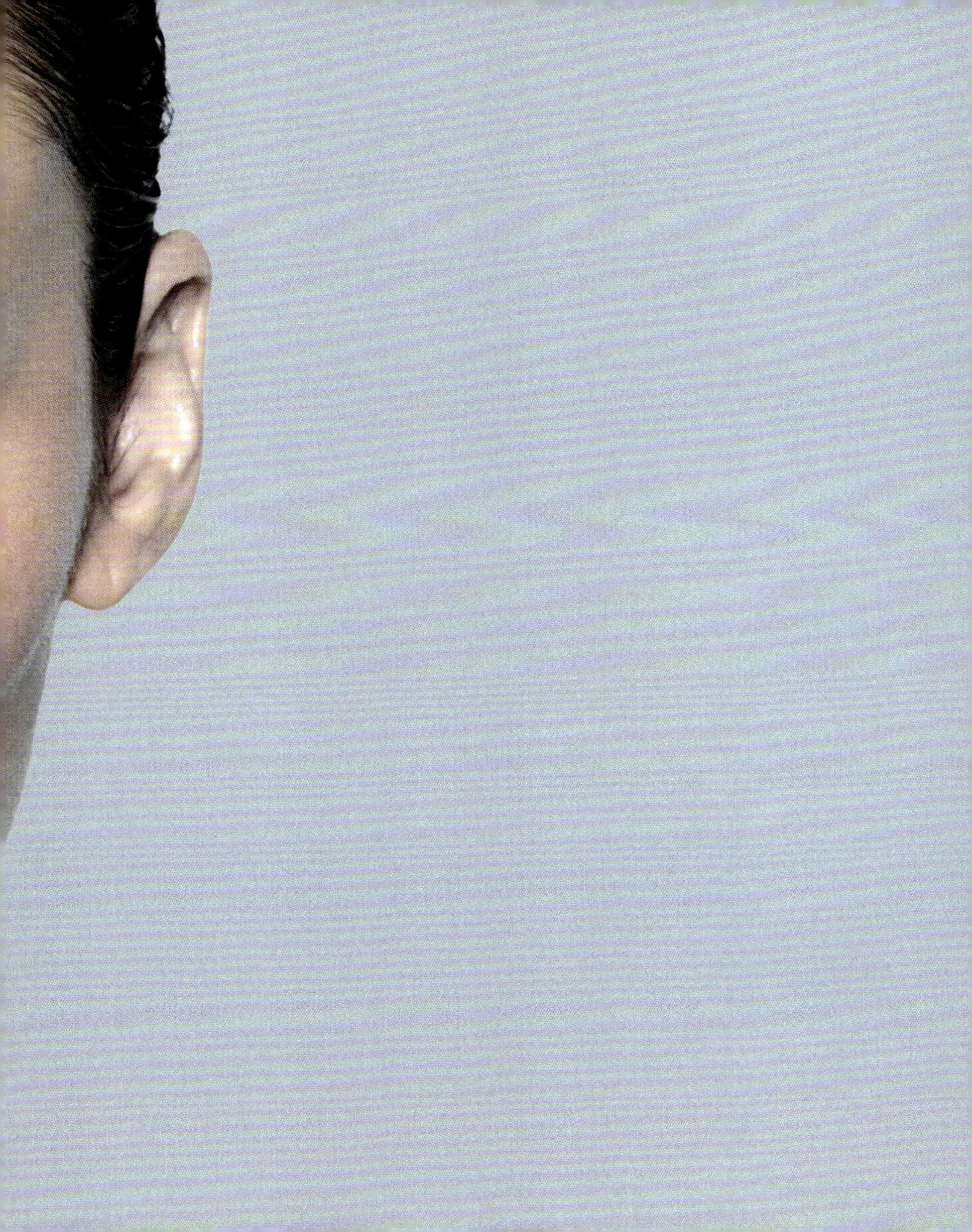

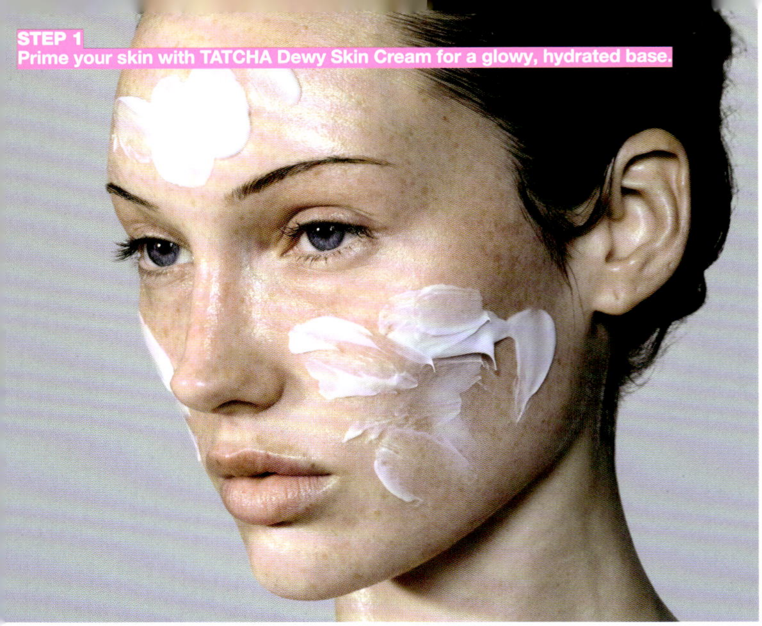

STEP 1
Prime your skin with TATCHA Dewy Skin Cream for a glowy, hydrated base.

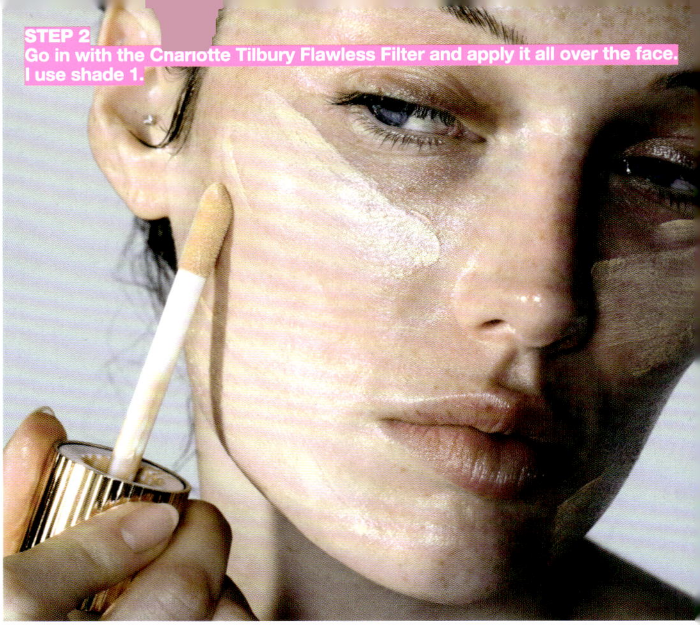

STEP 2
Go in with the Charlotte Tilbury Flawless Filter and apply it all over the face. I use shade 1.

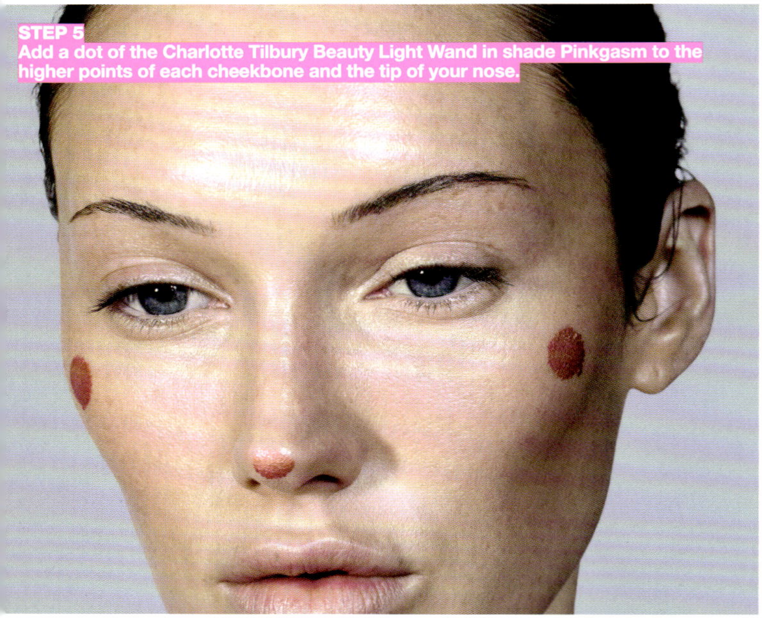

STEP 5
Add a dot of the Charlotte Tilbury Beauty Light Wand in shade Pinkgasm to the higher points of each cheekbone and the tip of your nose.

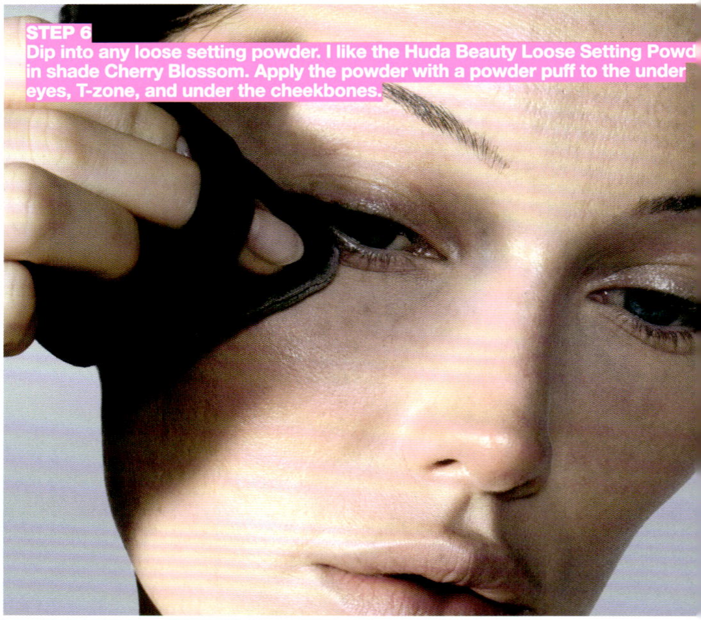

STEP 6
Dip into any loose setting powder. I like the Huda Beauty Loose Setting Powd in shade Cherry Blossom. Apply the powder with a powder puff to the under eyes, T-zone, and under the cheekbones.

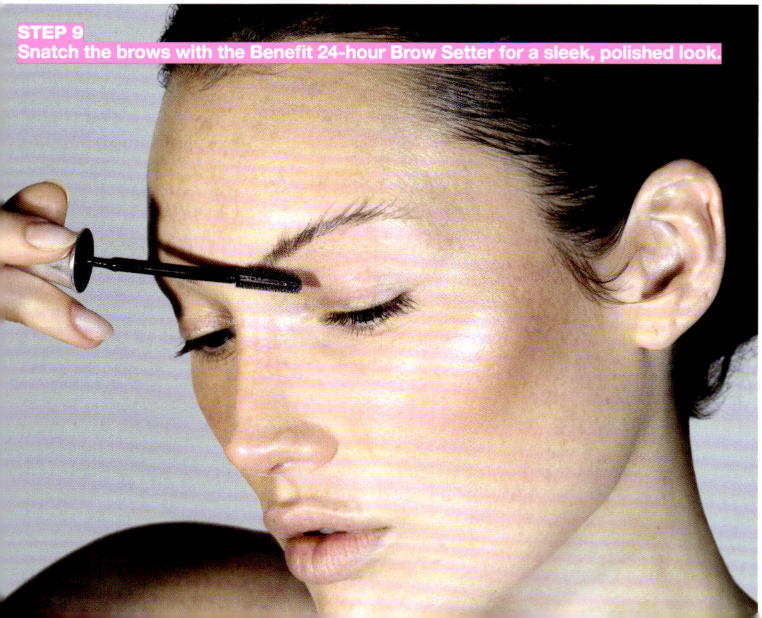

STEP 9
Snatch the brows with the Benefit 24-hour Brow Setter for a sleek, polished look.

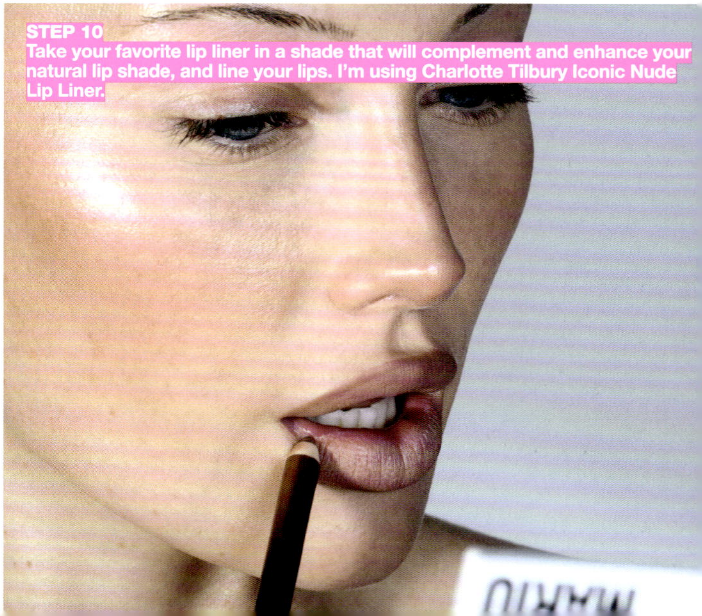

STEP 10
Take your favorite lip liner in a shade that will complement and enhance your natural lip shade, and line your lips. I'm using Charlotte Tilbury Iconic Nude Lip Liner.

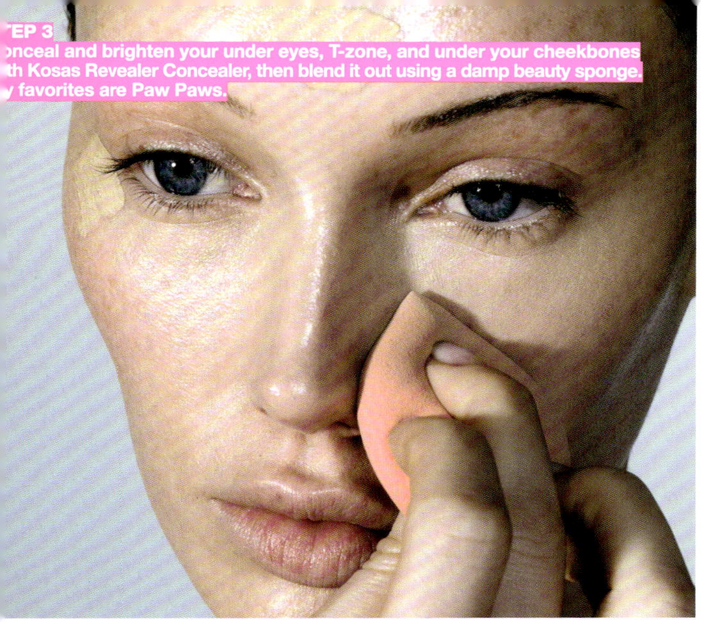

TEP 3
onceal and brighten your under eyes, T-zone, and under your cheekbones
th Kosas Revealer Concealer, then blend it out using a damp beauty sponge.
y favorites are Paw Paws.

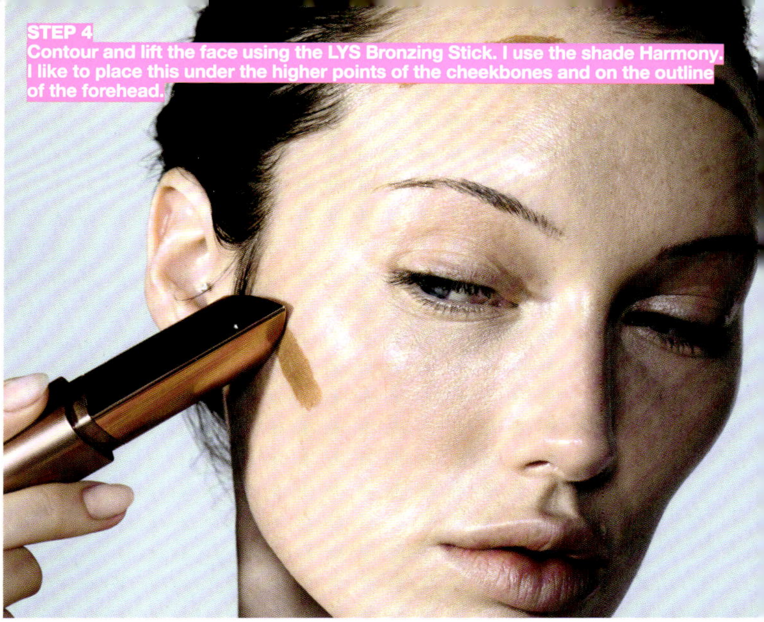

STEP 4
Contour and lift the face using the LYS Bronzing Stick. I use the shade Harmony. I like to place this under the higher points of the cheekbones and on the outline of the forehead.

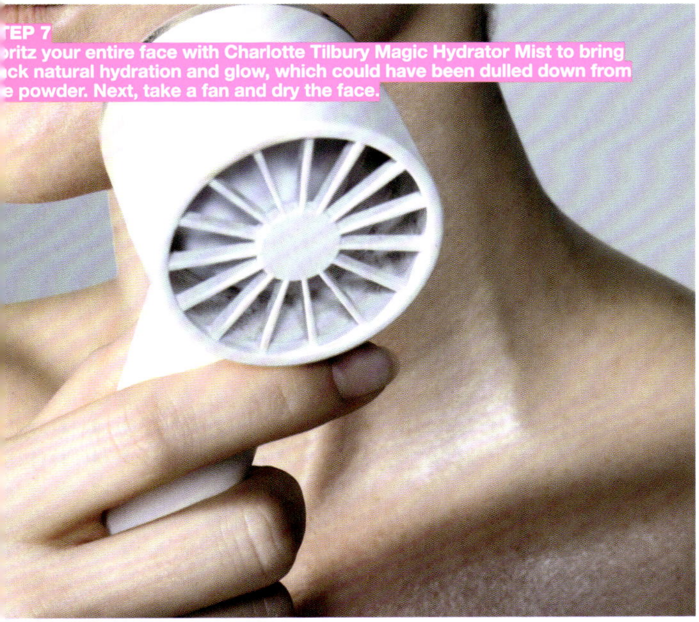

TEP 7
pritz your entire face with Charlotte Tilbury Magic Hydrator Mist to bring
ck natural hydration and glow, which could have been dulled down from
e powder. Next, take a fan and dry the face.

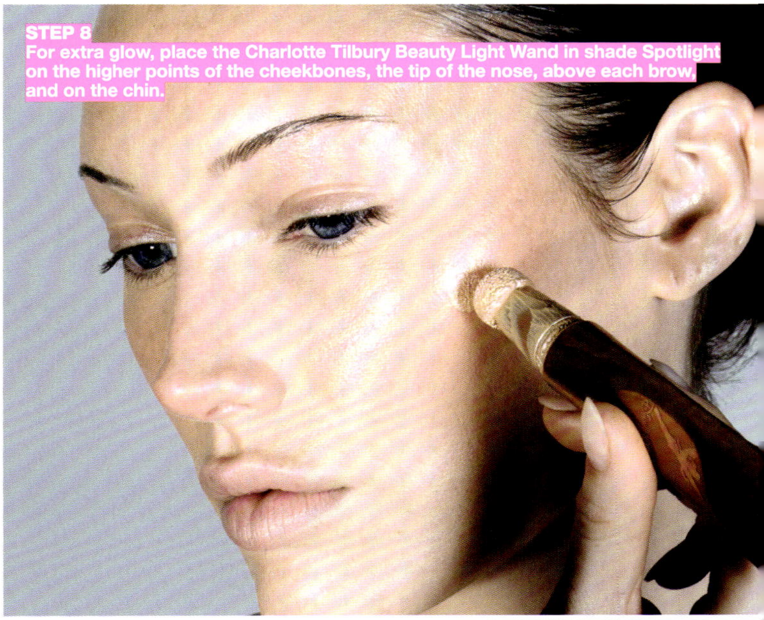

STEP 8
For extra glow, place the Charlotte Tilbury Beauty Light Wand in shade Spotlight on the higher points of the cheekbones, the tip of the nose, above each brow, and on the chin.

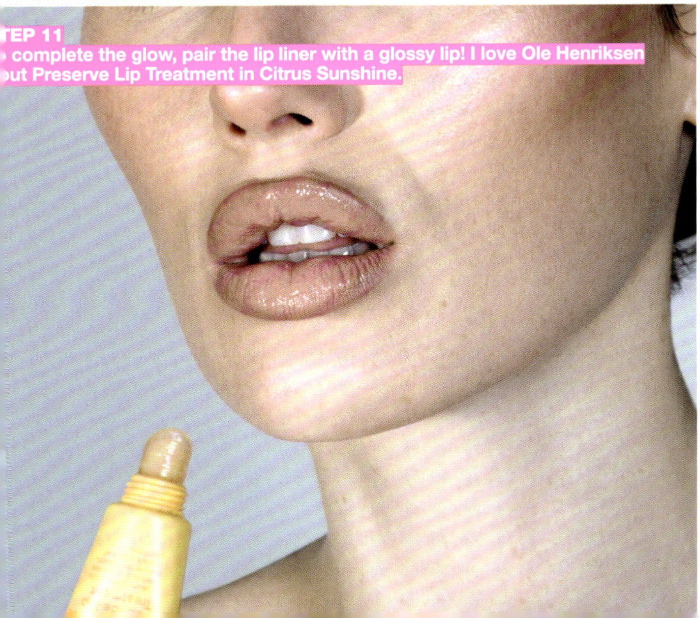

TEP 11
complete the glow, pair the lip liner with a glossy lip! I love Ole Henriksen
out Preserve Lip Treatment in Citrus Sunshine.

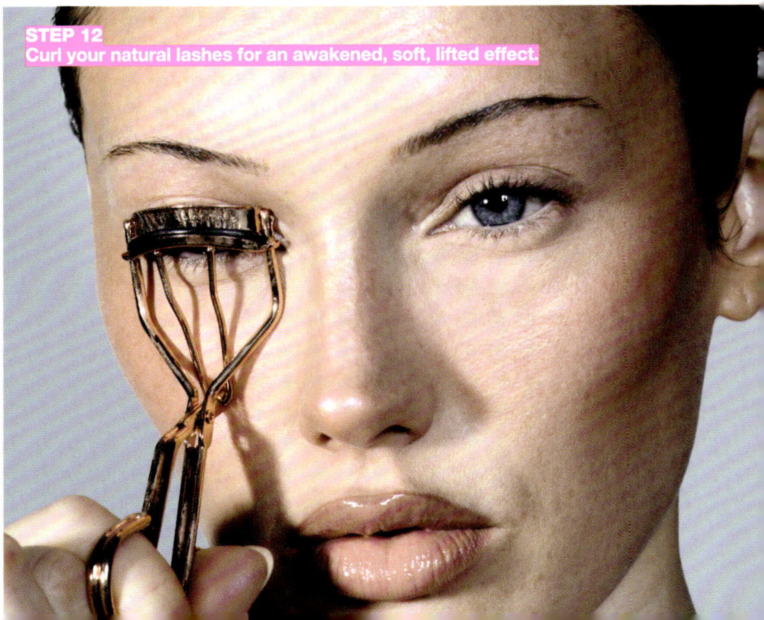

STEP 12
Curl your natural lashes for an awakened, soft, lifted effect.

HOW TO: OMBRÉ EYE

This is for the days when I want to be bolder and experiment with dimension and color. This technique is interchangeable with any colors that you desire, so play around and have fun with it!

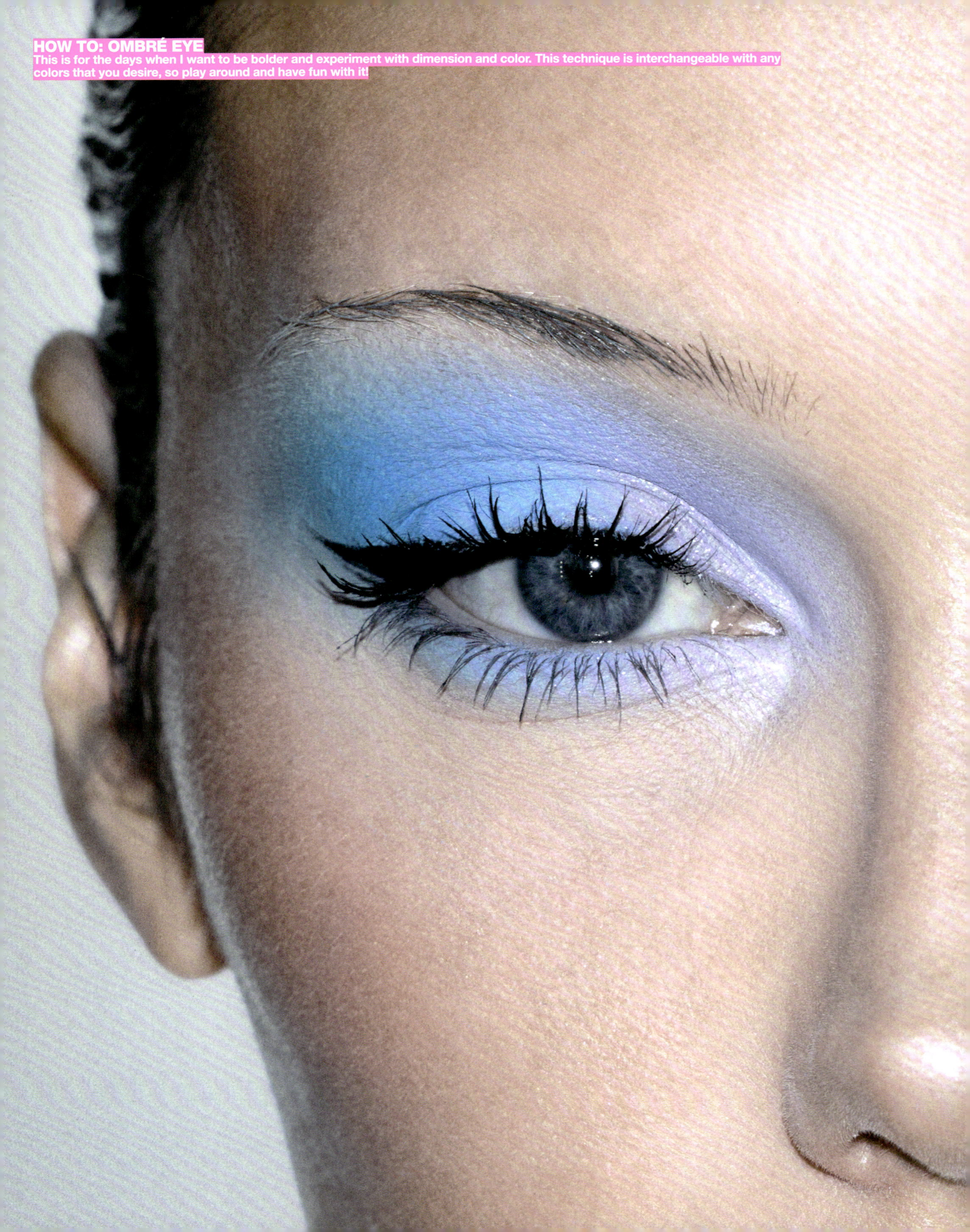

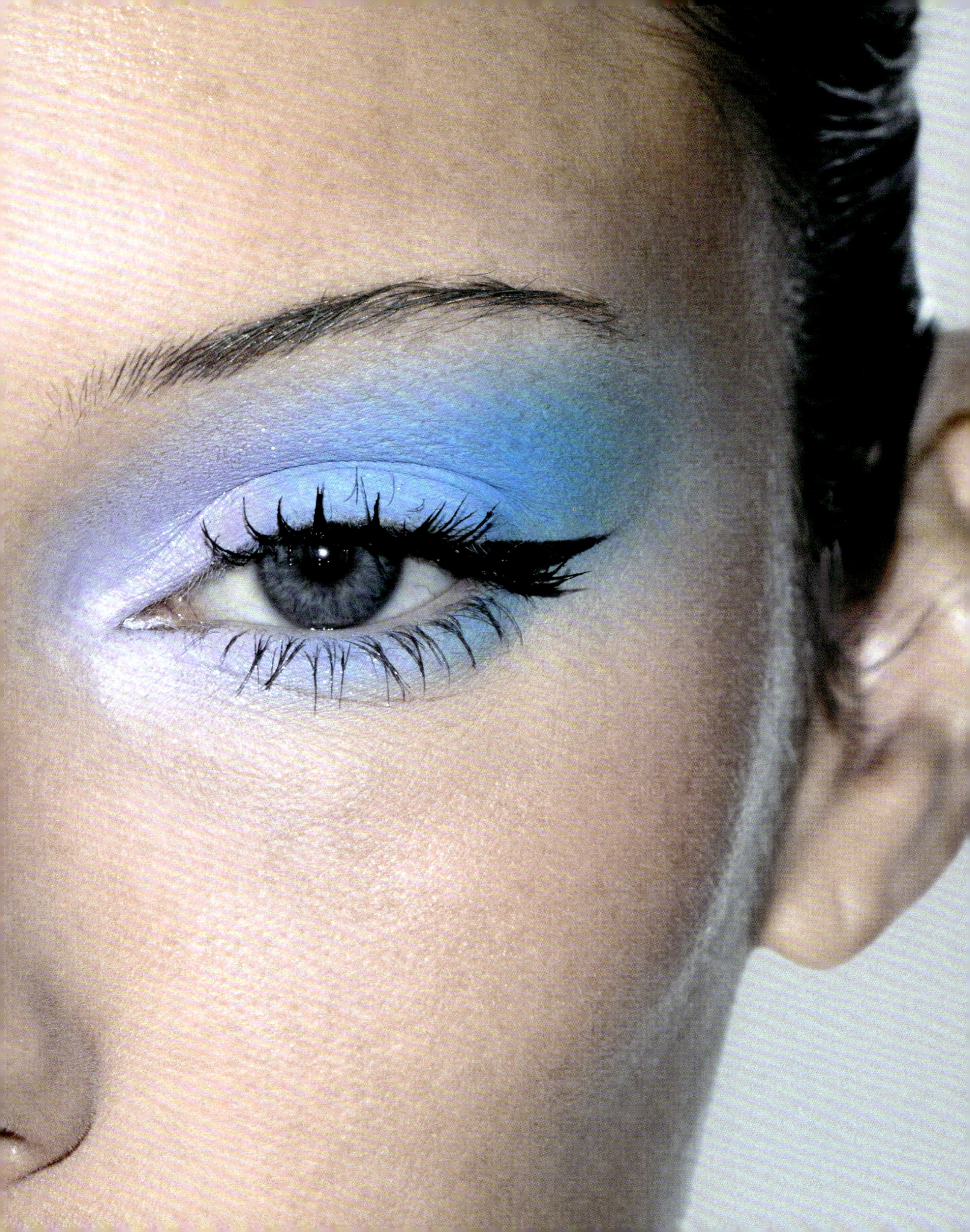

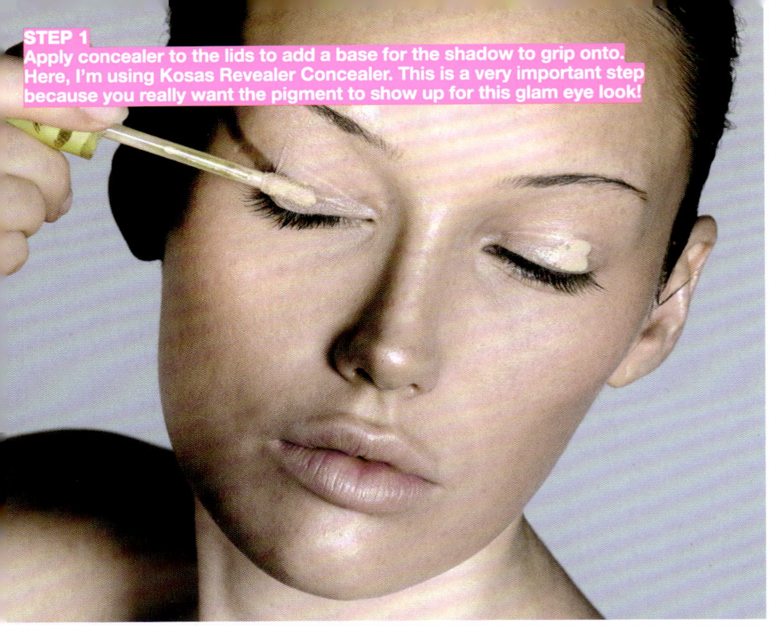

STEP 1
Apply concealer to the lids to add a base for the shadow to grip onto. Here, I'm using Kosas Revealer Concealer. This is a very important step because you really want the pigment to show up for this glam eye look!

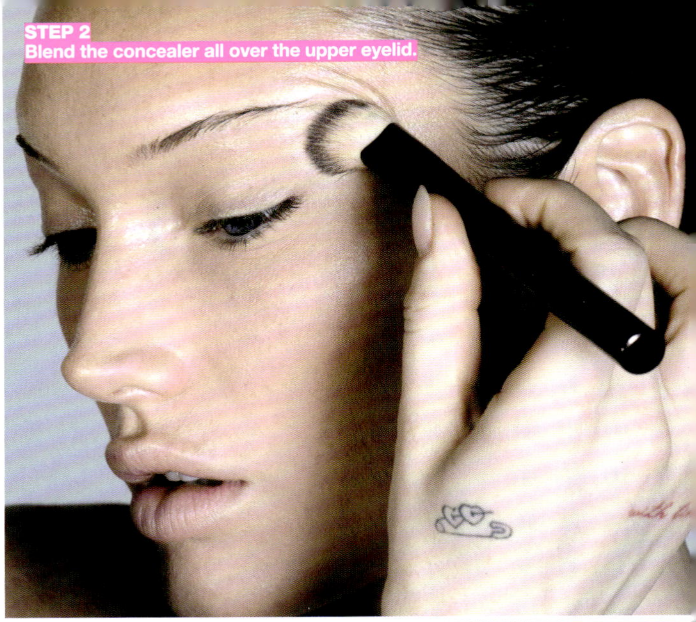

STEP 2
Blend the concealer all over the upper eyelid.

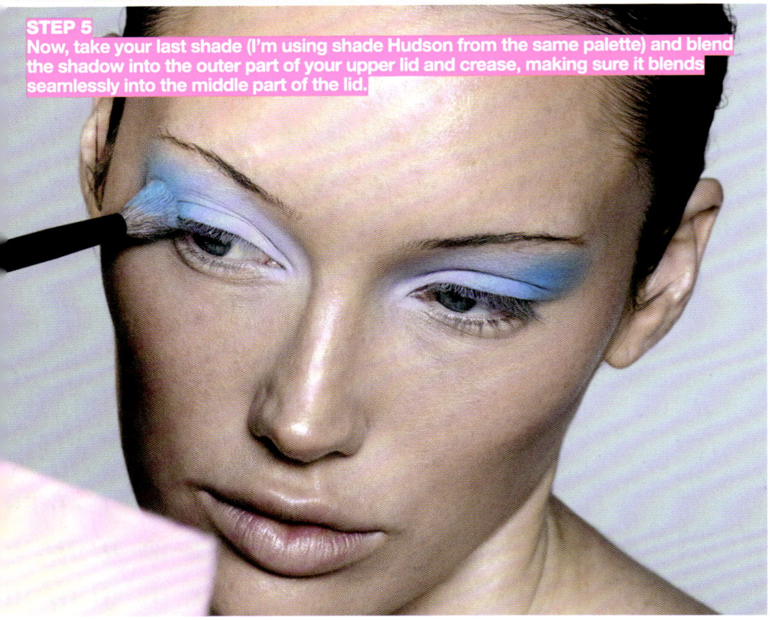

STEP 5
Now, take your last shade (I'm using shade Hudson from the same palette) and blend the shadow into the outer part of your upper lid and crease, making sure it blends seamlessly into the middle part of the lid.

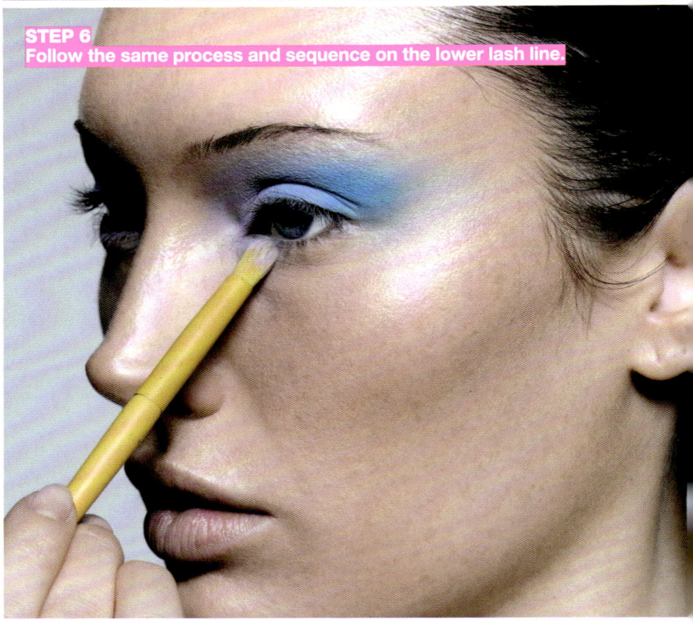

STEP 6
Follow the same process and sequence on the lower lash line.

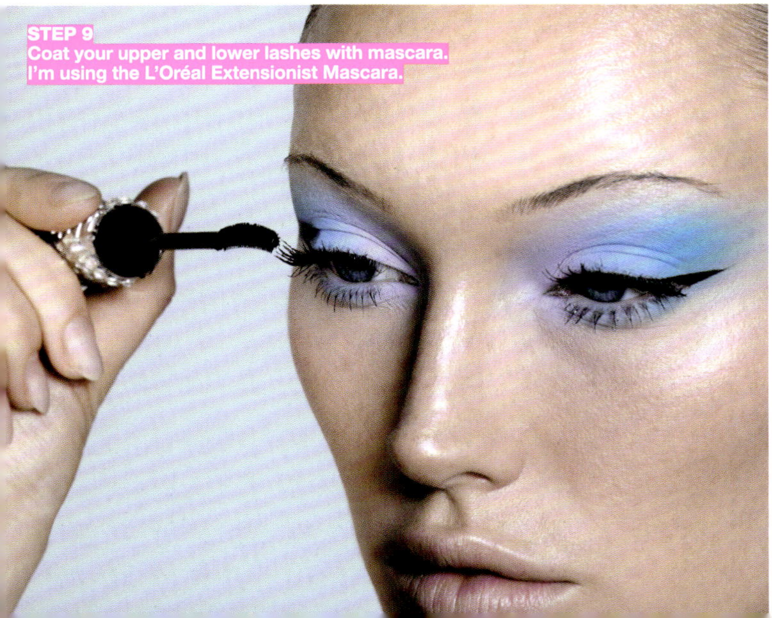

STEP 9
Coat your upper and lower lashes with mascara. I'm using the L'Oréal Extensionist Mascara.

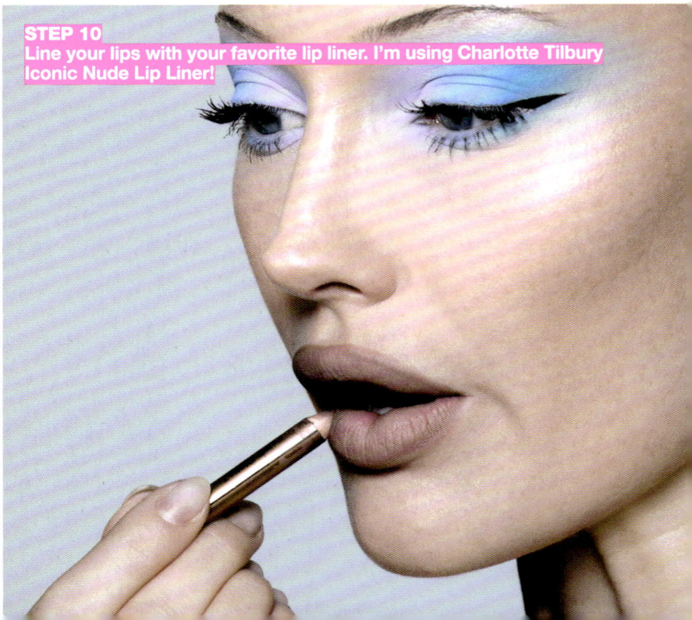

STEP 10
Line your lips with your favorite lip liner. I'm using Charlotte Tilbury Iconic Nude Lip Liner!

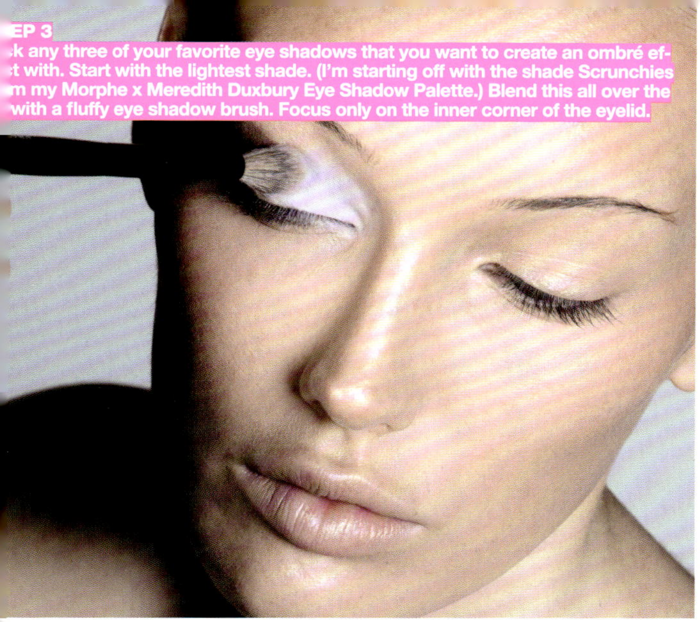

EP 3
ːk any three of your favorite eye shadows that you want to create an ombré ef-
ːt with. Start with the lightest shade. (I'm starting off with the shade Scrunchies
ːm my Morphe x Meredith Duxbury Eye Shadow Palette.) Blend this all over the
with a fluffy eye shadow brush. Focus only on the inner corner of the eyelid.

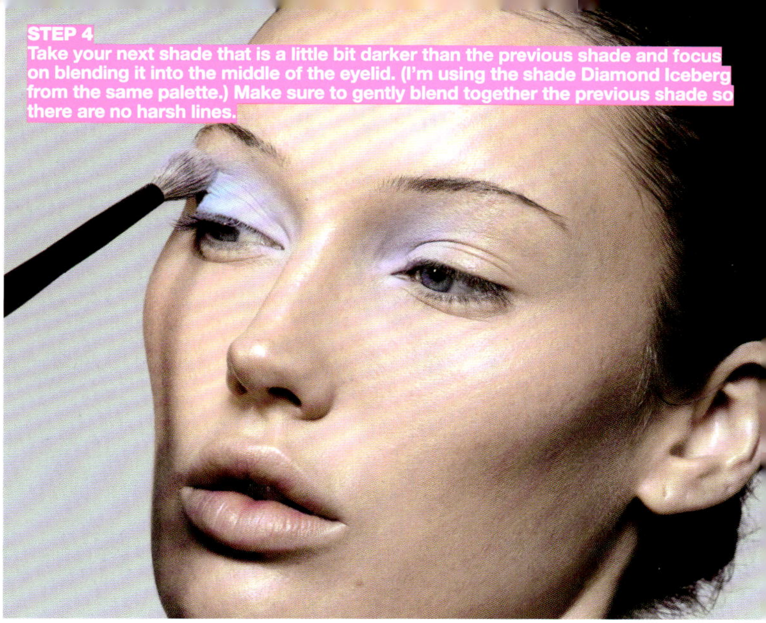

STEP 4
Take your next shade that is a little bit darker than the previous shade and focus on blending it into the middle of the eyelid. (I'm using the shade Diamond Iceberg from the same palette.) Make sure to gently blend together the previous shade so there are no harsh lines.

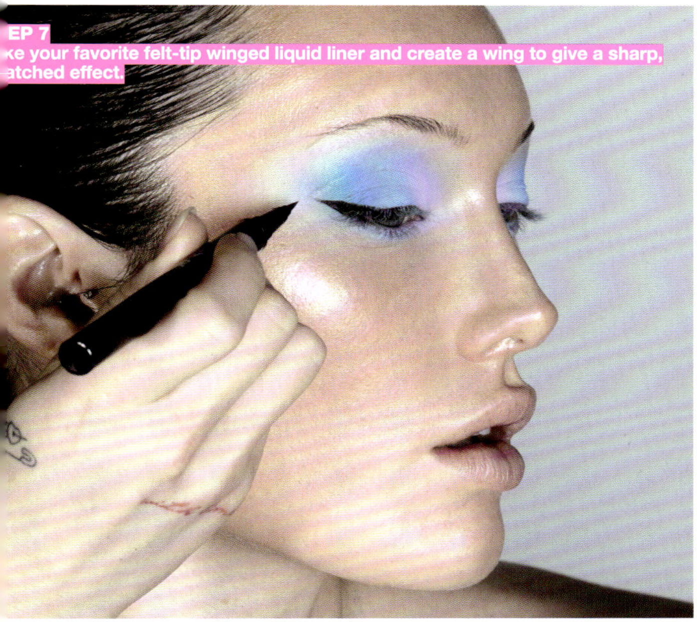

EP 7
ːe your favorite felt-tip winged liquid liner and create a wing to give a sharp,
atched effect.

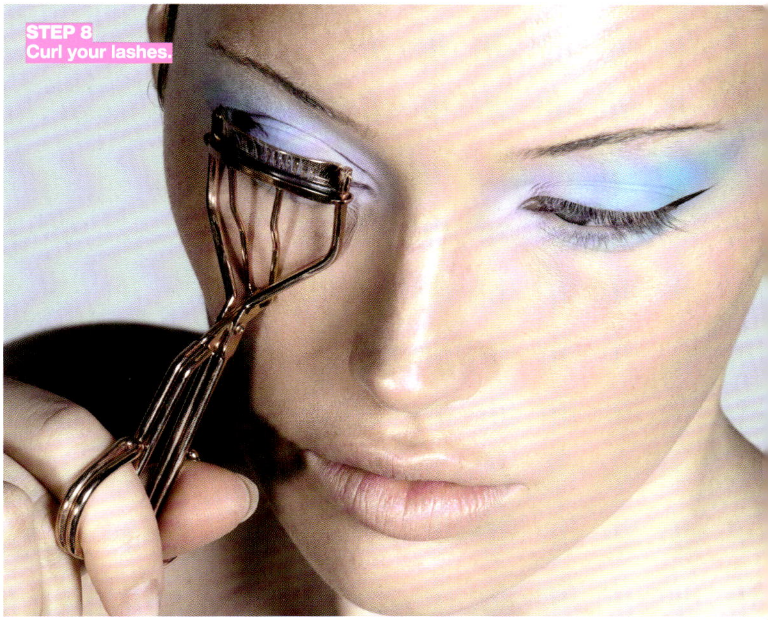

STEP 8
Curl your lashes.

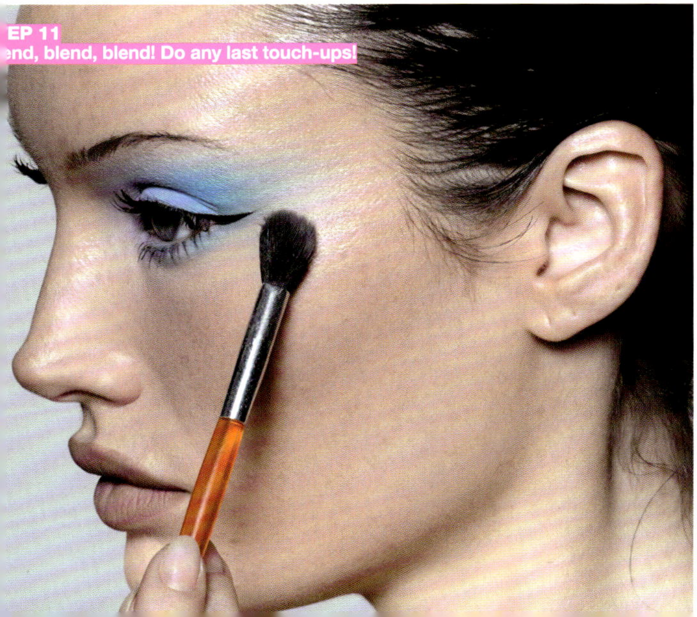

EP 11
end, blend, blend! Do any last touch-ups!

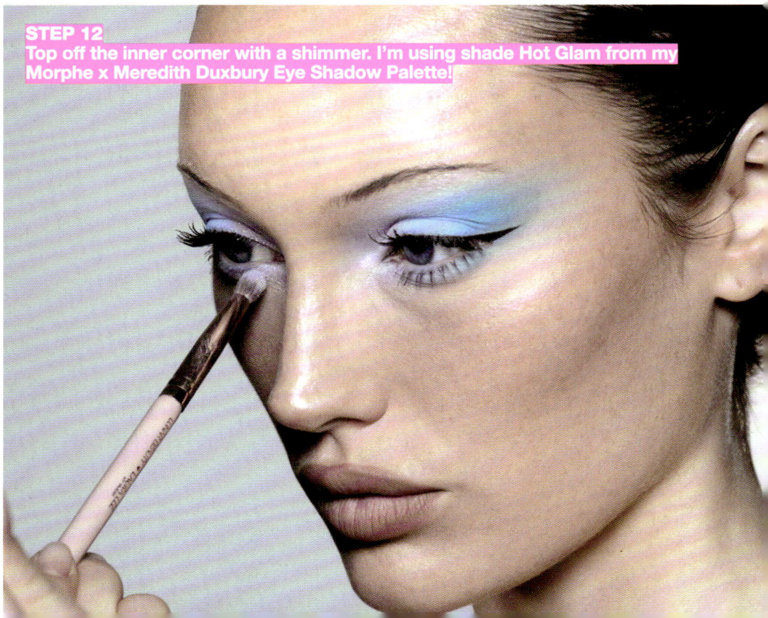

STEP 12
Top off the inner corner with a shimmer. I'm using shade Hot Glam from my Morphe x Meredith Duxbury Eye Shadow Palette!

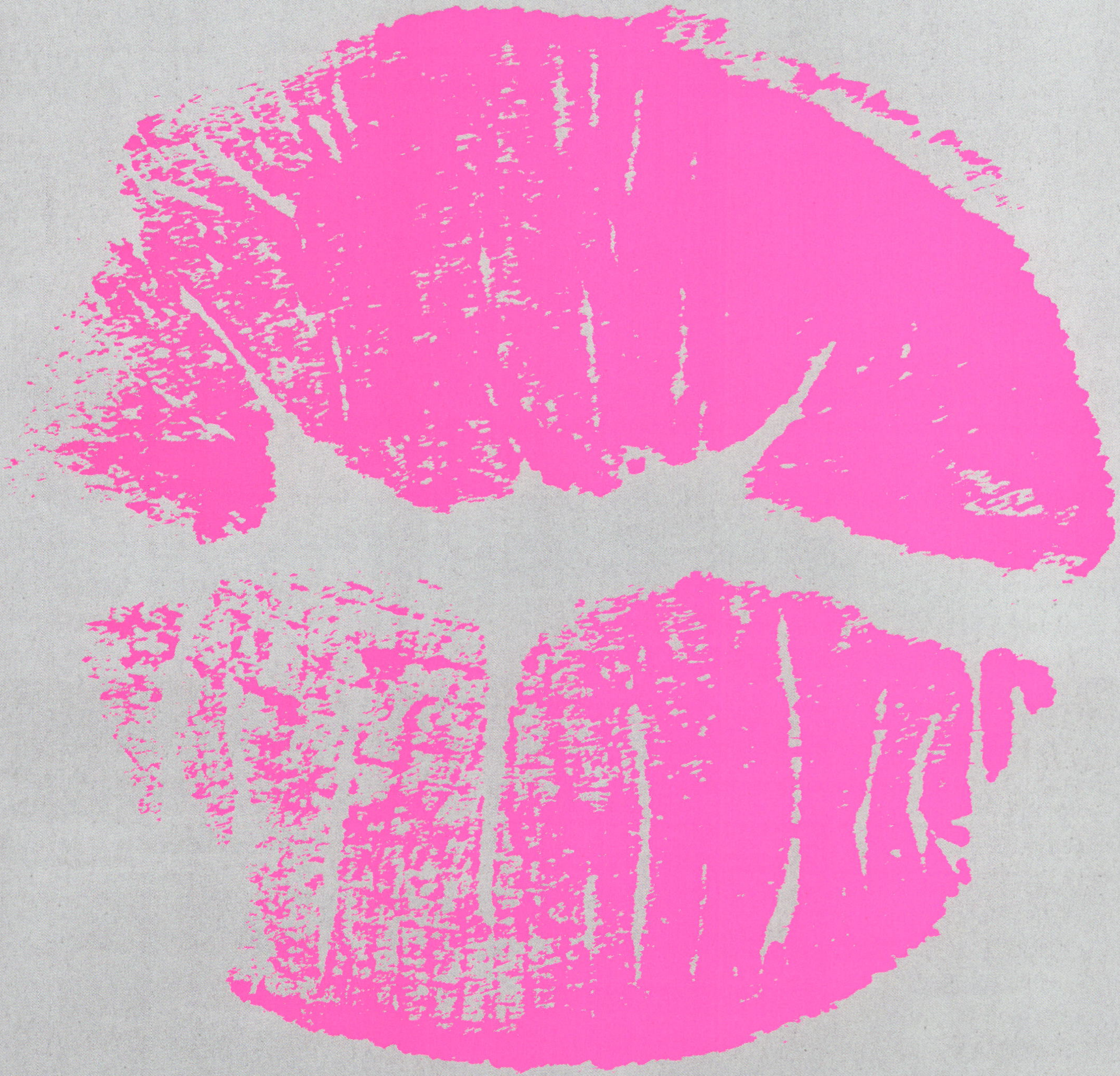

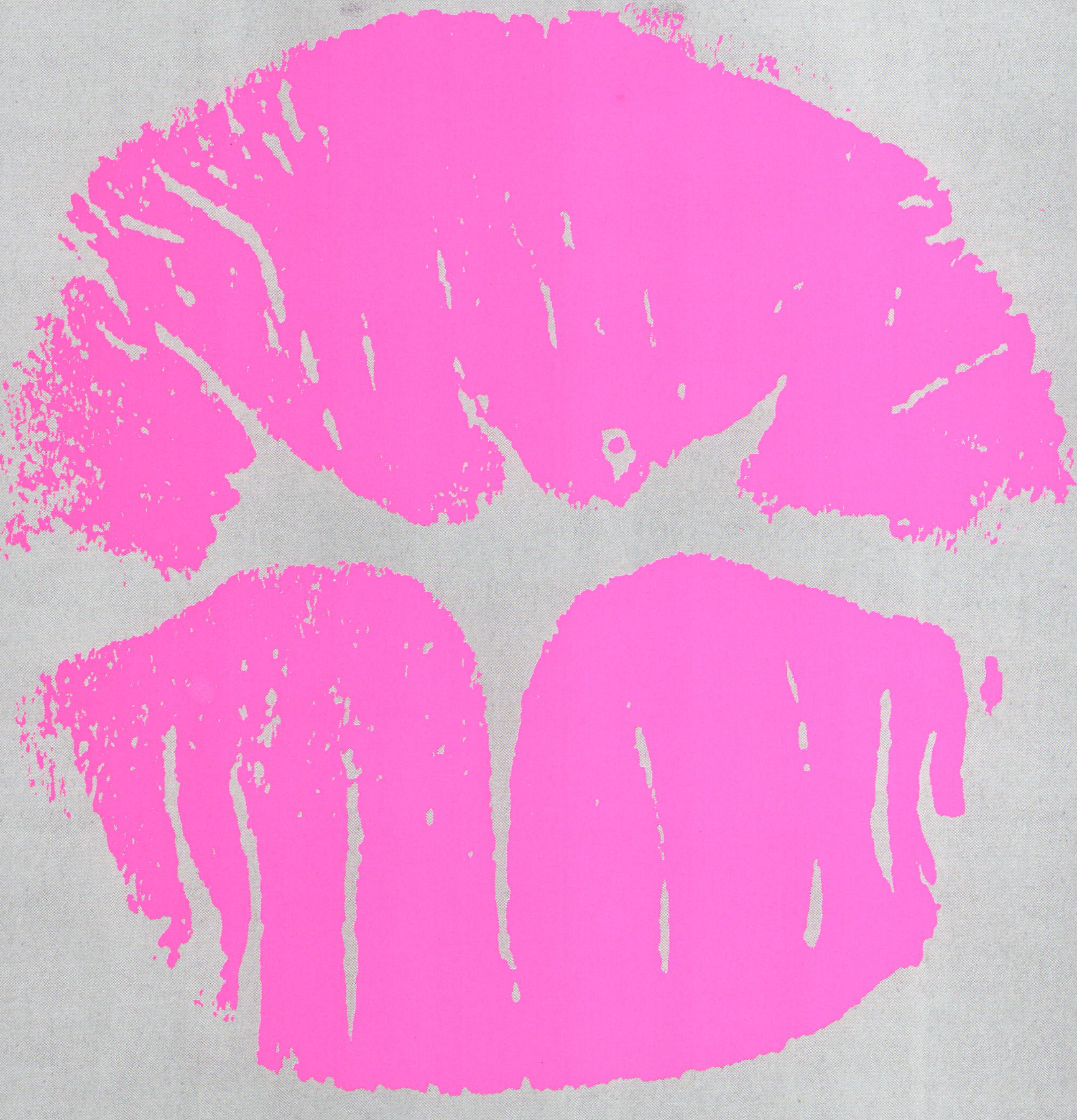

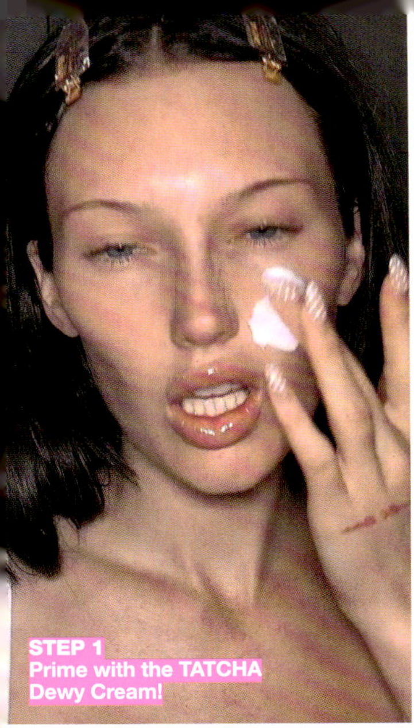

STEP 1
Prime with the TATCHA Dewy Cream!

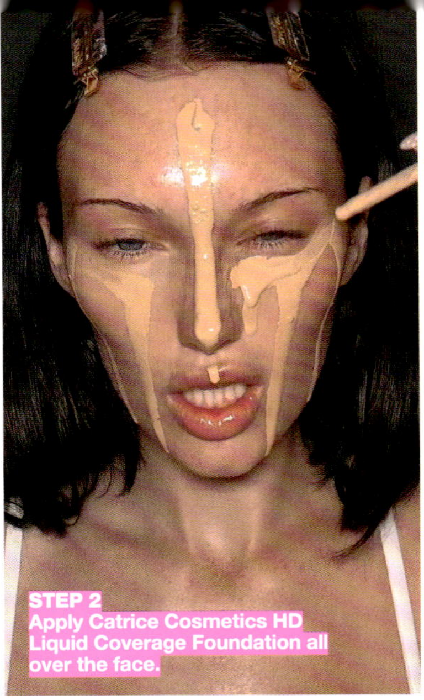

STEP 2
Apply Catrice Cosmetics HD Liquid Coverage Foundation all over the face.

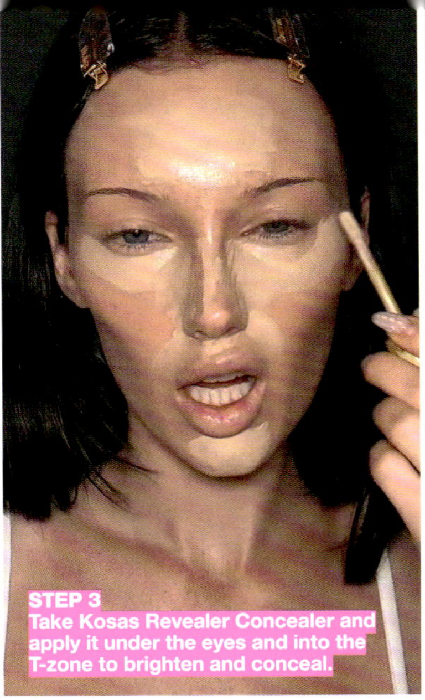

STEP 3
Take Kosas Revealer Concealer and apply it under the eyes and into the T-zone to brighten and conceal.

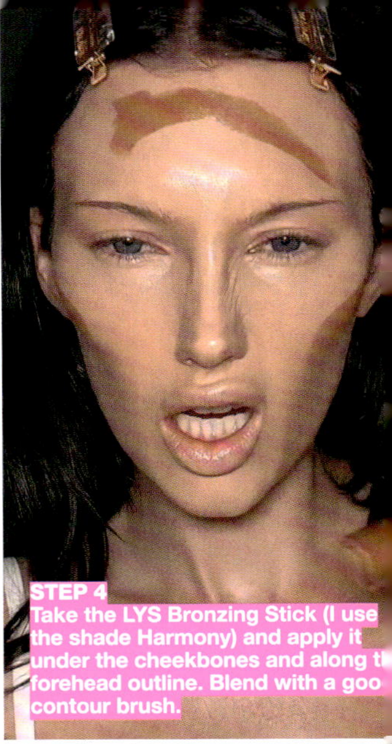

STEP 4
Take the LYS Bronzing Stick (I use the shade Harmony) and apply it under the cheekbones and along th forehead outline. Blend with a goo contour brush.

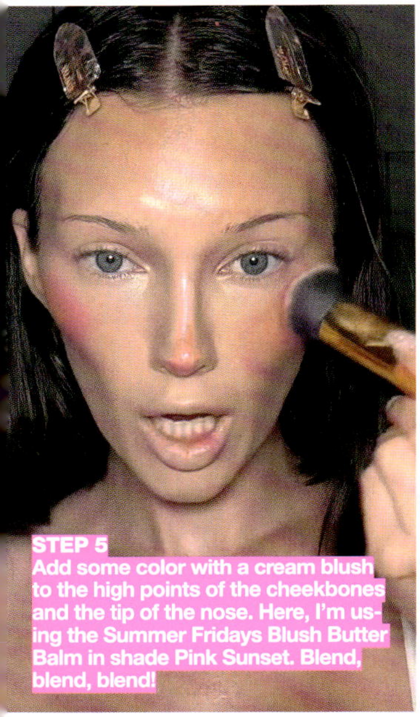

STEP 5
Add some color with a cream blush to the high points of the cheekbones and the tip of the nose. Here, I'm using the Summer Fridays Blush Butter Balm in shade Pink Sunset. Blend, blend, blend!

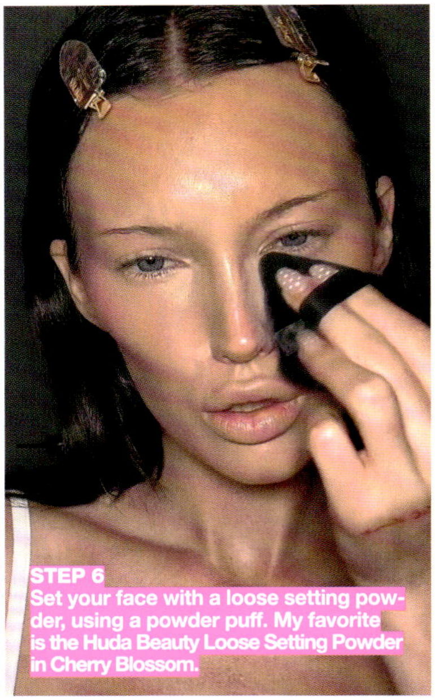

STEP 6
Set your face with a loose setting powder, using a powder puff. My favorite is the Huda Beauty Loose Setting Powder in Cherry Blossom.

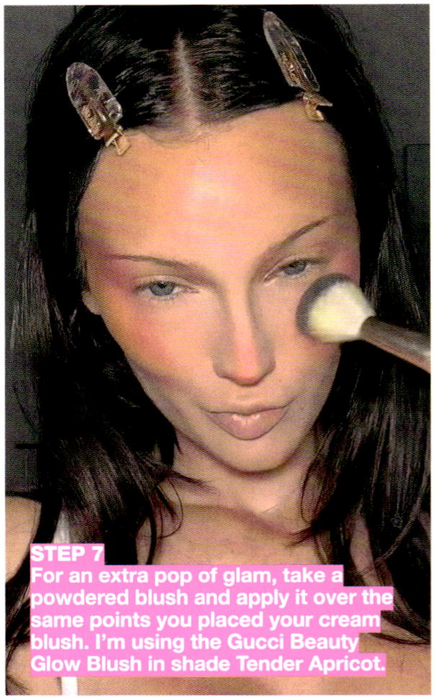

STEP 7
For an extra pop of glam, take a powdered blush and apply it over the same points you placed your cream blush. I'm using the Gucci Beauty Glow Blush in shade Tender Apricot.

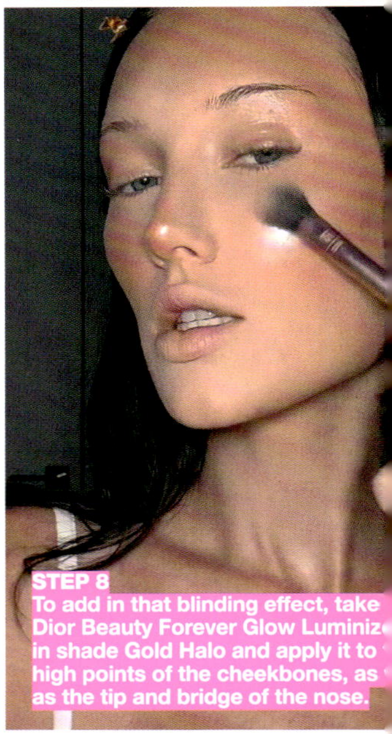

STEP 8
To add in that blinding effect, take Dior Beauty Forever Glow Luminize in shade Gold Halo and apply it to high points of the cheekbones, as as the tip and bridge of the nose.

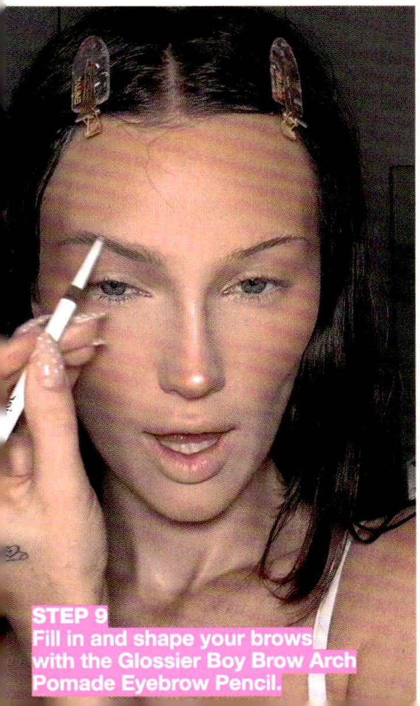

STEP 9
Fill in and shape your brows with the Glossier Boy Brow Arch Pomade Eyebrow Pencil.

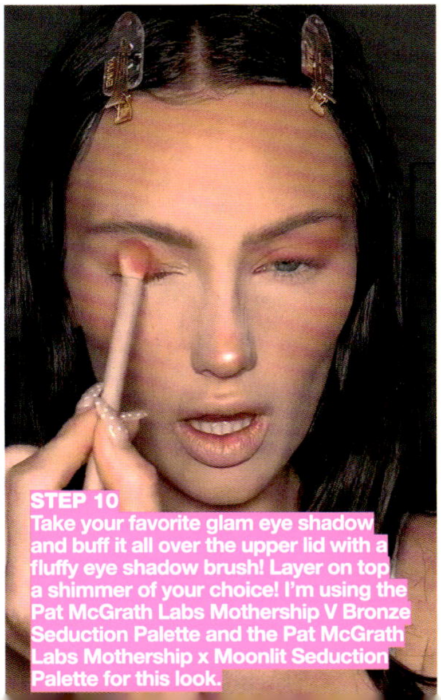

STEP 10
Take your favorite glam eye shadow and buff it all over the upper lid with a fluffy eye shadow brush! Layer on top a shimmer of your choice! I'm using the Pat McGrath Labs Mothership V Bronze Seduction Palette and the Pat McGrath Labs Mothership x Moonlit Seduction Palette for this look.

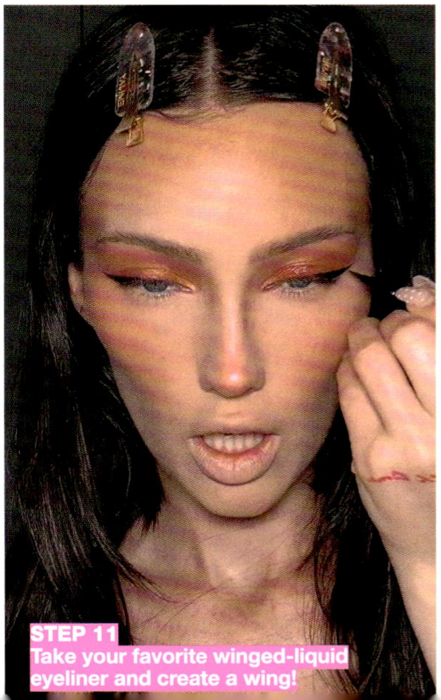

STEP 11
Take your favorite winged-liquid eyeliner and create a wing!

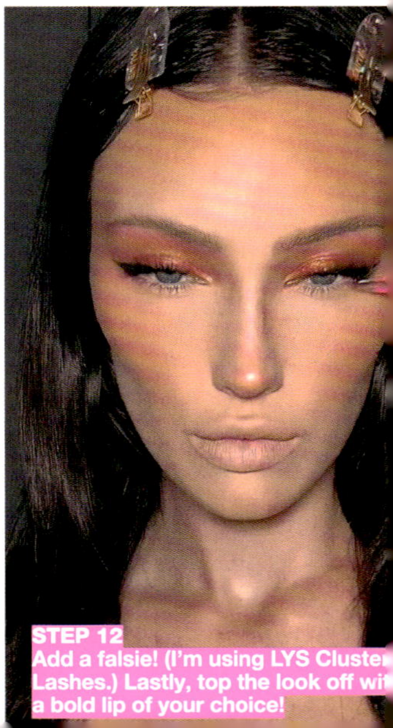

STEP 12
Add a falsie! (I'm using LYS Cluste Lashes.) Lastly, top the look off wi a bold lip of your choice!

HOW TO: RED CARPET GLAM

I love this glam when I want to reach outside my usual comfort zone. A red lip is a great way to do that, it's easy to create and looks beautiful on everyone!

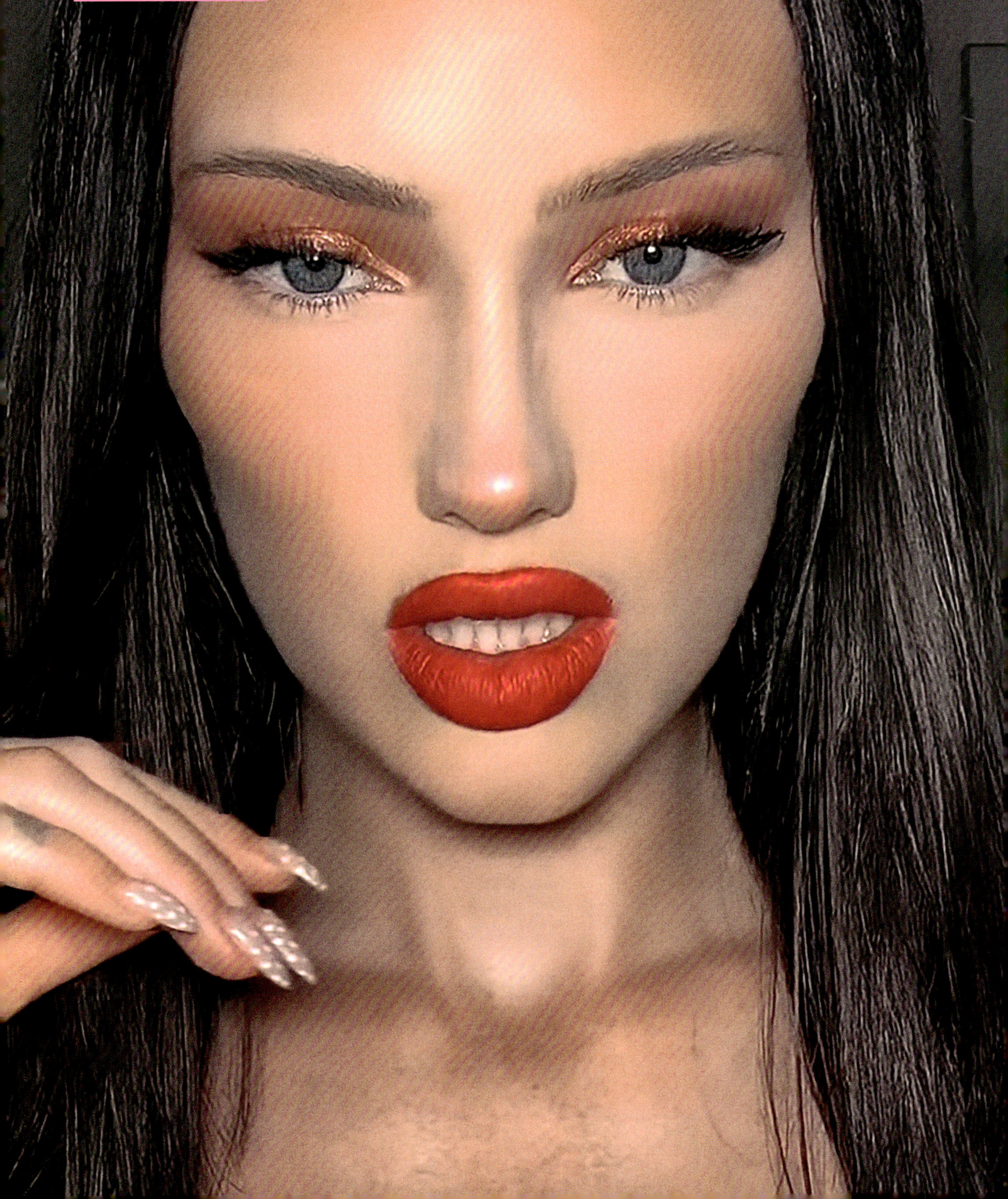

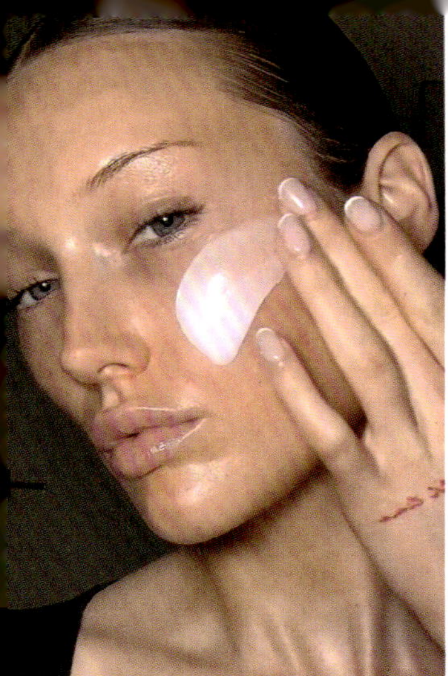

STEP 1
Prime with the TATCHA Dewy Skin Cream.

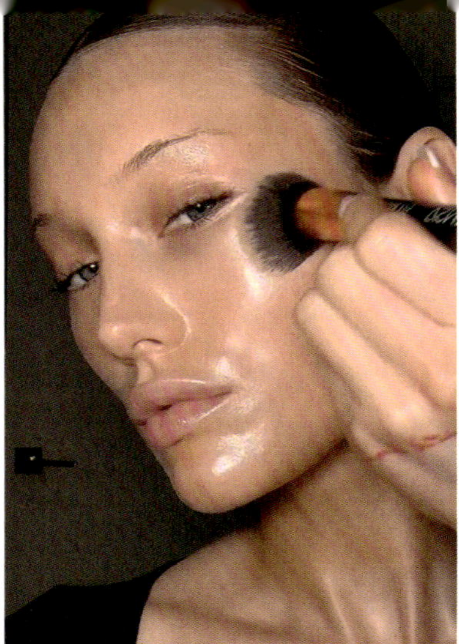

STEP 2
Apply Charlotte Tilbury Flawless Filter all over the face and blend.

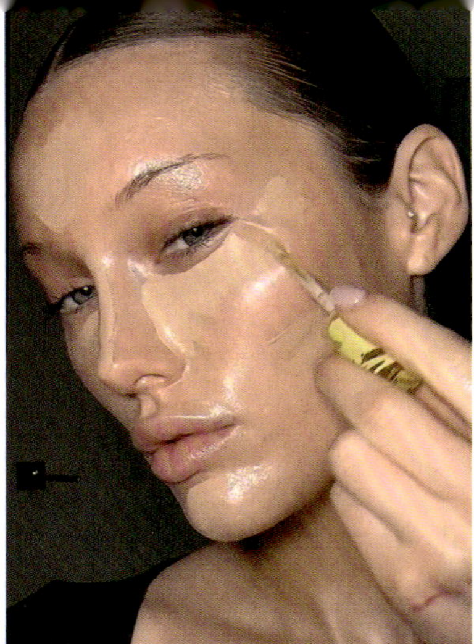

STEP 3
Conceal and brighten with the Kosas Revealer Concealer under the eyes and all over the T-zone!

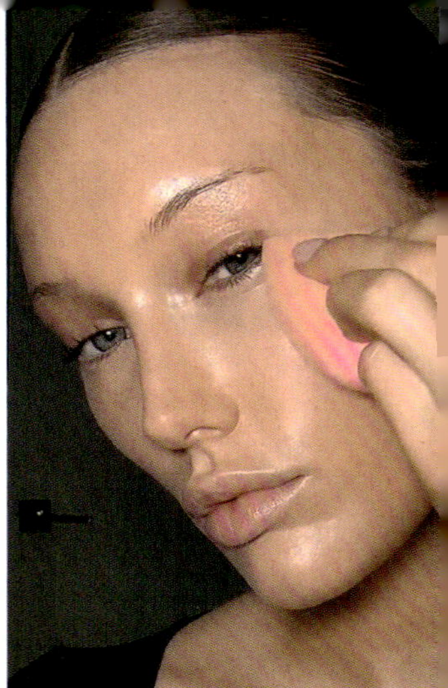

STEP 4
Blend out with a damp beauty sponge by tapping—not pulling or rubbing!

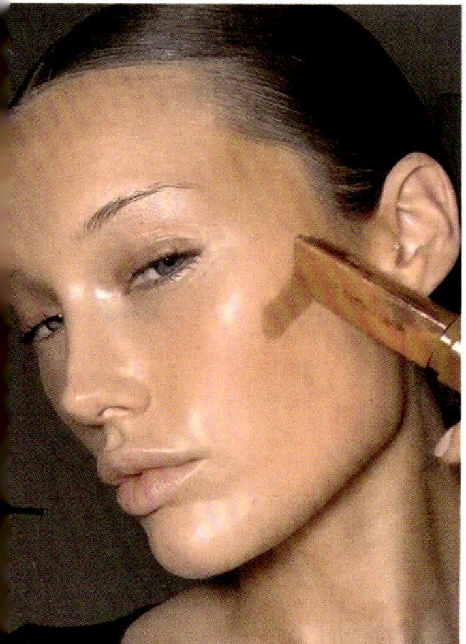

STEP 5
Contour with the LYS Bronzing Stick. Apply higher up under the cheekbones for a more lifted, chiseled effect. Blend!

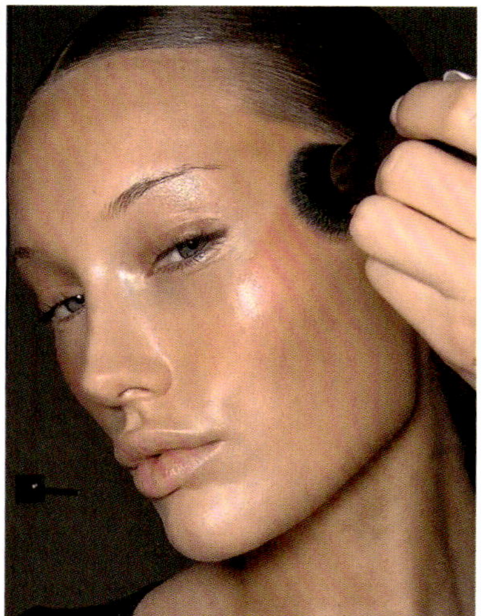

STEP 6
Take the Charlotte Tilbury Beauty Light Wand in shade Pinkgasm and apply it to the higher points of the cheekbones. Blend upward.

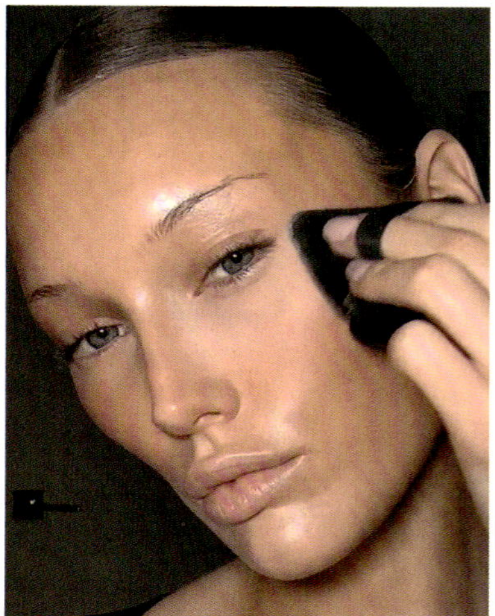

STEP 7
Set the under eyes and T-zone with a setting powder of your choice using a powder puff. I'm using Huda Beauty Loose Setting Powder in shade Cherry Blossom.

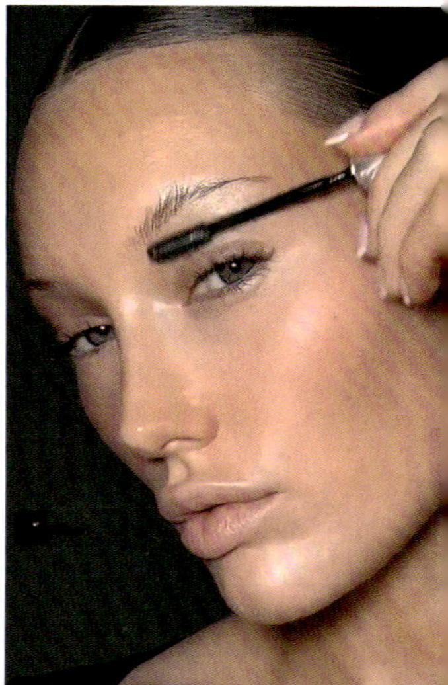

STEP 8
Brush up and sculpt the brows with a brow gel. My favorite is the Benef 24-hour Brow Setter.

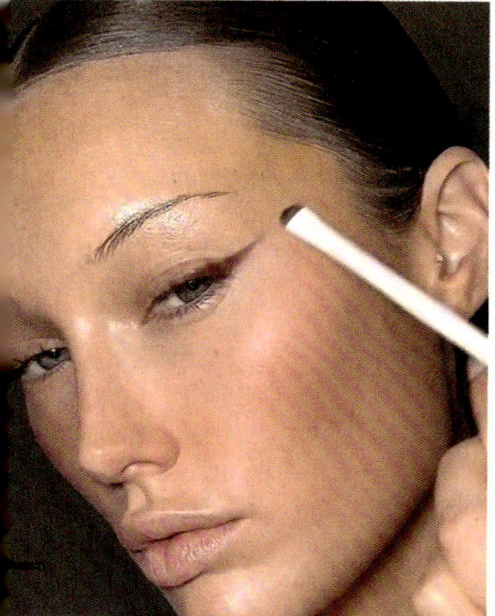

STEP 9
Take a detail smudger brush and dip it into a mauvy purple shade. Create a winged line from the outer edge of your upper lash line, and pull outward. I'm using the Pat McGrath Labs Mothership IX Huetopian Dream Palette.

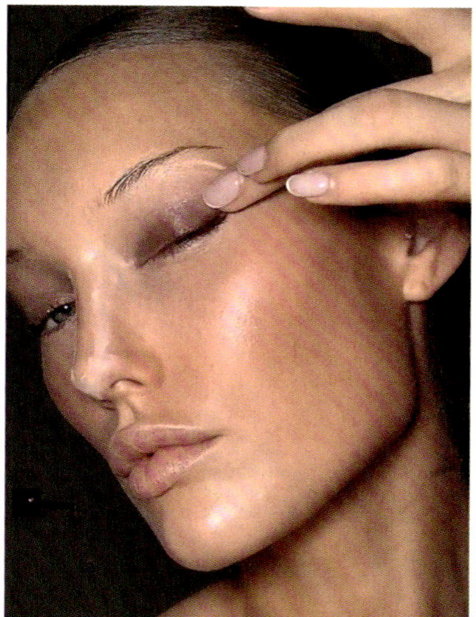

STEP 10
Then dip into the same palette, taking a shimmer and lightly dusting that all over the upper lid with your finger.

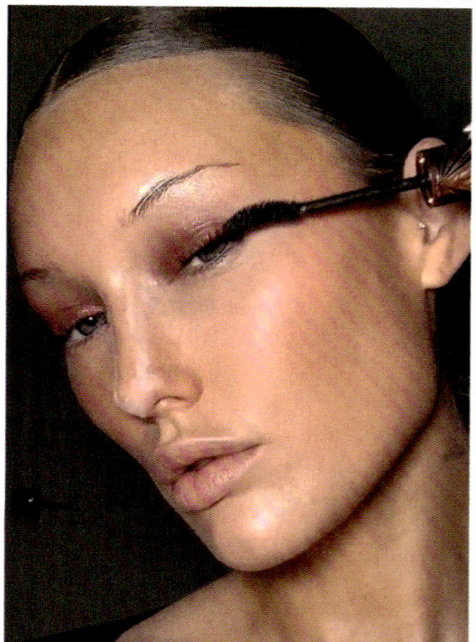

STEP 11
Curl and top off your lashes with a coat of mascara. I'm using Charlotte Tilbury Exagger-eyes Volume Mascara.

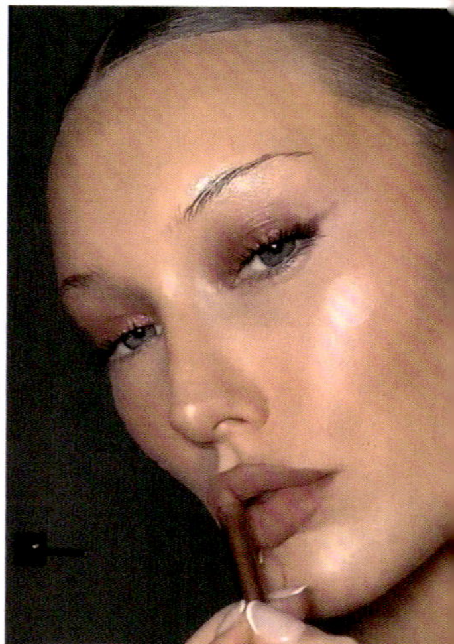

STEP 12
Line your lips with Charlotte Tilbury Iconic Nude Lip Liner, then top it off with the Fenty Beauty Gloss Bomb Stix High-Shine Gloss Stick in shade Hot Chocolit!

HOW TO: GLOWY SHIMMER GLAM WITH A BOLD LIP

This look is my take on a sculpted, high-gloss glam with radiant, glass-like skin. The focus is on the luminosity of the skin and eyes, while pairing it with a bold, cool-toned dark lip!

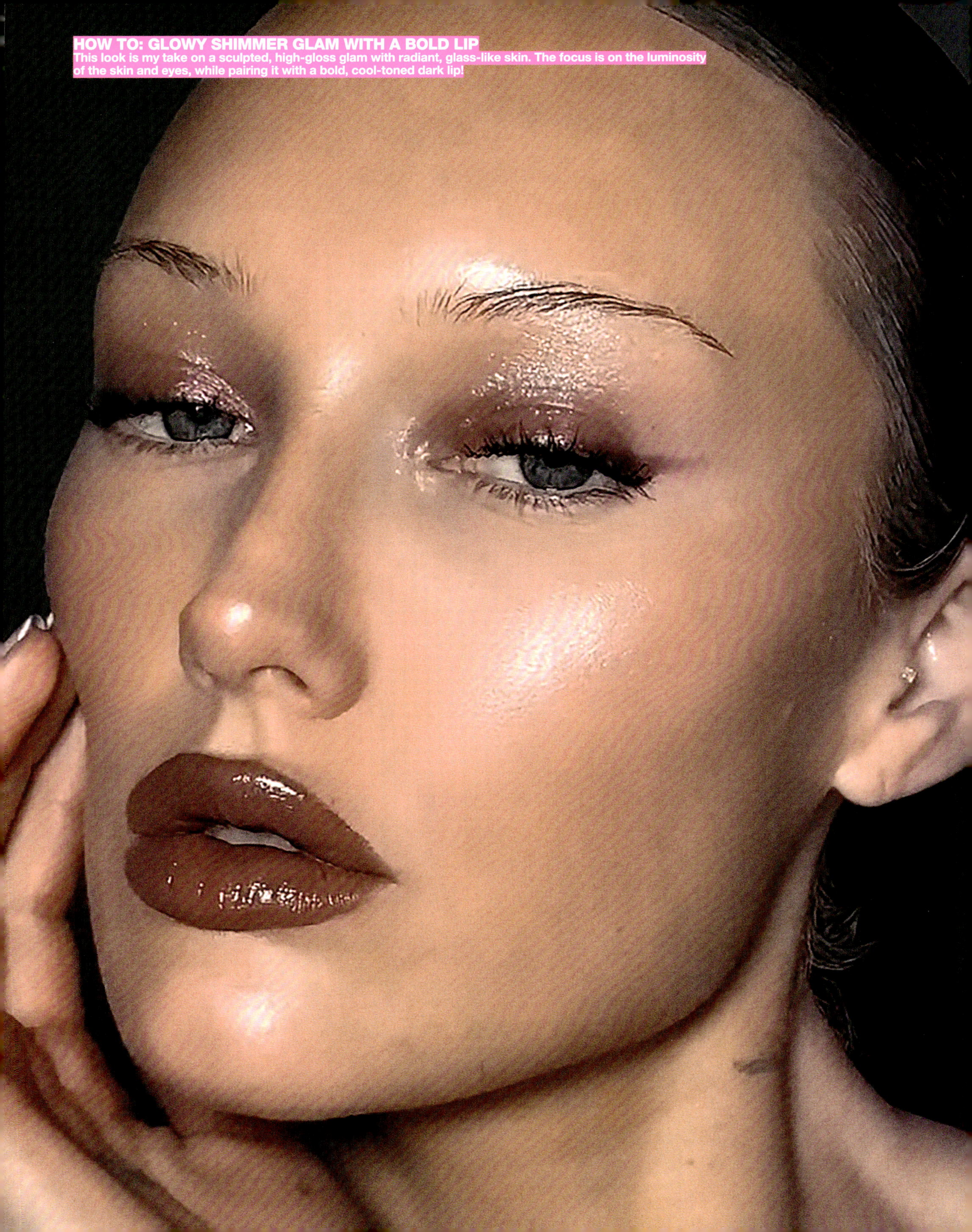

FASHION

3

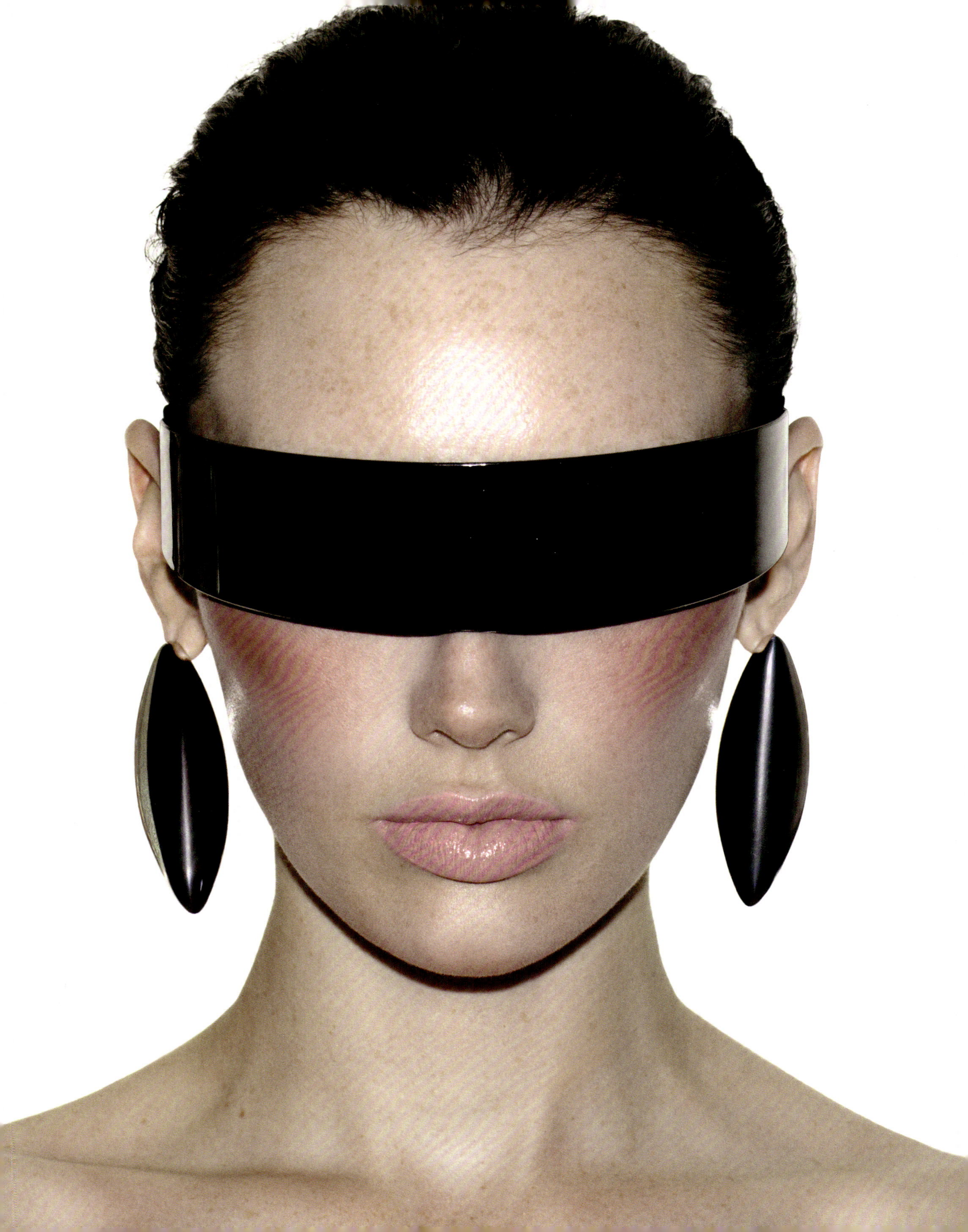

When I first entered the world of fashion, it felt intimidating yet welcoming at the same time. I knew it was more traditional than the beauty industry, but it was a challenge I wanted to take. It can be scary to enter into an industry that you're not a pro in. I didn't have a clear idea of my style, which made me question what I was offering to this new audience. The thing is, you don't have to have it all figured out. Your sense of style is going to forever evolve, and you don't need to put yourself in a box. People will appreciate your journey way more when you're vulnerable and honest, rather than pretending like you have it all figured out.

Modeling, for me, was another way to understand the fashion industry from another point of view. Seeing the creative directors working in real time on the collections and them pinning pieces of fabric to you during fittings is so cool. You get to see those torn-up pieces of fabric turn into their unique finalized designs that eventually hit the runway. I got to see IRL how much creativity goes into it by being there in those moments that lead up to that finalized collection.

When I walked into my first casting, I was so nervous. I tried to keep telling myself that I deserved to be in this room and I have a place in it…but when an environment feels so new, your mind tends to panic. What I realized is you have to feel a little bit of discomfort in order to grow and learn and become better. Life is all about taking risks and challenging yourself to try something new. What good ever comes out of being complacent?

The first time a designer dressed me, I felt so honored that they trusted me with their vision. There is so much thought that goes into each design, and to have that trust was everything to me. It felt like all my hard work within the fashion industry was finally paying off. Getting recognition from such a respected brand and designer meant I was doing something right.

Fashion, for me, is the experience of stepping into new rooms, new eras, and new versions of myself—never fully knowing what's coming, but always willing to evolve. It's not about perfection; it's about the courage to show up as myself, again and again, while creating throughout the process of it all.

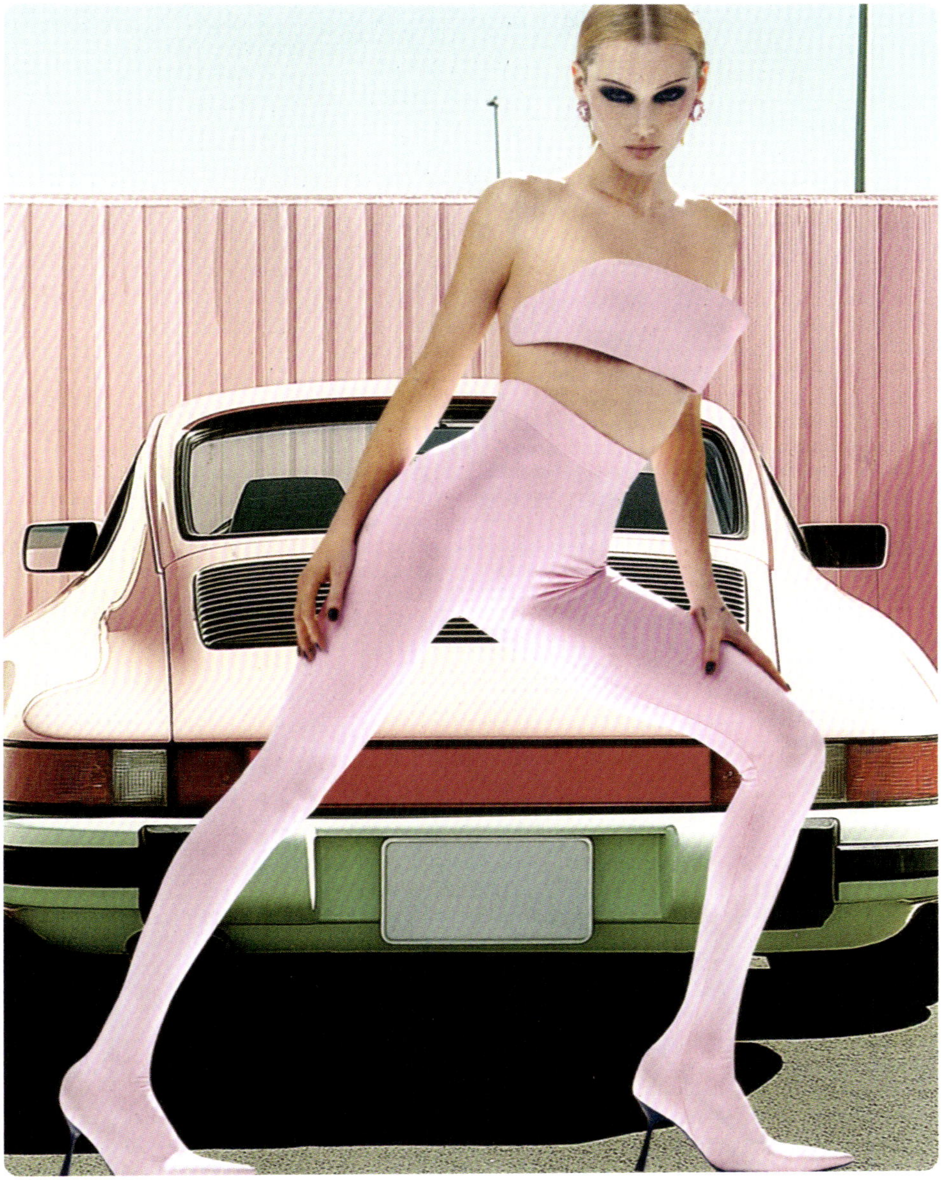

This was an editorial shoot for *V Magazine*. I was styled in a full Balenciaga look. I loved how it turned out! I was pretty new to modeling here and remember being so nervous about how I was going to pose, but it ended up working!

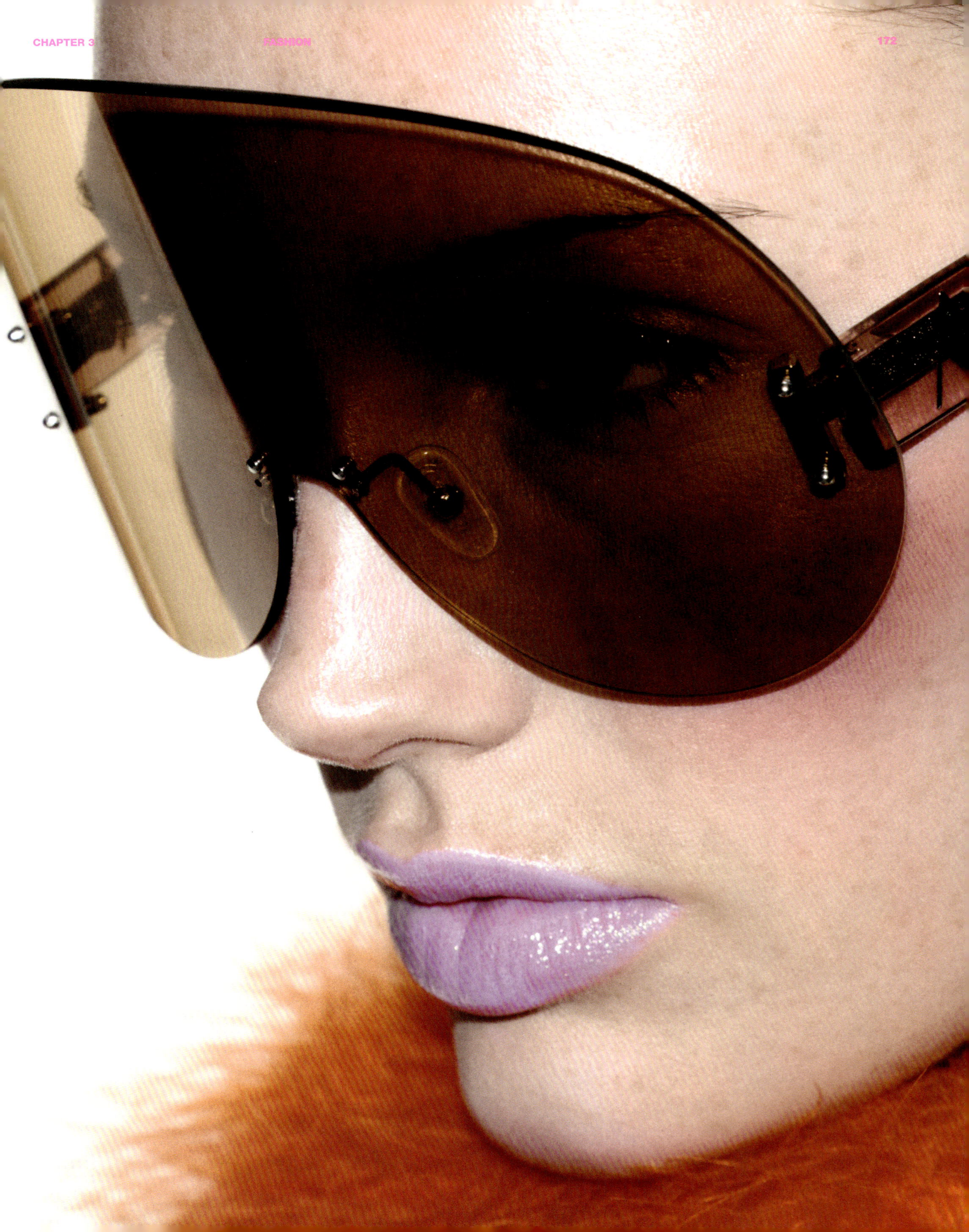

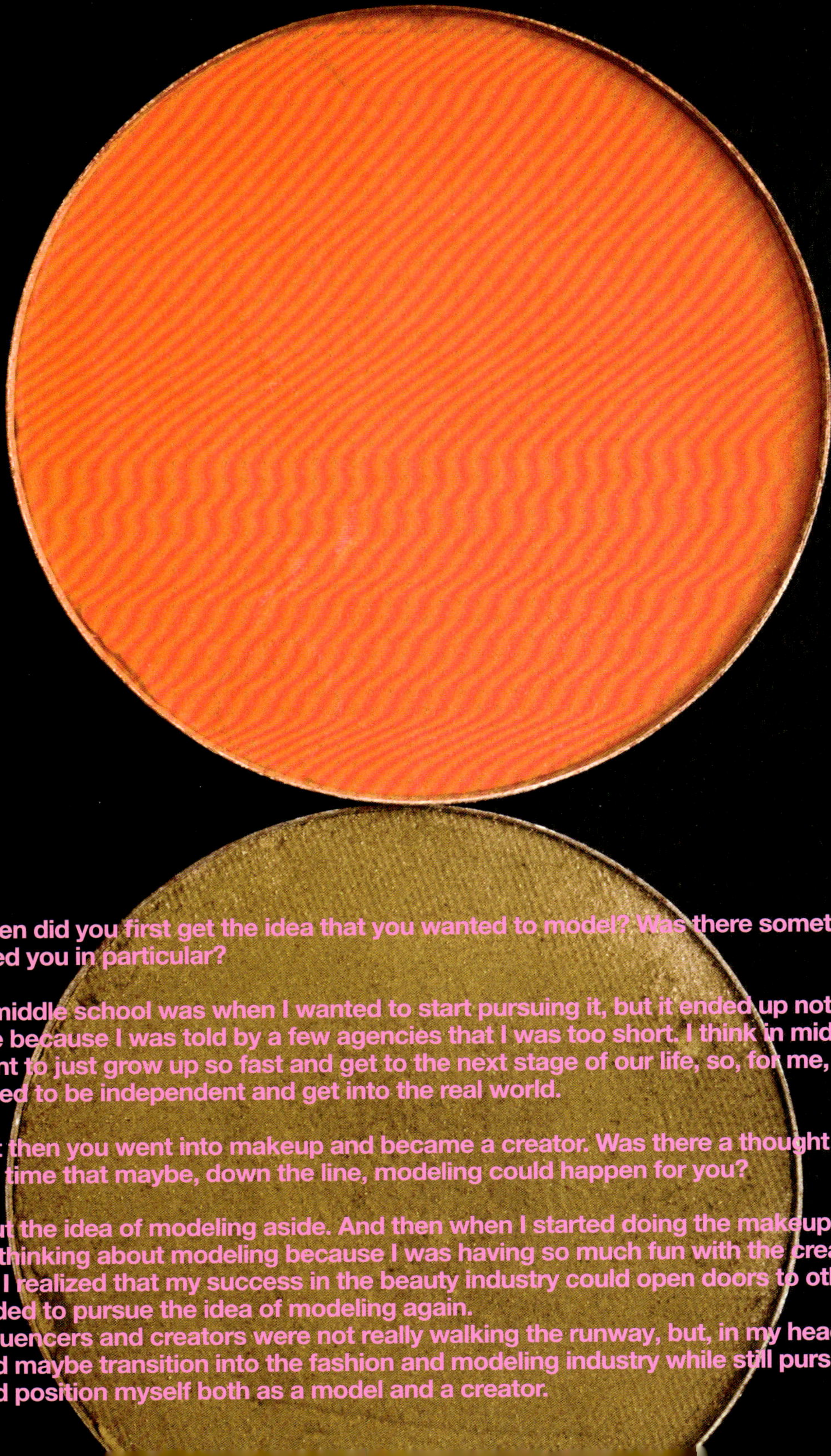

Q When did you first get the idea that you wanted to model? Was there something that inspired you in particular?

A In middle school was when I wanted to start pursuing it, but it ended up not working out for me because I was told by a few agencies that I was too short. I think in middle school we all want to just grow up so fast and get to the next stage of our life, so, for me, this was that. I wanted to be independent and get into the real world.

Q But then you went into makeup and became a creator. Was there a thought in your head the whole time that maybe, down the line, modeling could happen for you?

A I put the idea of modeling aside. And then when I started doing the makeup, I wasn't even really thinking about modeling because I was having so much fun with the creativeness of it all. When I realized that my success in the beauty industry could open doors to other industries, I decided to pursue the idea of modeling again.

Influencers and creators were not really walking the runway, but, in my head, I thought I could maybe transition into the fashion and modeling industry while still pursuing beauty. I could position myself both as a model and a creator.

Q How did it feel to say it out loud that you wanted to pursue modeling?

A pair of sunnies can add so much to your whole look. These are a vintage Tom Ford pair I found. If you know me, you know this burnt-orange color is one of my faves.

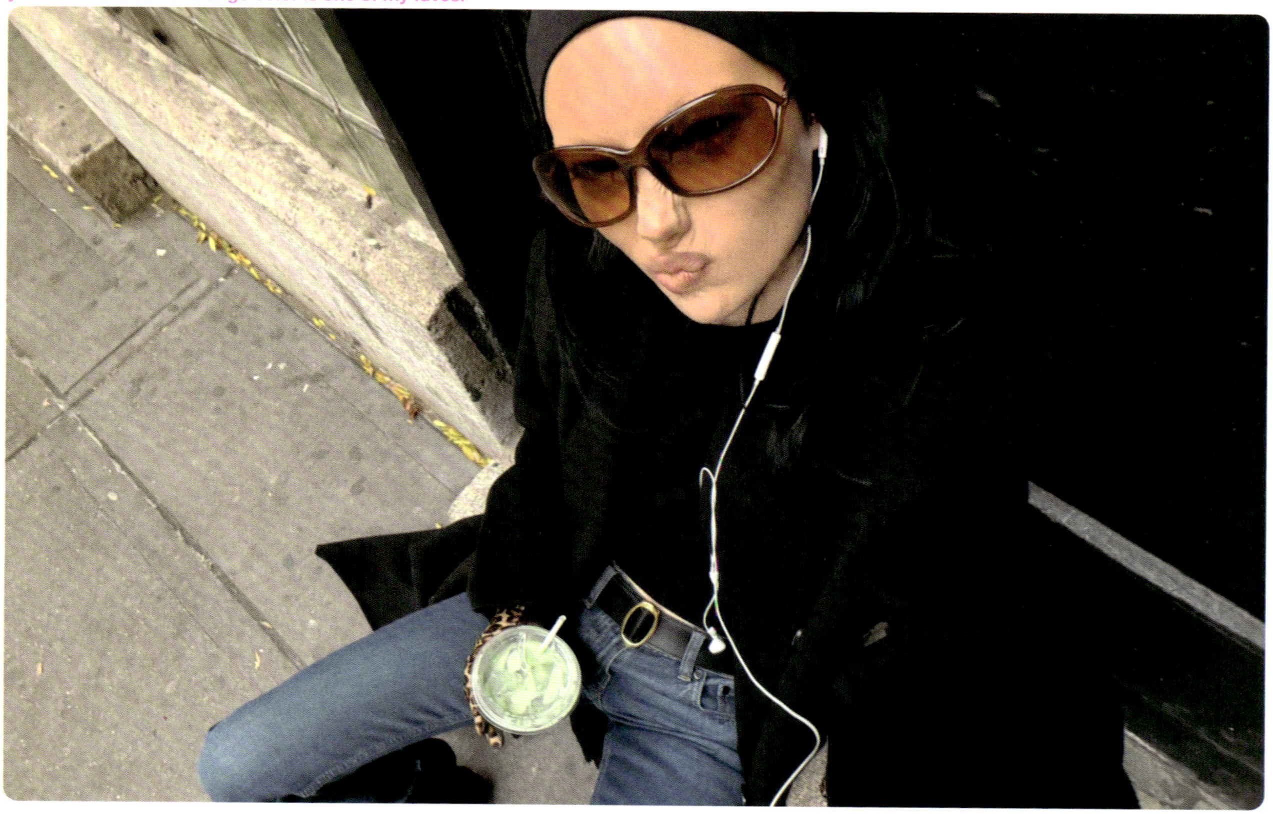

A It was scary, I didn't know if people were going to take me seriously because I'm not a traditional model.

Q Did you feel intimidated because you were coming from the creator space into the fashion industry?

A One hundred percent! As much as fashion and beauty go hand in hand, the industries and expectations in both are completely different.

In beauty, there is more room for error, I feel. In fashion, there are some rules. So it took a lot of finding my own personal sense of style before I felt comfortable in the industry and what content I was providing.

Q What steps did you take to feel like when you walked into a casting, people would take you seriously?

A I knew going into castings, I had to be barefaced. When you walk into a casting, they are not going to take you seriously if you wear a full face of makeup. The casting directors want to see the "raw" version of you because they want to see how you can be a chameleon, if you can adapt to different styles and looks.

I have definitely walked into a casting and been surrounded by very tall traditional models, and I did not feel like I fit in. But I had to remind myself that I have a place in the room, and all I can do is show up, be myself, and give it my all.

Q Tell me about the first moment that you felt like, "Wait, I'm actually becoming a part of the fashion industry," before you even walked the runway.

A I felt that way the first time I was gifted clothing or loaned clothing from a luxury brand.

I remember Valentino was one of the first major luxury fashion houses to loan me. The fact that they were willing to loan me their outfits that were so expensive and trust me with them, and also trust that I could create a vision aligned with their brand, felt incredible to me because it meant I was doing something right. It reassured me that I was on the right path, that people enjoy my content, and there is, indeed, a space for me.

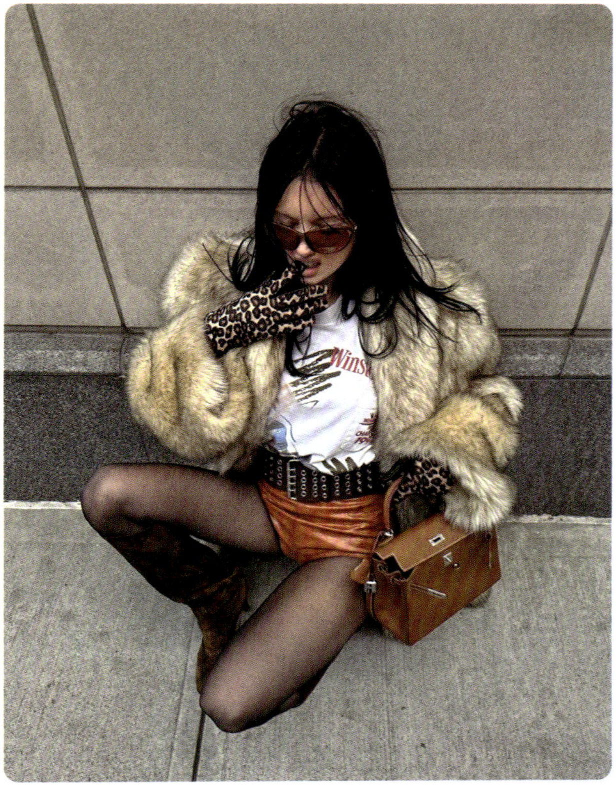

I love dressing up, styling a look, and taking pics with my friends! Noting it was 20 degrees here, but I think I can confidently say that we got the shot.

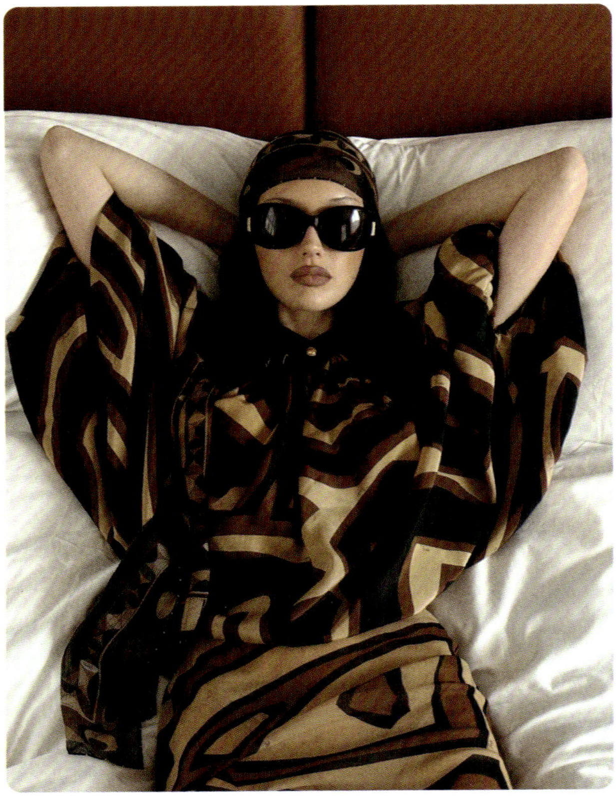

This is what napping looks like during Fashion Week, lol.

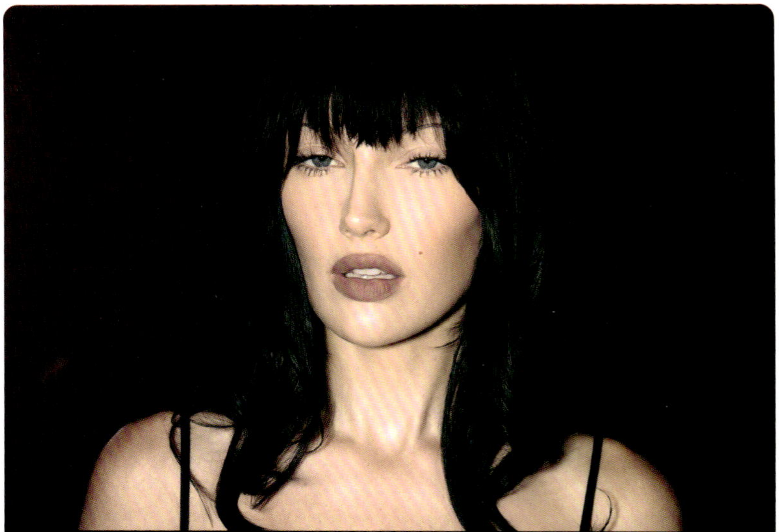

A fave fashion week glam moment. PRO TIP: I had a stubborn pimple that wouldn't go away, so I created a little beauty mark on top with a brown liner to hide it. You would never know!

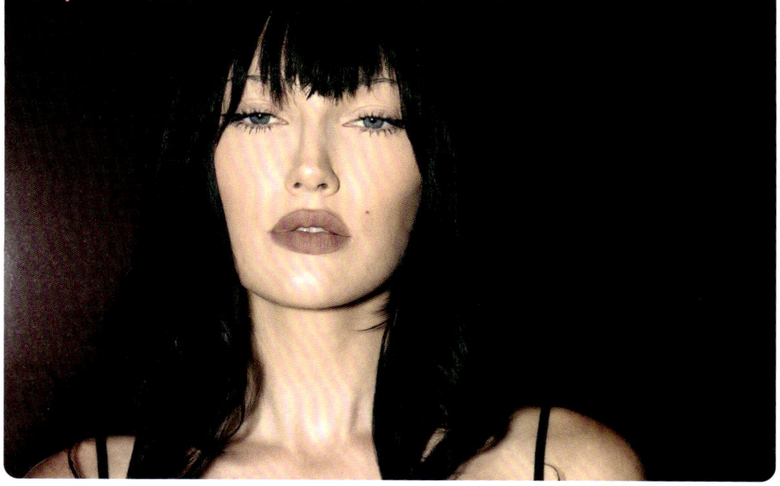

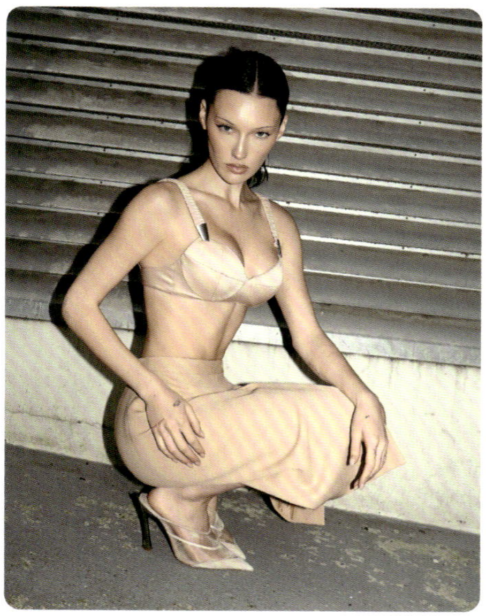

Archival Mugler that I wore to their runway show. A top favorite for sure!

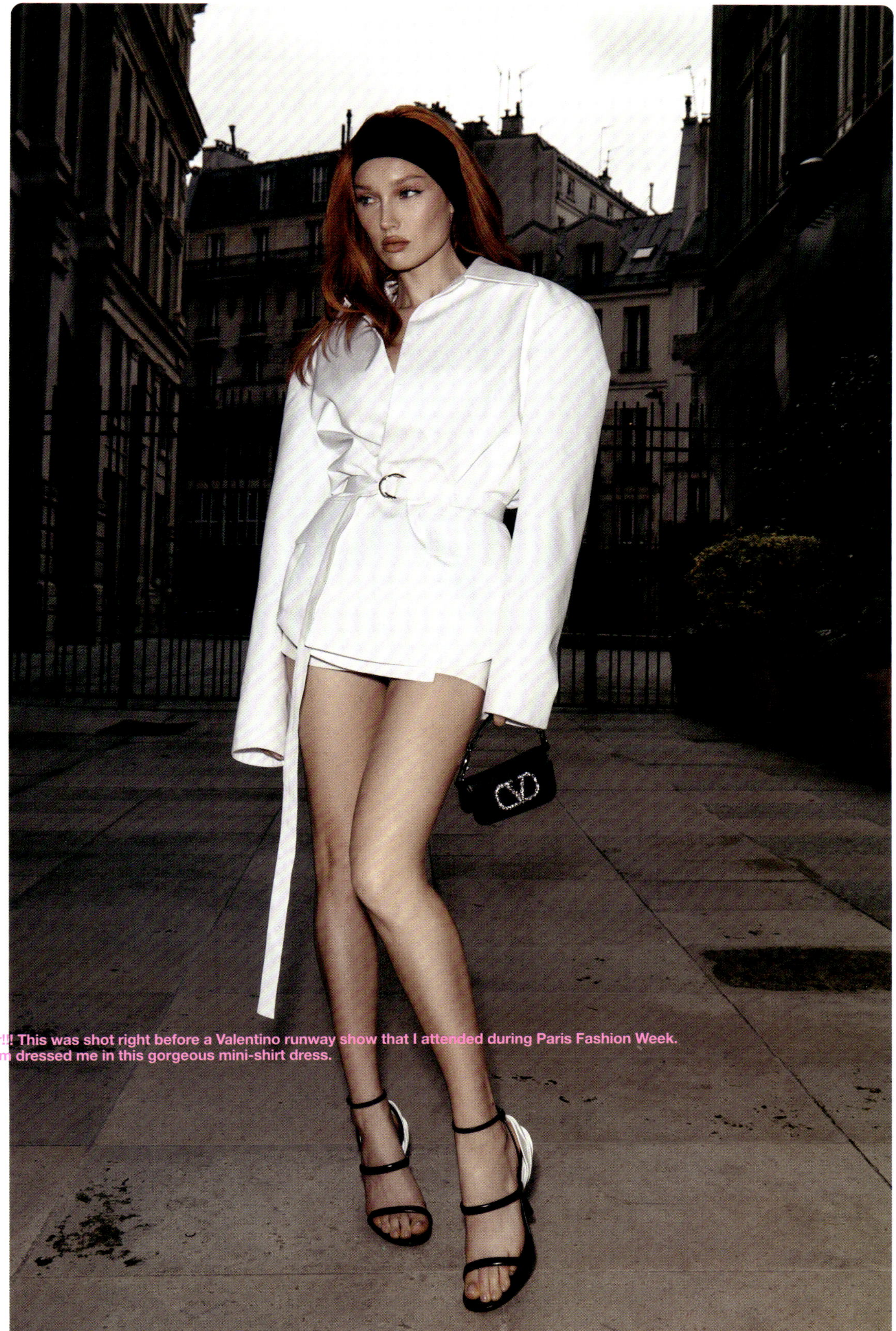

I miss my red hair!!! This was shot right before a Valentino runway show that I attended during Paris Fashion Week. The Valentino team dressed me in this gorgeous mini-shirt dress.

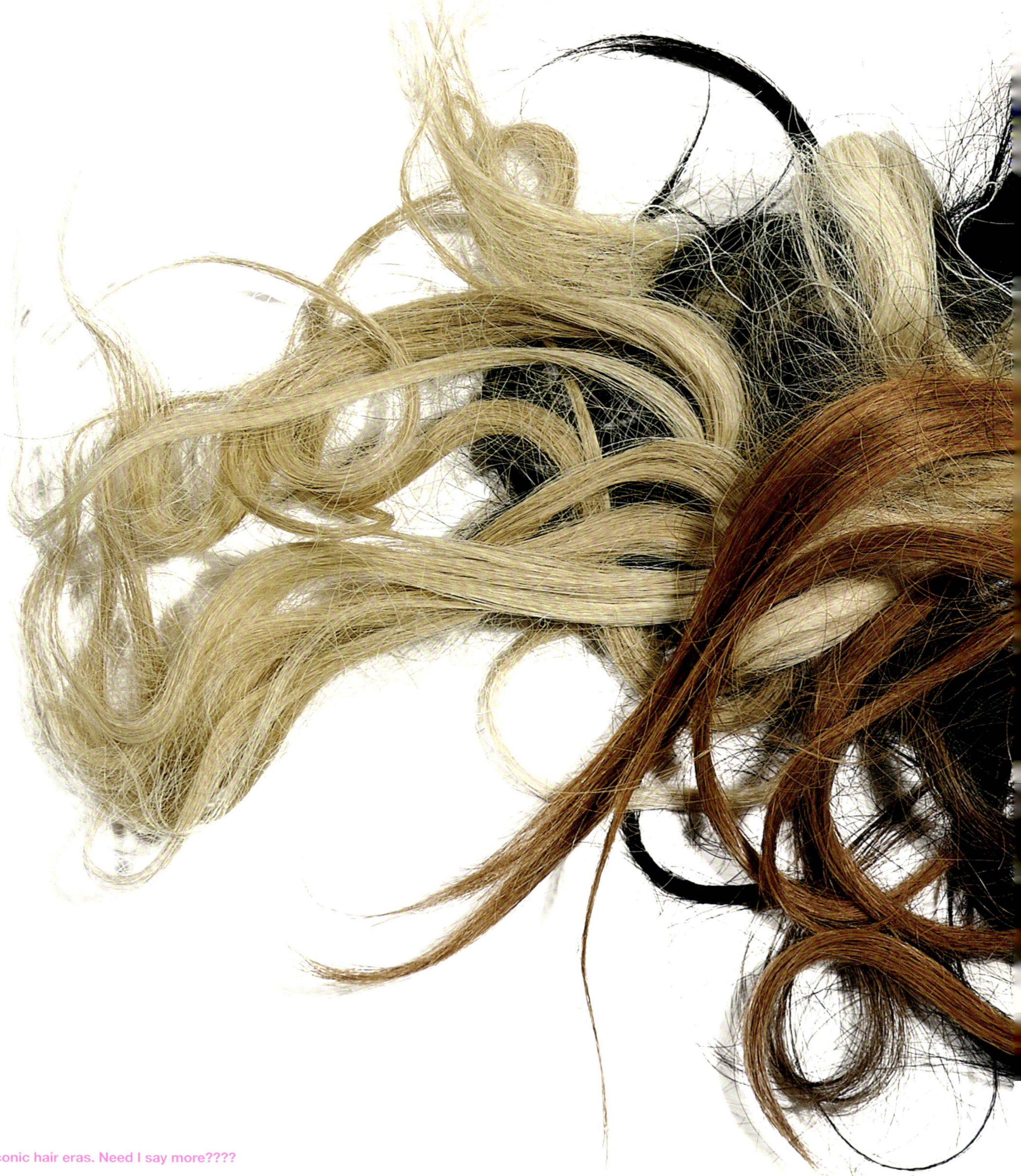

My iconic hair eras. Need I say more????

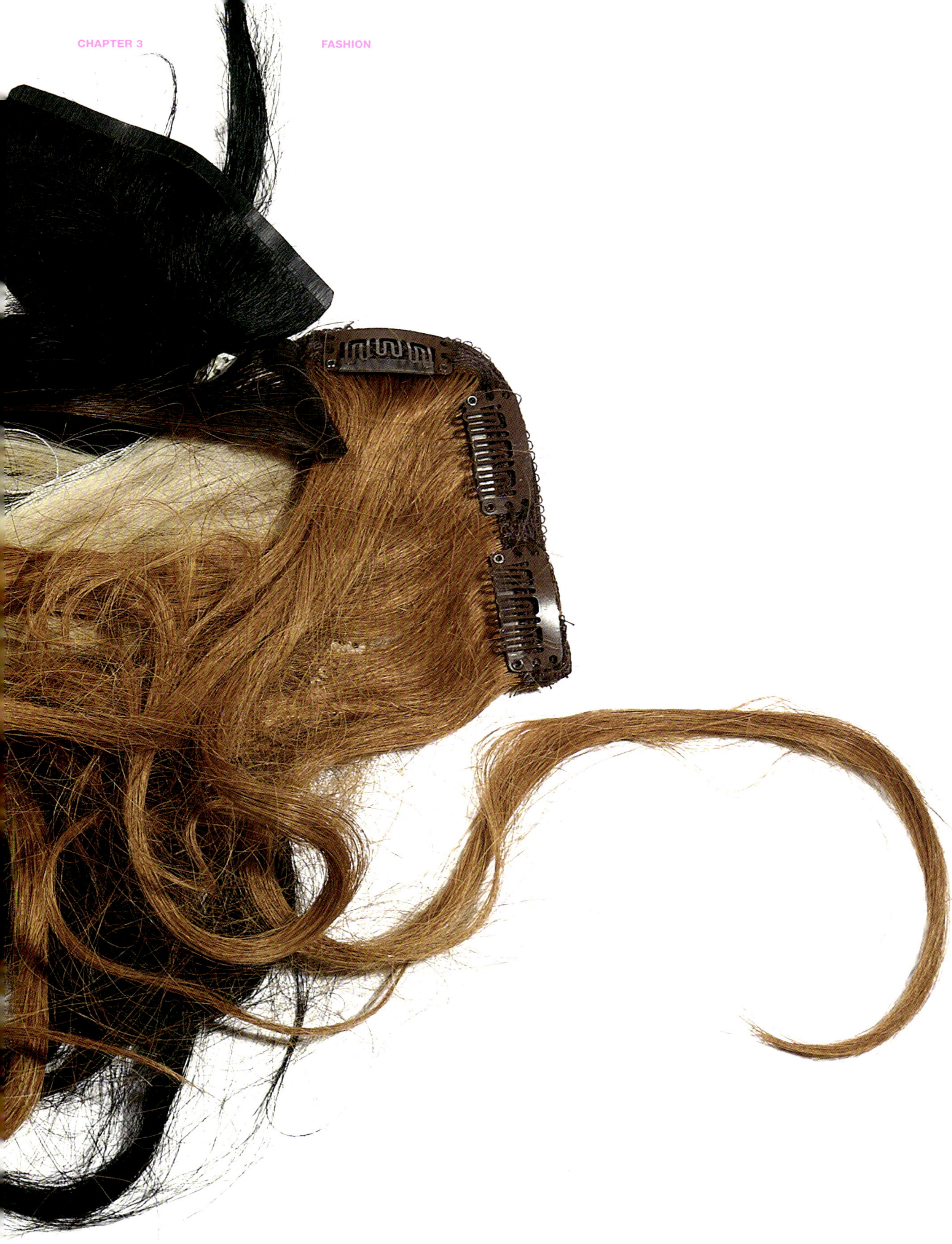

It was definitely challenging at first. Getting to this point was not easy, coming from a full-glam beauty guru.

Q As you started to document your entrance into the fashion industry, how did your followers react?

A They were so supportive! They love being on the journey with me and getting to be a part of it all.

As I became more and more committed to modeling, I spent about a year really stripping back my full glam for it. I already had so many eyes on me for my foundation videos that I knew I had to go into this new industry as a blank slate so that these brands could see me as someone other than "the foundation girl."

It sucks to have to pull yourself back, but at the same time, I do understand, because brands need to uphold the vision they've created for the brand. If they turn me down, it's not that they didn't like me or my personality. It's just that I didn't fit with the brand at that time. So, yeah, it was hard for me to pull back, but I also learned from it. It was a challenge for me, and I always love a good challenge. I can be "foundation Meredith," and I can be this and that, too.

My followers liked that I was entering the fashion industry, but as time went on and I was wearing a lot of natural makeup, they questioned where the old Meredith had gone. They said, "We still want to see that." And that's when it started to feel upsetting to me, because I still wanted to give them the content they originally fell in love with.

Q You said you had to strip back your personality a little bit. What does that mean?

A It meant stripping back my energy to come across as softer and also putting aside the full-glam looks where I would try to emulate certain bold personas or characters through my tone and personality. In a lot of my videos, I have this big, loud, kind of chaotic energy doing crazy looks. I can be a very loud personality in my content, and that doesn't fit with every brand.

Miu Miu created an entire Miu Miu beach club at the Cannes Film Festival. It was such a beautiful pop-up in the South of France. It's always so fun getting to experience these moments in different parts of the world!

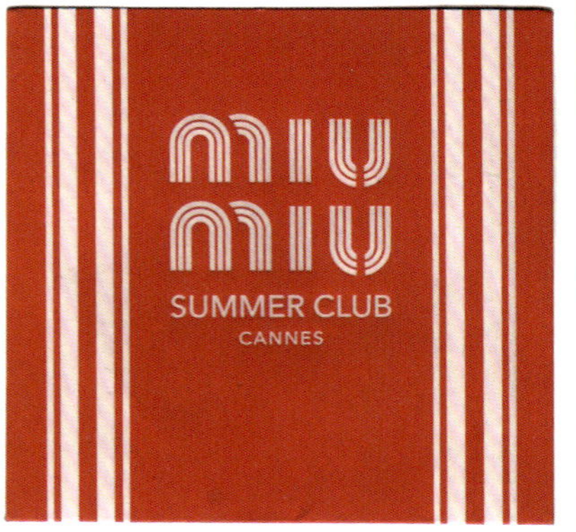

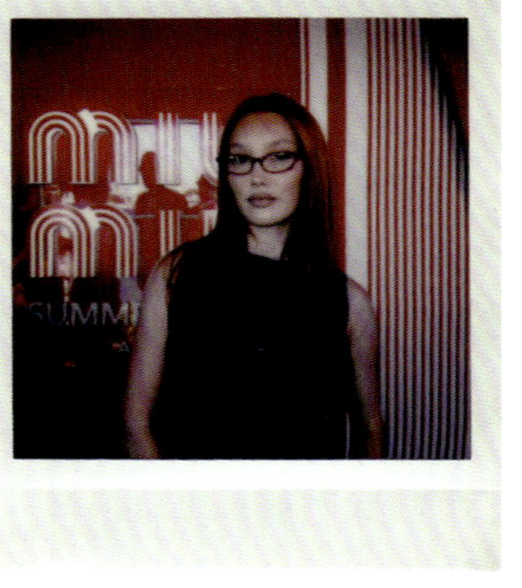

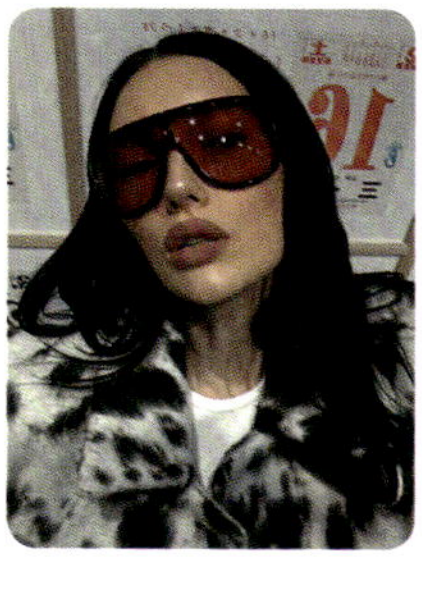

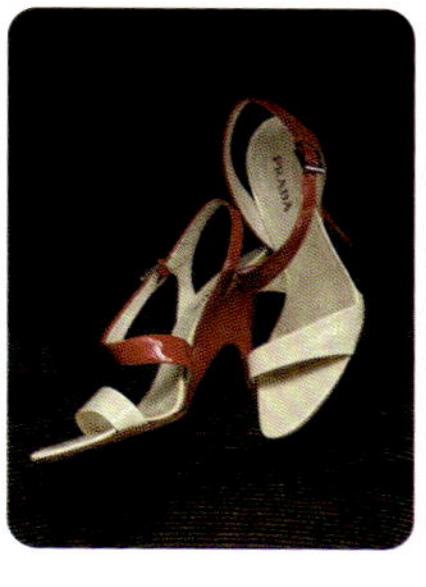

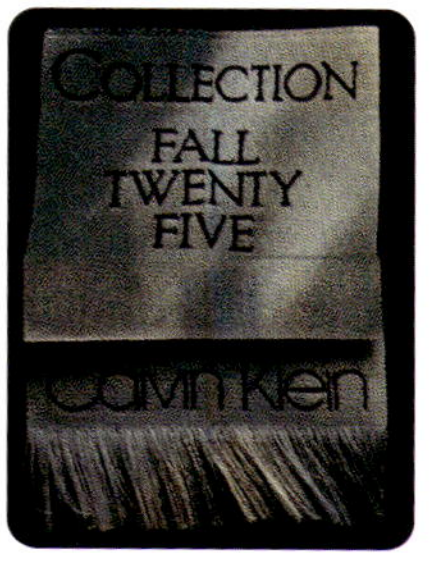

Fun little fashion moments: iconic selfies, vintage shoes, and show invitations.

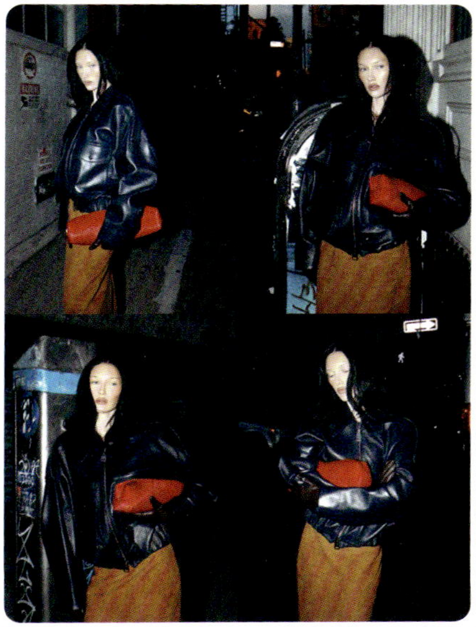

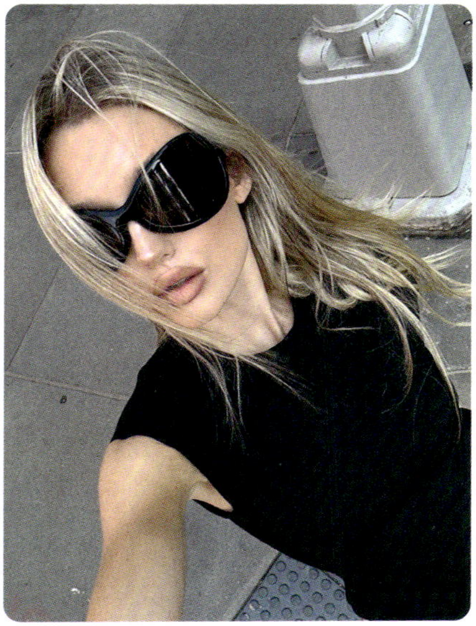

LEFT: Going to the Khaite show at New York Fashion Week. RIGHT: One of my favorite accessories is a big pair of black sunnies. These are from Acne Studios.

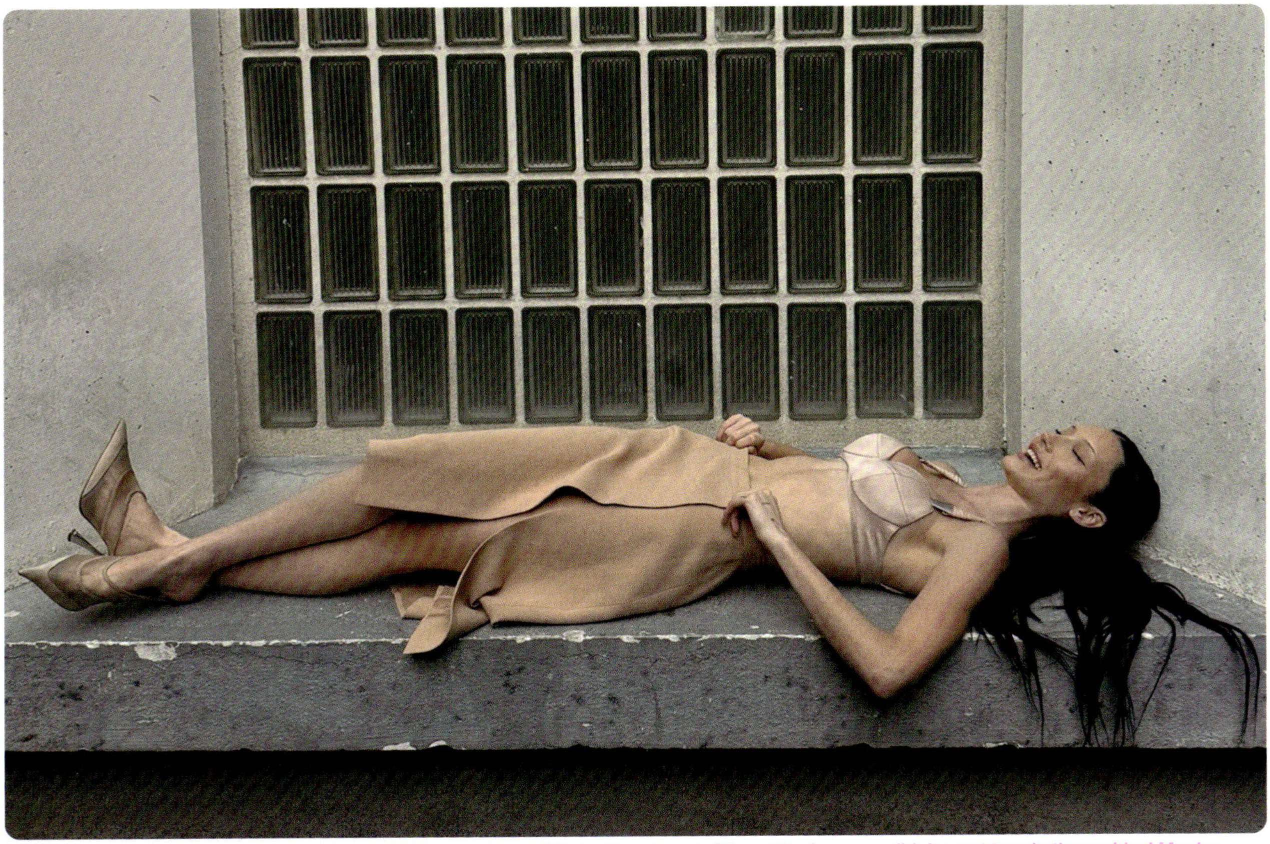

A reminder that not everything is as it seems! This bench was filled with ash and dirt, and I, of course, didn't want to ruin the archival Mugler outfit. This was an interesting experience, but we got the shot!

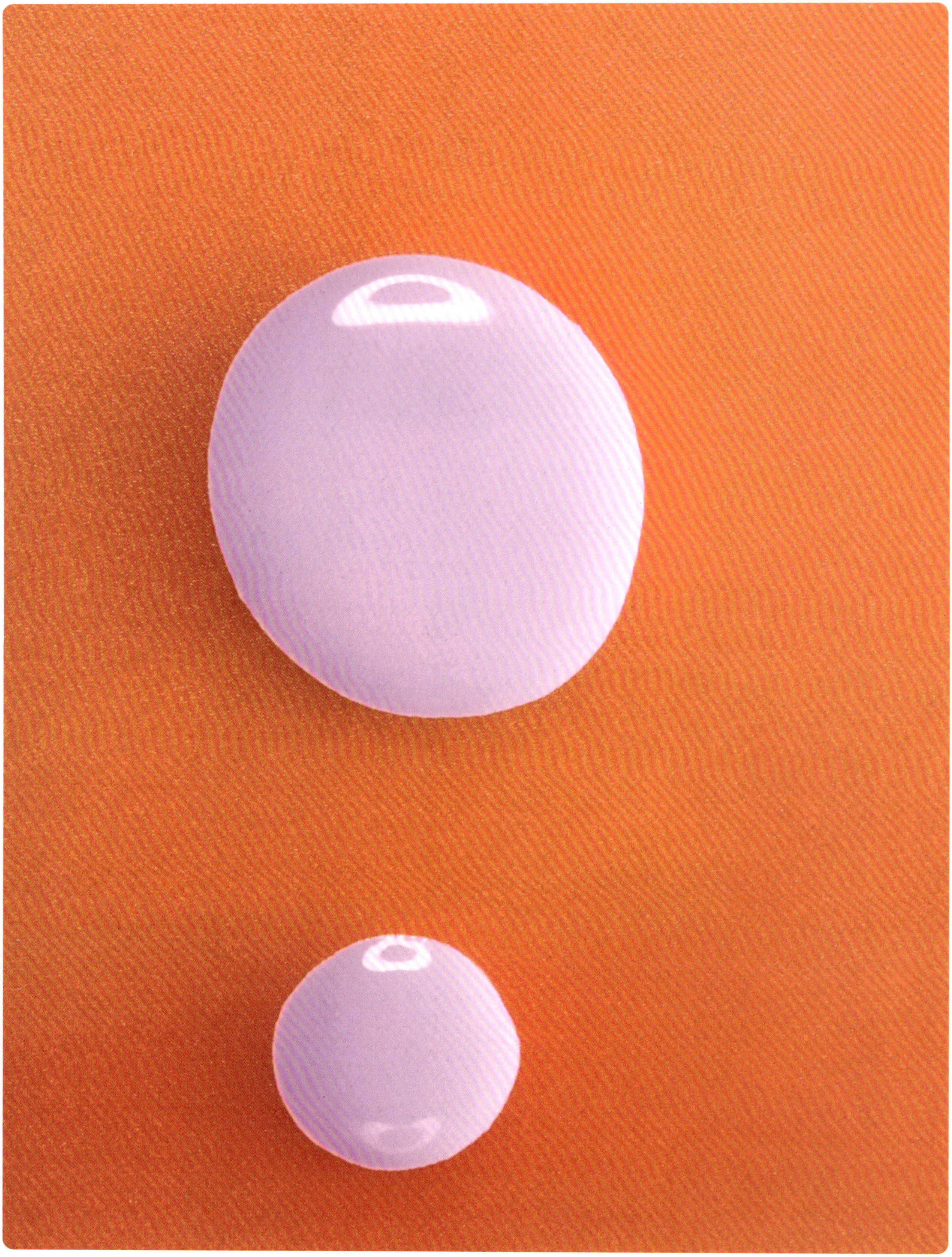

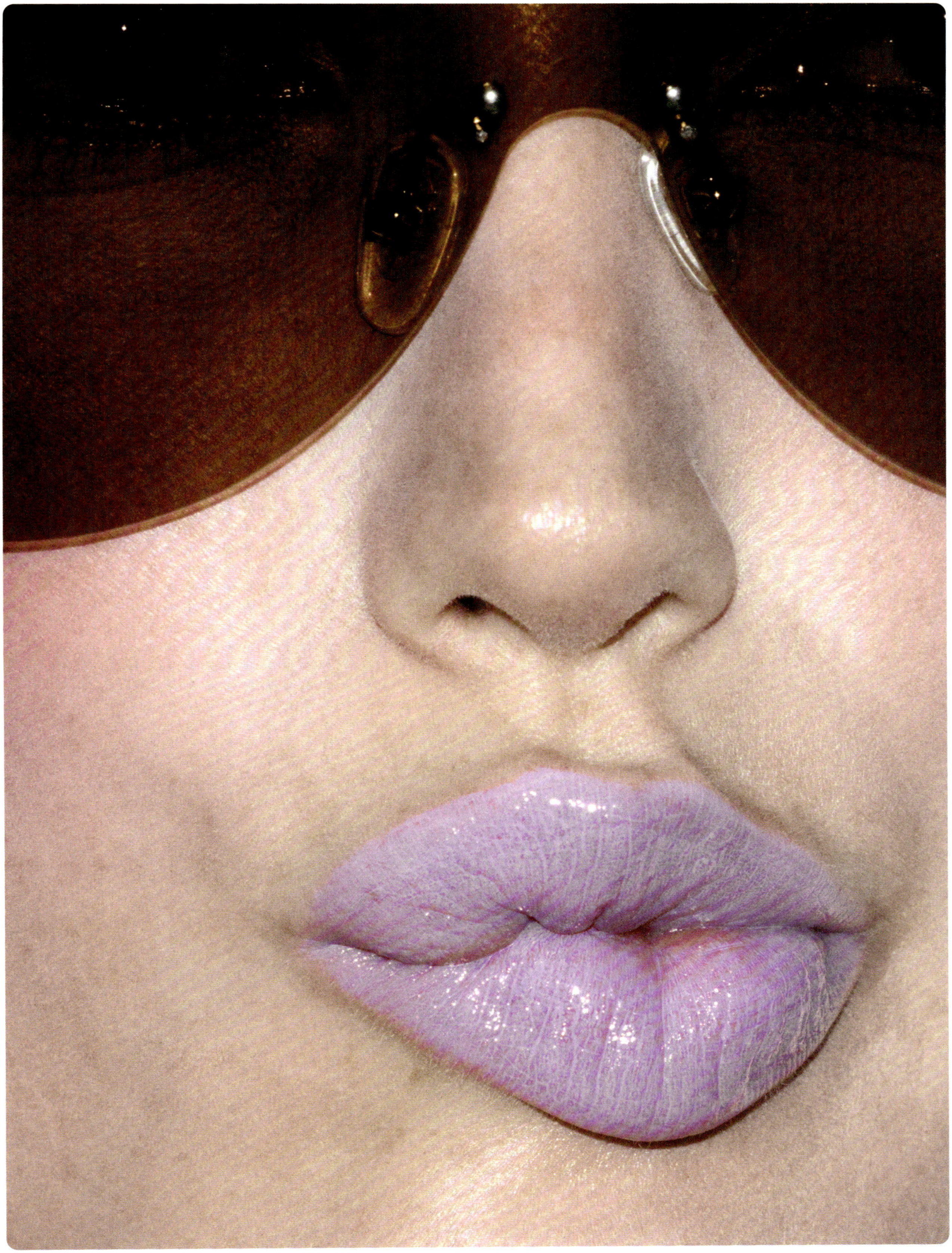

Q You talked a bit about how some of your followers asked where the old Meredith was. Is there a comment that kind of lives rent-free in your mind?

A People are always so quick to comment negative things when they see a slight change in numbers and views; they use it as fuel to bash the creator. To me, numbers don't define my success in life. There is a lot offline that I'm working on that are huge goals of mine and things I could only have dreamt of.

When I came back to doing the foundation videos again, people would be like, "Oh, she's so washed up, her views are so low, so she has to resort to doing this again." But no, it was always the plan for me to come back to glam once I made some more growth in modeling and fashion. Those people took my return to making foundation videos as if the modeling didn't go so well, but that isn't the case.

If that's their idea and perception of me, then fine. Everyone is entitled to their own opinion, and they can live with that. I don't really care because I know my truth.

Q What is something that surprised you about the modeling industry?

A Over the past year and a half, I've really seen personality and fun come back into runways; for example, for Demna's debut runway show at Gucci, I loved how he created characters within his collection, the clothes made you feel as if you wanted to be whoever that character was walking down the runway. Each model had their own walk, attitude, vibe. I was lucky enough to walk that runway show, and it was really inspiring to see the whole creative process of it and how many countless hours he and his team dedicated to it.

Diesel and some of the more edgy brands are really bringing that back into shows as well, which I love and I think is so important. They are really embracing personality and the personality of the individual models. Models are so much more than pretty faces on a runway—they're creatives, they're funny, they're cool, they're hardworking, they're unique. And I love that we're seeing that come across in how brands are doing their marketing, where the model-as-personality really shines through.

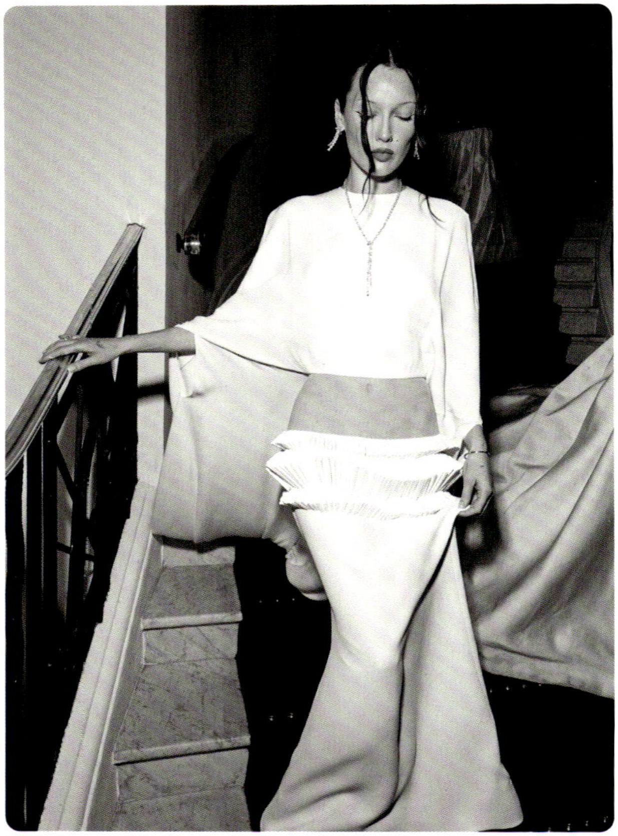

TOP: Cannes Film Festival with L'Oréal! I felt like a princess this day and loved my gown. I wanted to go for something unexpected and different. The waistband was made out of ceramic chips! OPPOSITE PAGE: I love a good subway photo shoot. This was a Burberry look that I wore to the US Open. So chic! Always make sure you're having fun, whatever you're doing!

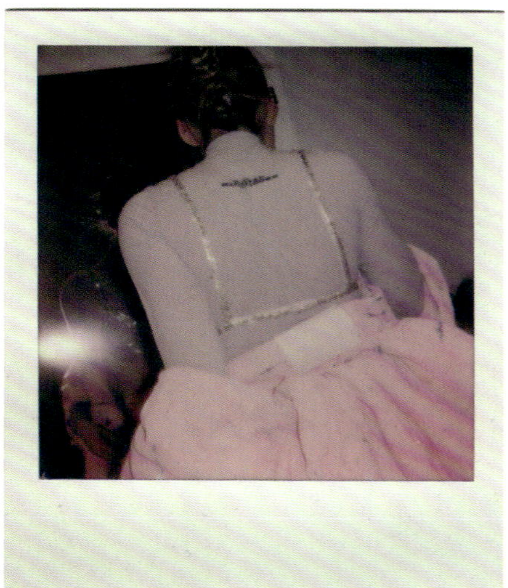

A behind-the-scenes shot of me getting ready for a Marc Jacobs runway show!

Q What is the most fashion industry moment you have had so far?

A I ran into Anna Wintour backstage at the Versace show, and we were wearing the same jacket. I walked by her, and I thought, "Oh, my God! Oh, my God! Just look forward. Don't bother her." And then she said, "Nice jacket!" It was so cute. Sometimes the industry can feel really intimidating, and I never want to bother anyone. But a lot of the time, they are very open and want to connect with the people around them.

Q I think she has much more of a sense of humor than people give her credit for.

A And then ten steps later, I run into Pat McGrath, and she introduces me to Donatella Versace, who tells me, "I love your makeup! Thank you for being here."

Little me would just scream because it's insane to have such iconic people standing in front of me. Having such amazing interaction with them is so memorable.

Q Let's talk a bit about your first casting.

A It was very, very nerve-racking. I'm the type of person who wants to have a vision and a layout in my head for how a situation is going to be.

In a casting situation, everything's out of your control except for you showing up and presenting yourself. So I remember walking into my first casting, but I didn't know who to speak to. I didn't know which way to turn. I didn't know if I should put on my heels right away or wait.

Q What did the casting actually look like? Did you walk for them?

A Yeah, I walked for them. I walked in, and they had me wait in a line. Then they called my name, and they asked me where I was from, my age, and where I was living now.

Q You walked in front of the other models?

A Yeah. If there's a line of people waiting behind you, you're walking in front of them, which can be very nerve-racking.

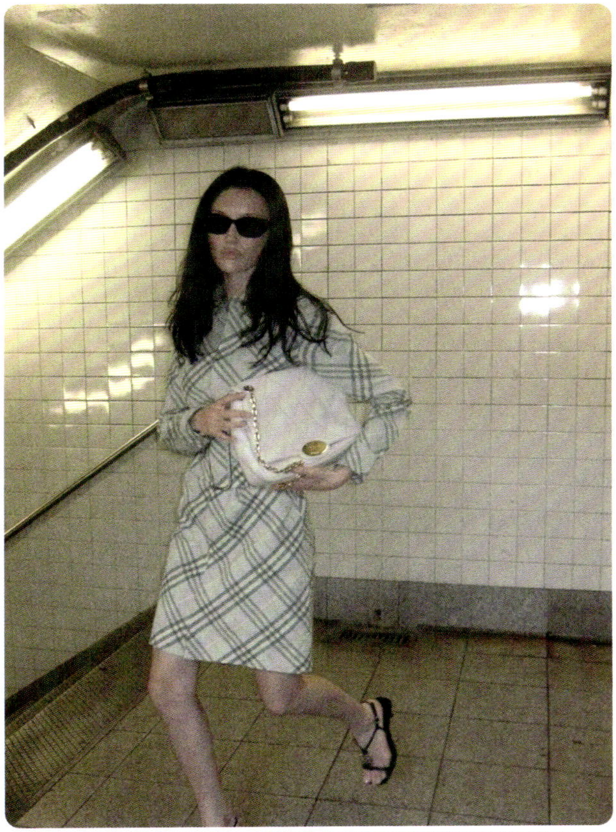

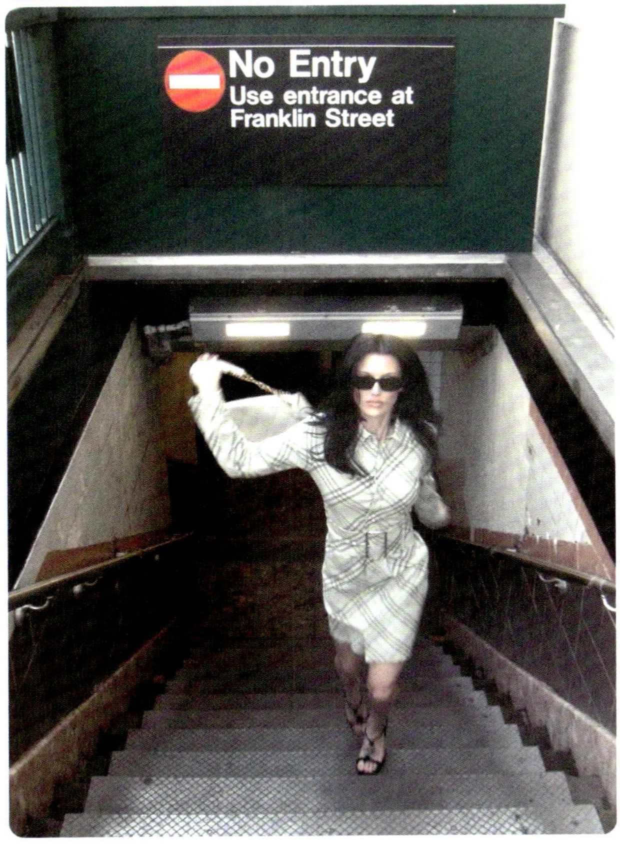

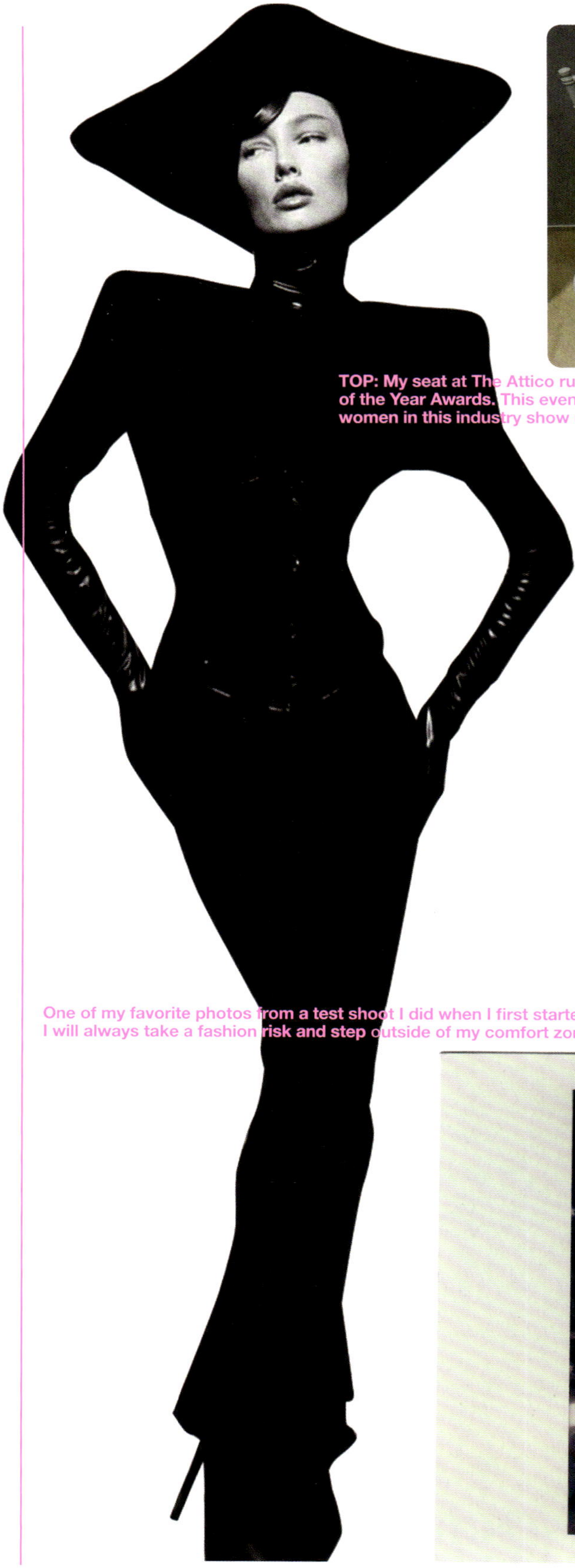

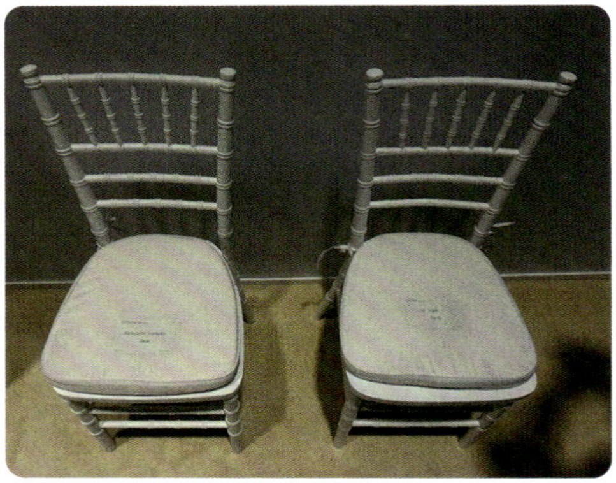

TOP: My seat at The Attico runway show. CENTER RIGHT: A little memento from the 2025 Glamour Women of the Year Awards. This event was so special to attend. It was amazing to see all the powerful, hardworking women in this industry show up to support one another and uplift each other, including mother Pat McGrath.

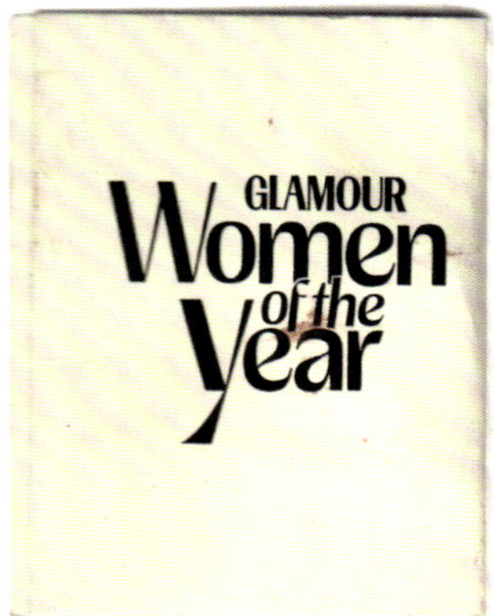

One of my favorite photos from a test shoot I did when I first started to dip into modeling. How cool is this styling! One thing about me: I will always take a fashion risk and step outside of my comfort zone. This neon pink Marc Jacobs skirt below definitely was one for the books!

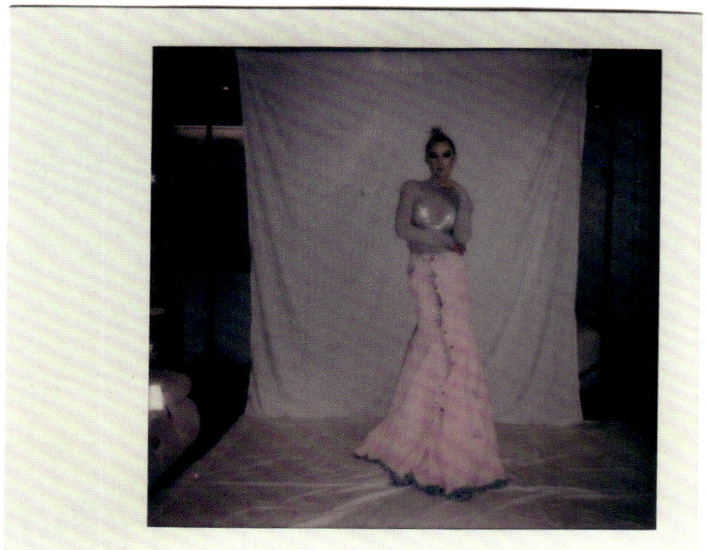

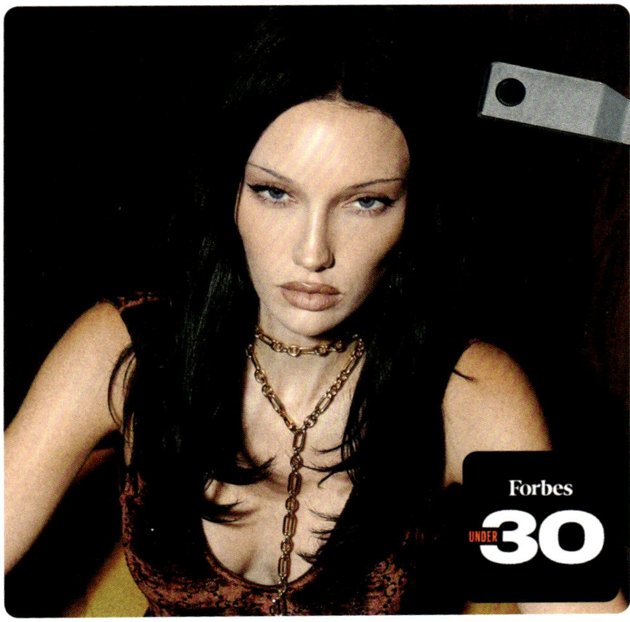

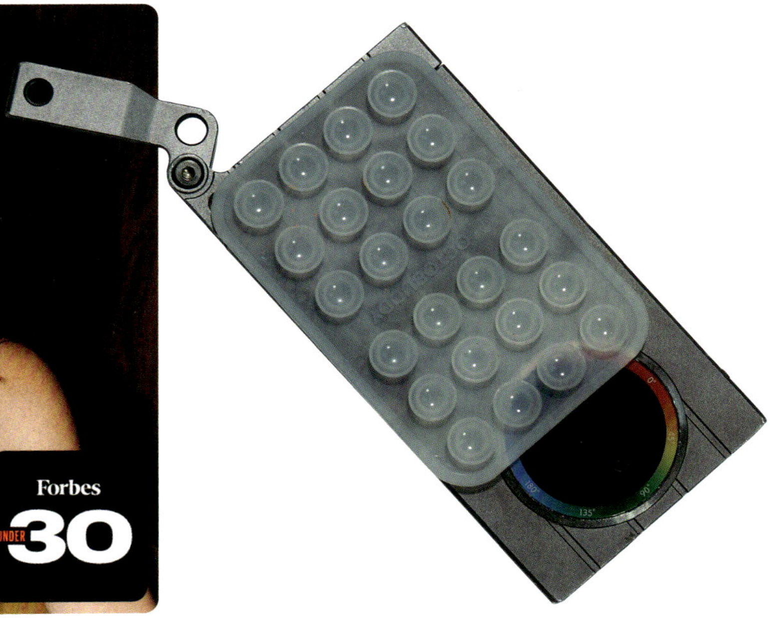

LEFT: To be in the Forbes 30 under 30 class of 2025 was such a privilege and felt like a dream come true. RIGHT: Best filming light in the game: Godox RGB Mini Creative M1 LED Light. BELOW: Being named alongside some of the most talented creators and leaders in the industry was a huge pinch-me moment. I felt so incredibly honored to be recognized for my work in the fashion space.

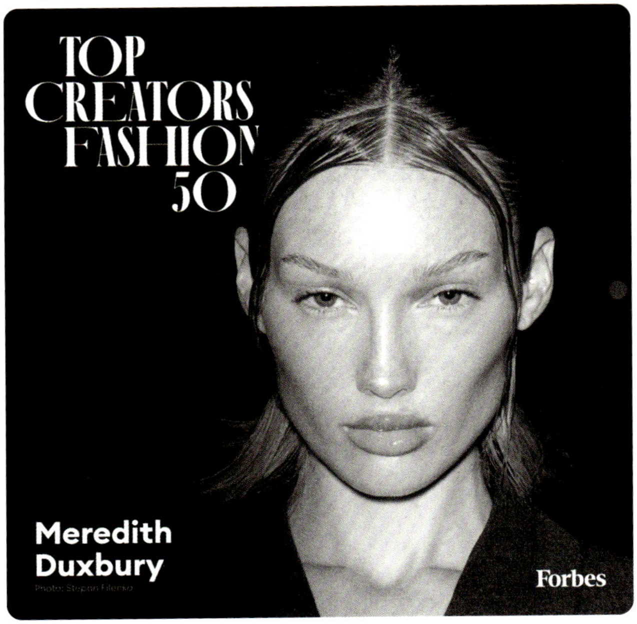

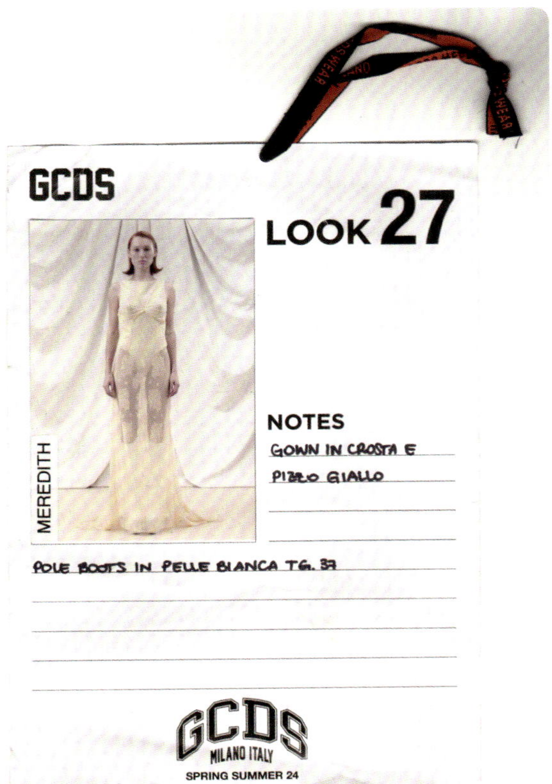

I love keeping a paper trail of all my runway moments. They are so special to me. This is the card that hangs on the rack with your look when you arrive backstage.

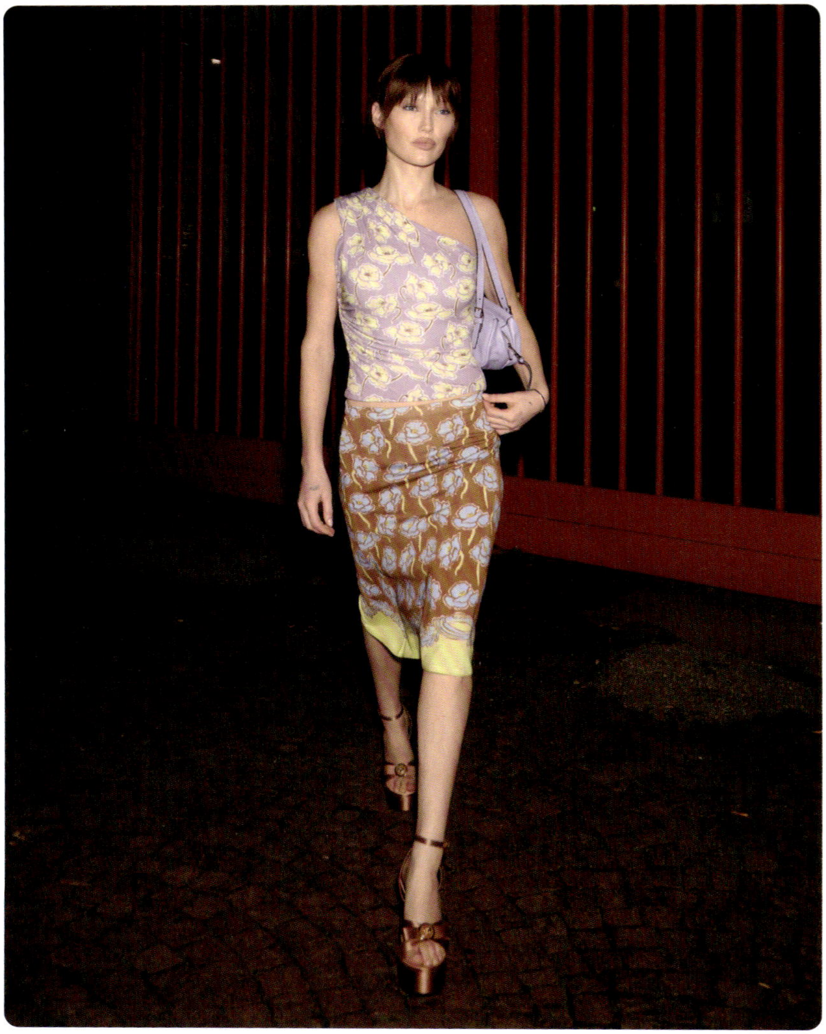

The Versace Fall/Winter 2025 runway show. I did a faux bang for this look, which is one of my favorites.

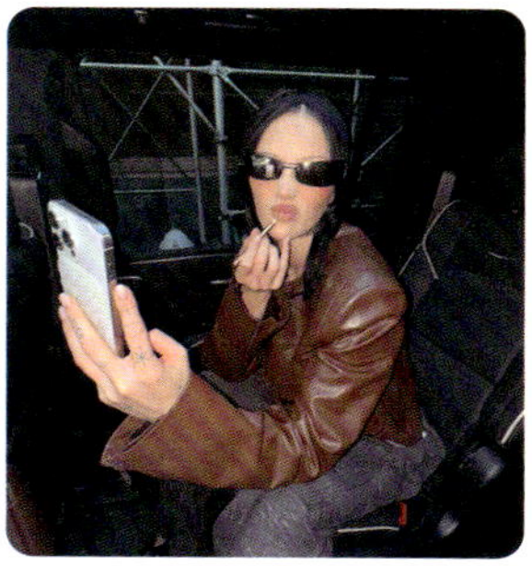

Before the show, behind-the-scenes photos are always the best. They show what really goes on! In this case, I was just doing a quick lip touch-up before arriving at the Tory Burch runway show during New York Fashion Week.

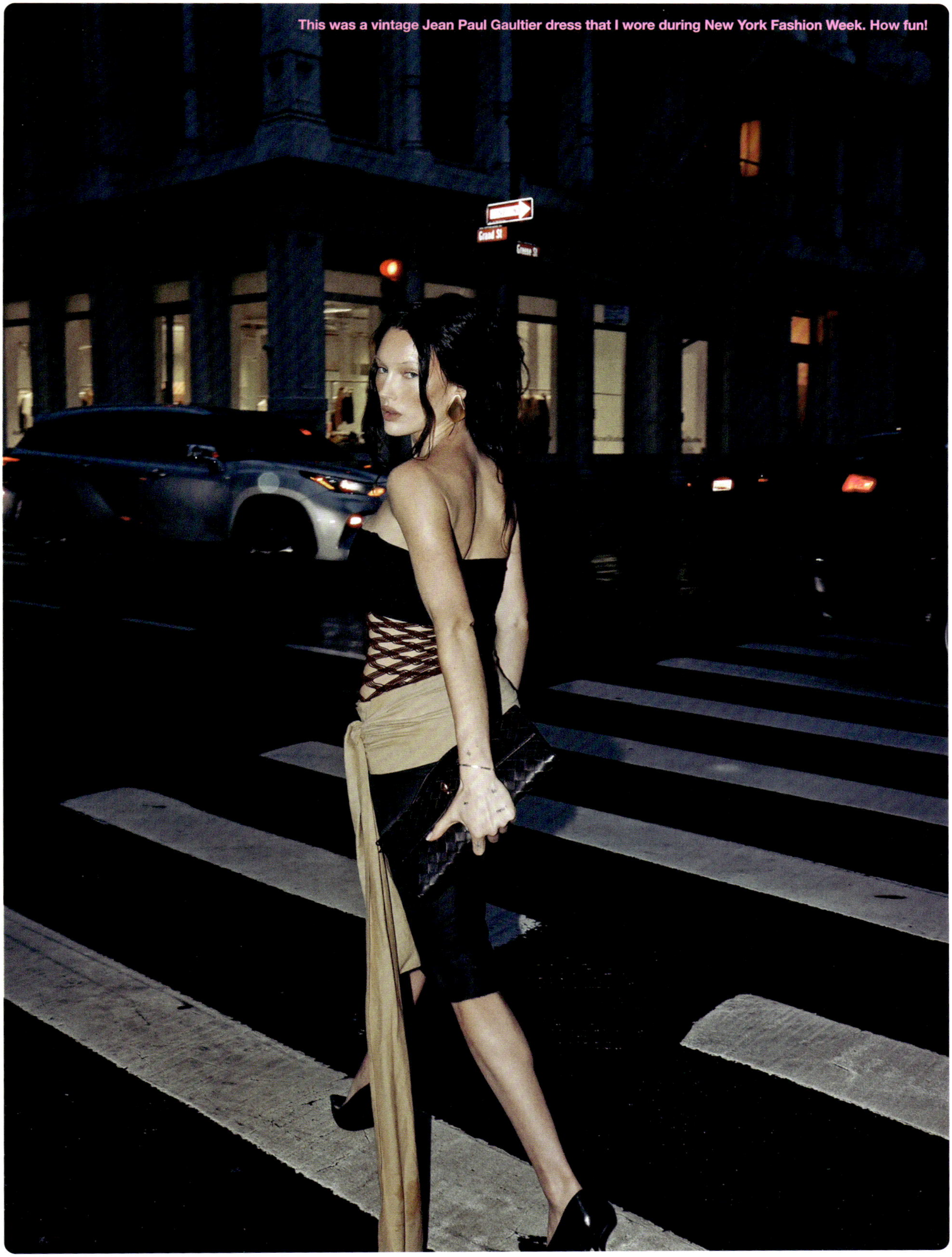

This was a vintage Jean Paul Gaultier dress that I wore during New York Fashion Week. How fun!

Q How did you come up with your walk?

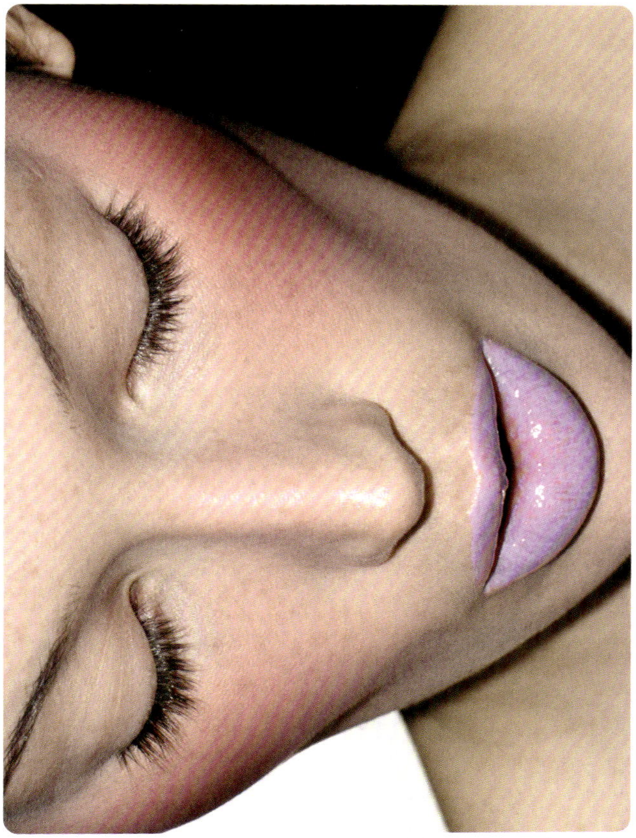

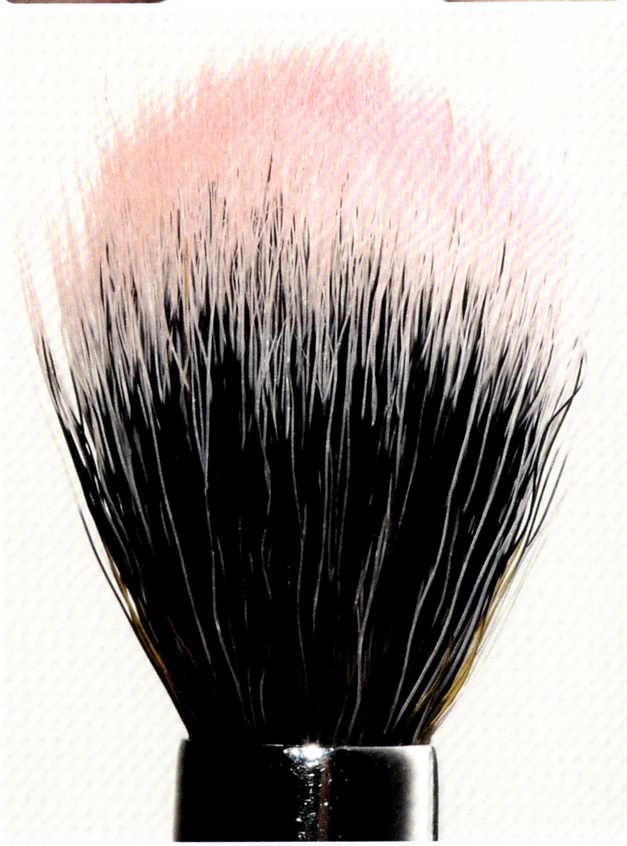

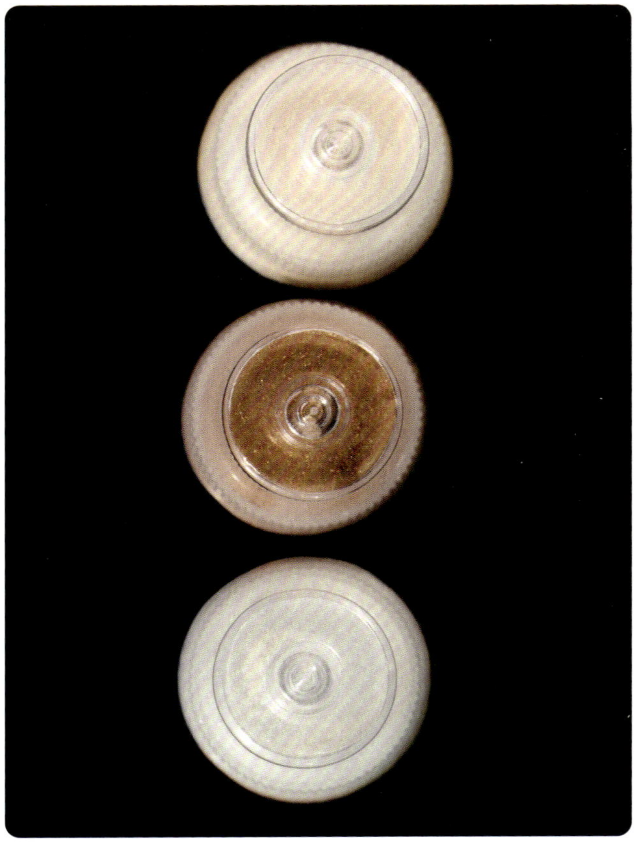

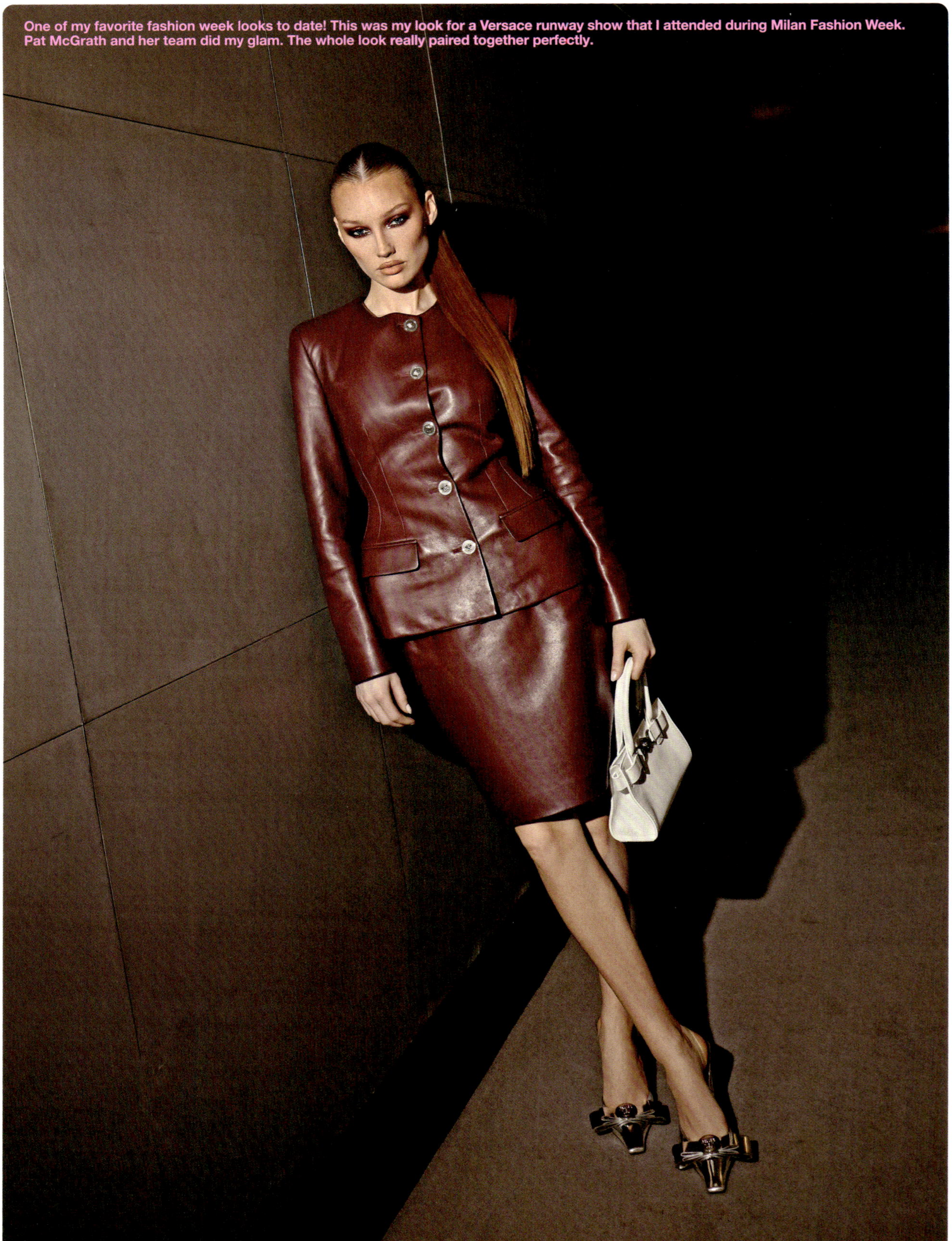

One of my favorite fashion week looks to date! This was my look for a Versace runway show that I attended during Milan Fashion Week. Pat McGrath and her team did my glam. The whole look really paired together perfectly.

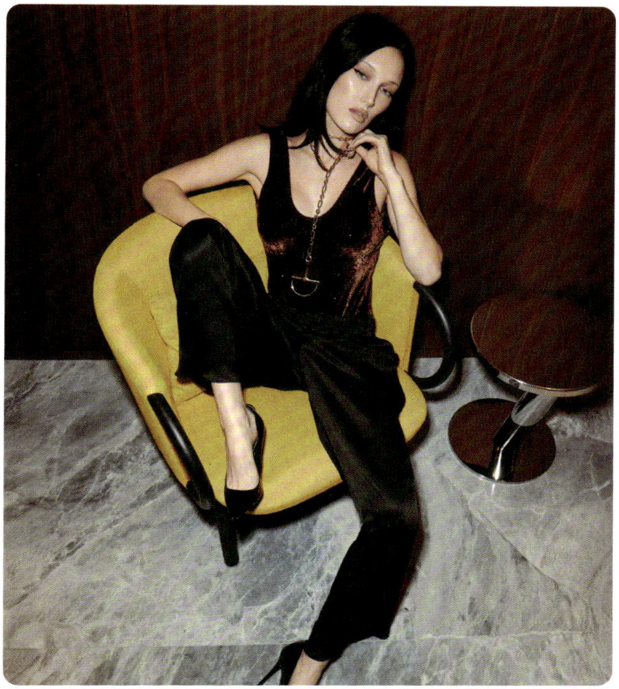

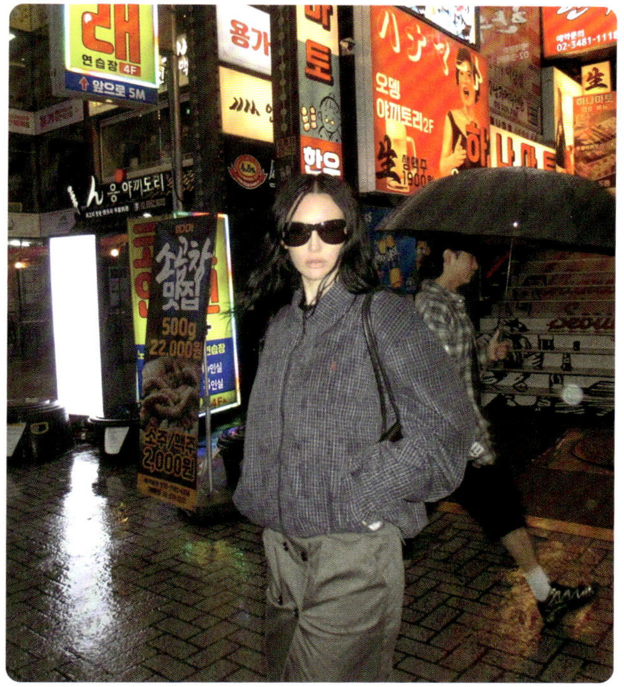

A I kind of just pretended like I was on a fun night out with my friends, strutting in my heels! I also met up in Paris with Coco Rocha for a fun little walking sesh and got some tips and tricks from her!

Once you walk into casting, you kind of black out. You forget about which way your body is moving. I remember I did my walk and the casting director asked me to walk again, but a little faster the second time, and I was like, "Oh no! Did I mess up my whole shot?"

Q You were probably wondering, "Did I walk wrong the first time?"

A You kind of just have to be delulu and fake it until you make it.

Q Do you remember any other advice Coco Rocha gave you?

A She said modeling requires confidence. If you have a shitty walk, you just have to be confident about it. Maybe it'll be viewed as an interesting walk, not a bad one. They could be like, "Oh, we love the horsey-stomp walk."

You never know if someone could take what you consider a weakness of yours and turn it into something that's different and cool. It always goes back to just being yourself.

TOP LEFT: Wearing Gucci in Milan...this was me manifesting walking the Gucci show before I even knew it! TOP RIGHT: Different cultures and environments really inspire my style, so visiting Seoul, Korea, was super fun. I got to experiment a lot with street style and found some amazing vintage shops there as well.

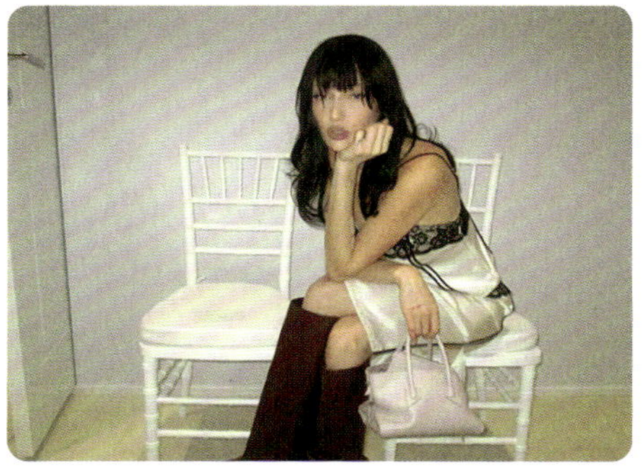

The Attico! I adore this brand so much. They really love to have fun with color and silhouettes. I always look forward to their runway shows!!

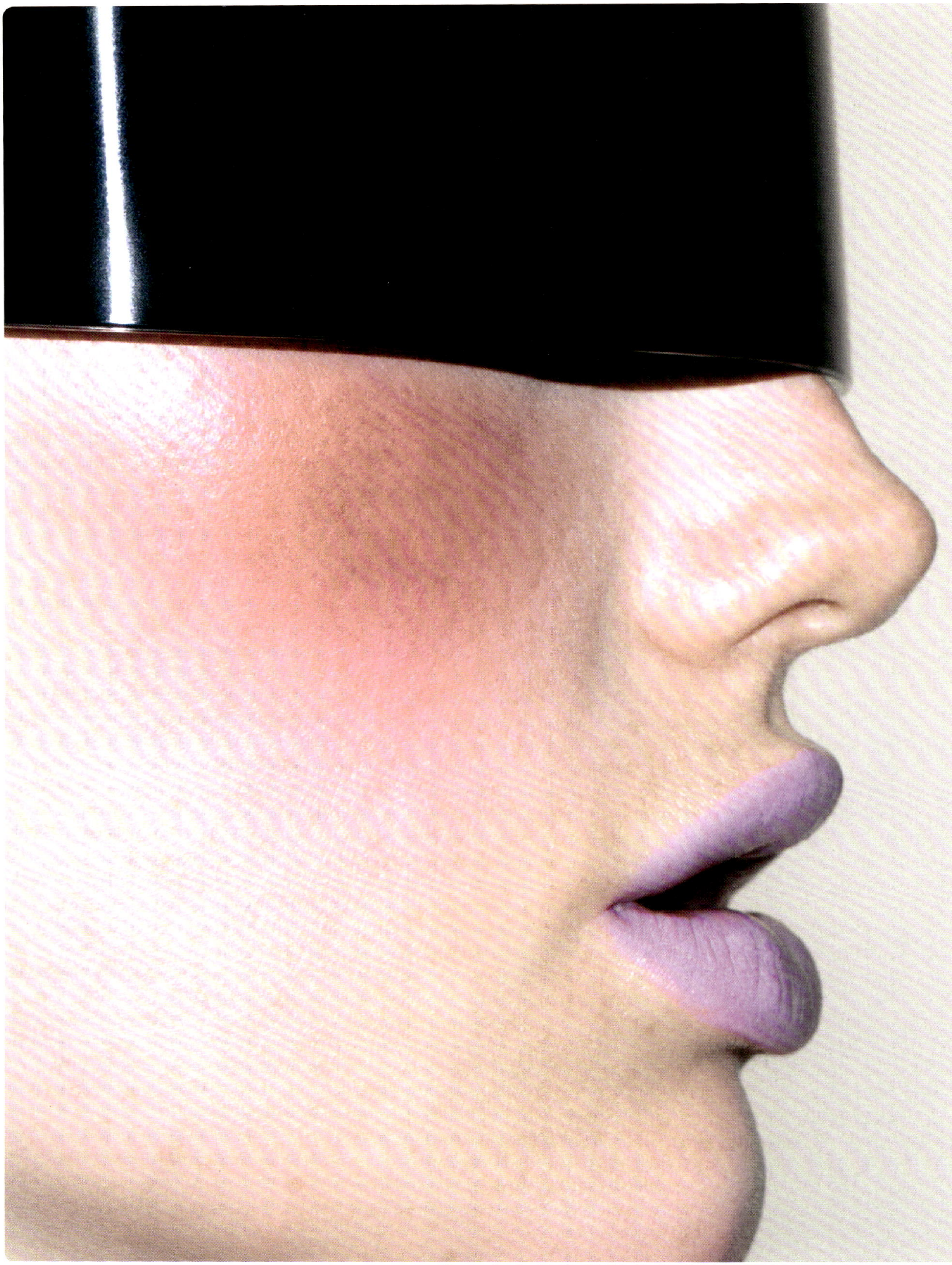

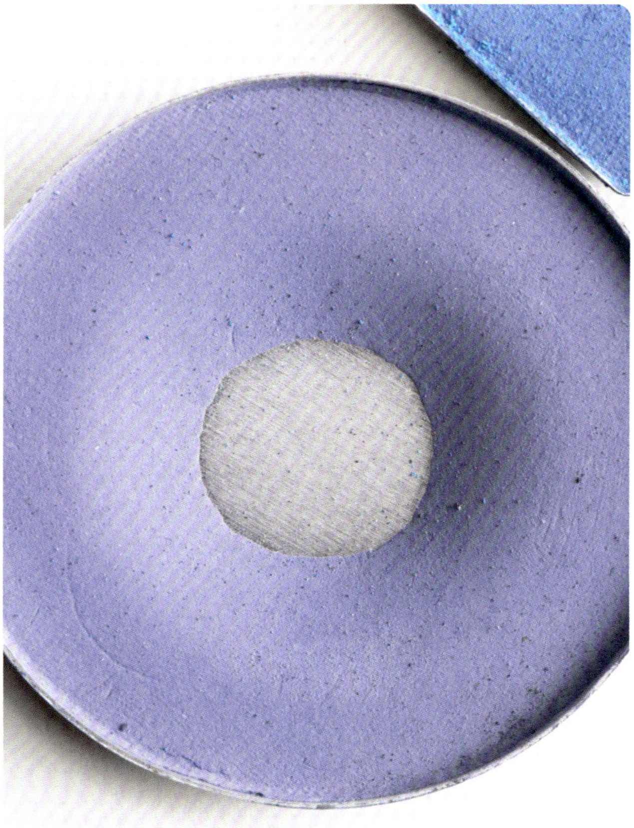

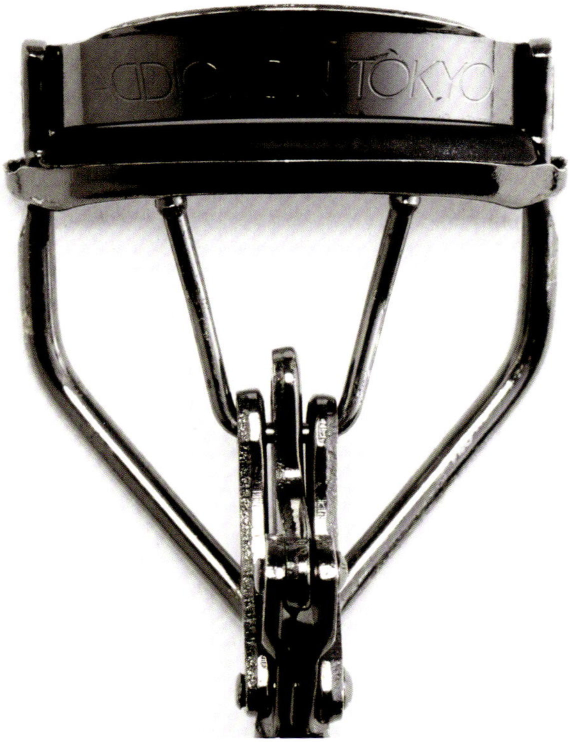

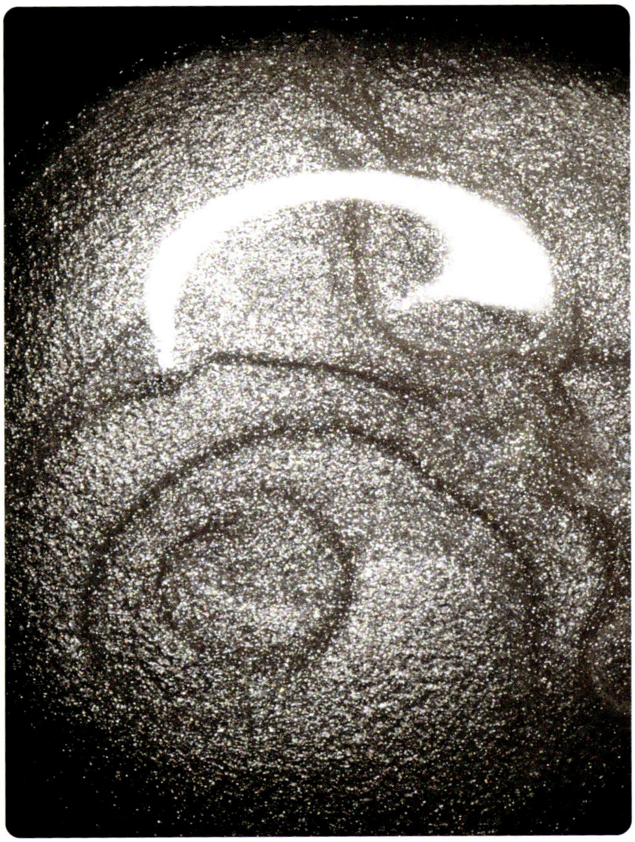

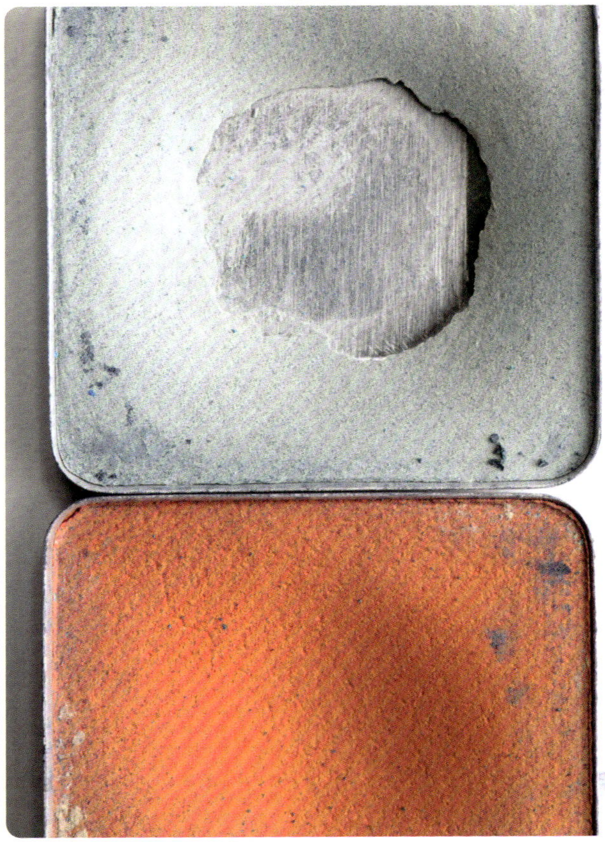

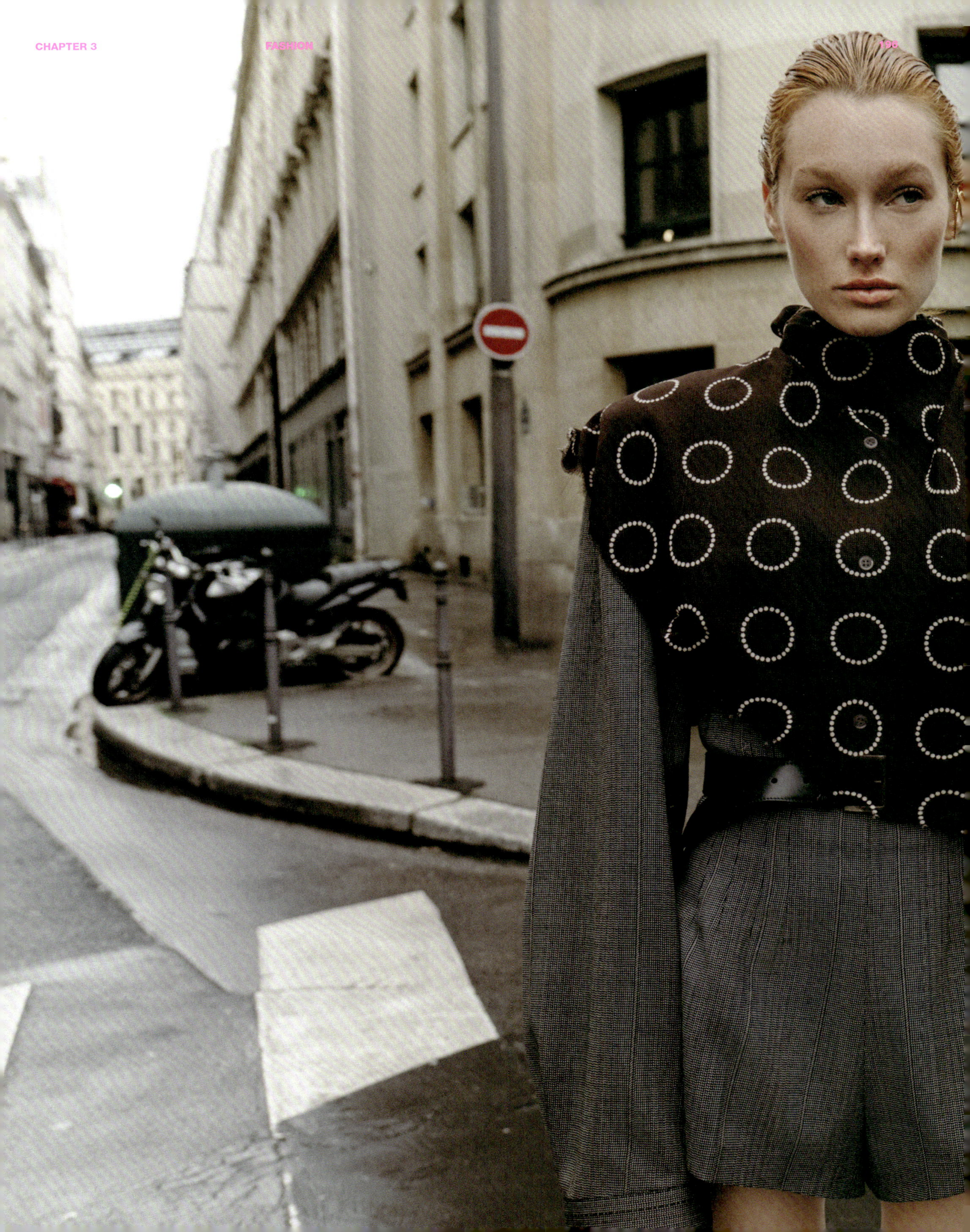

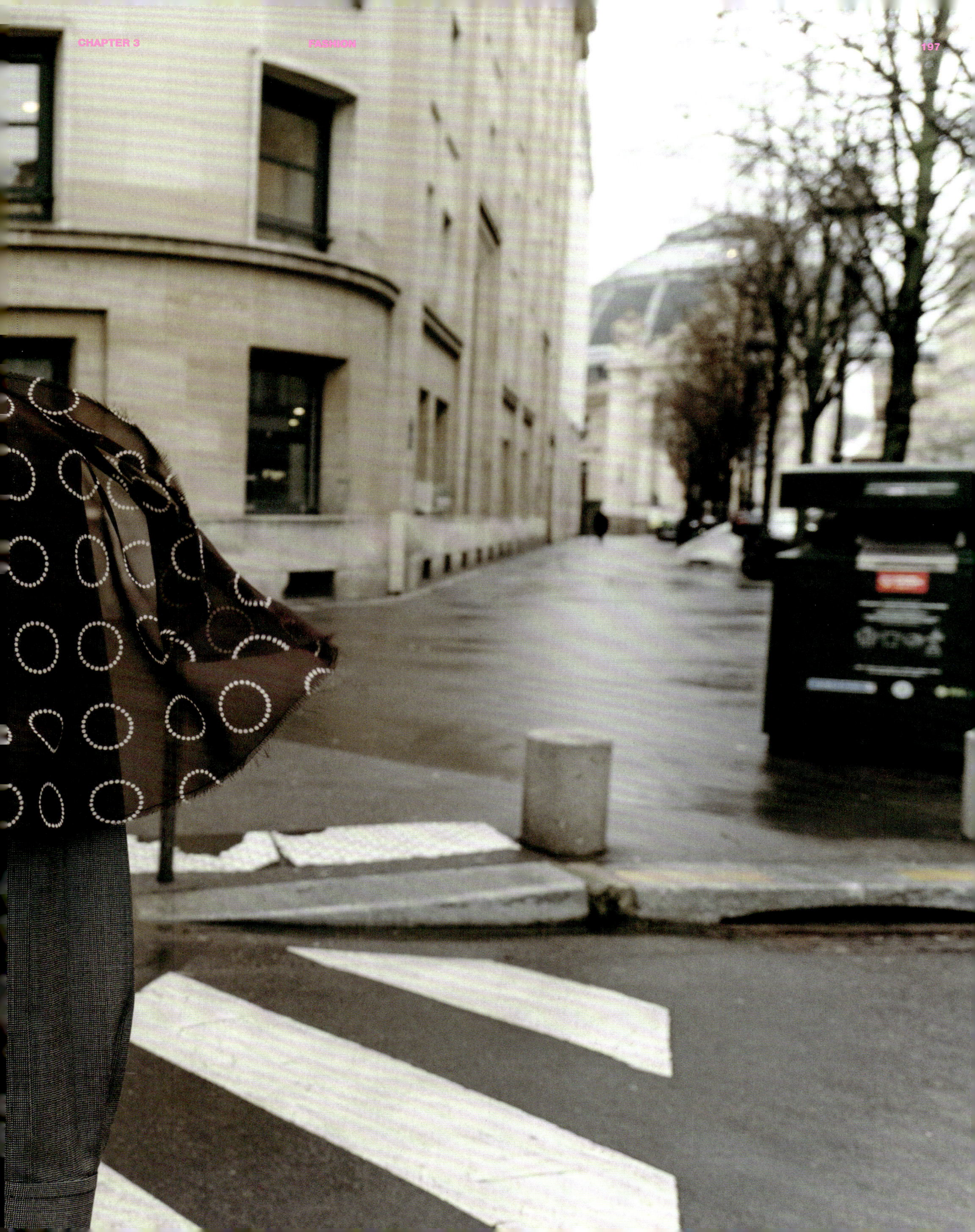

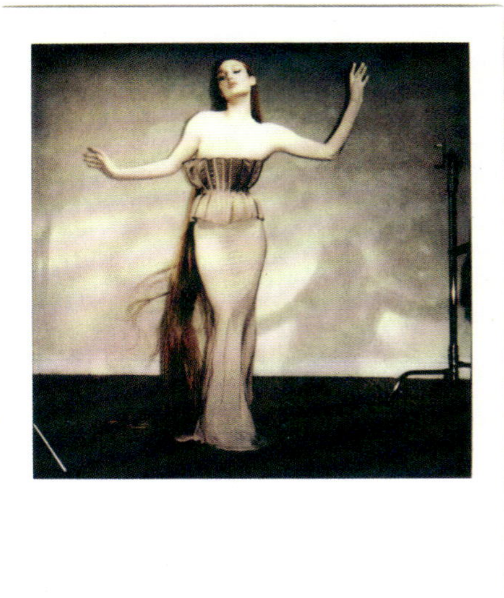
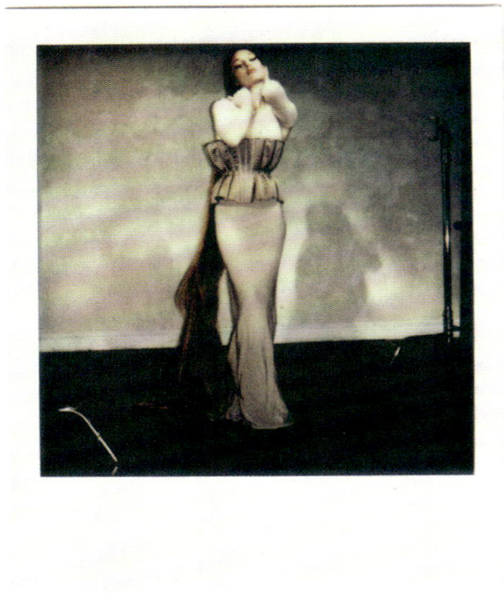
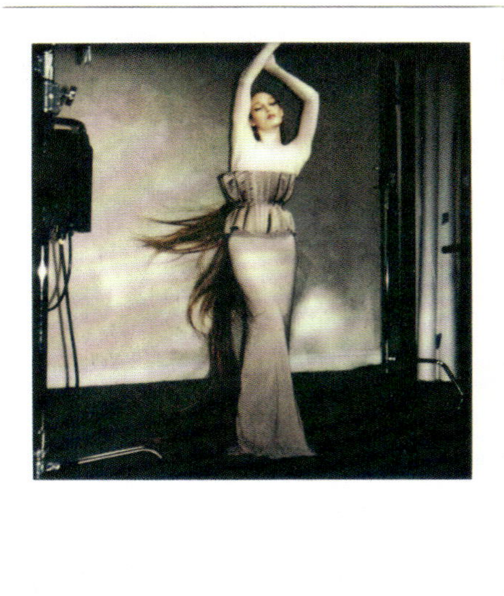
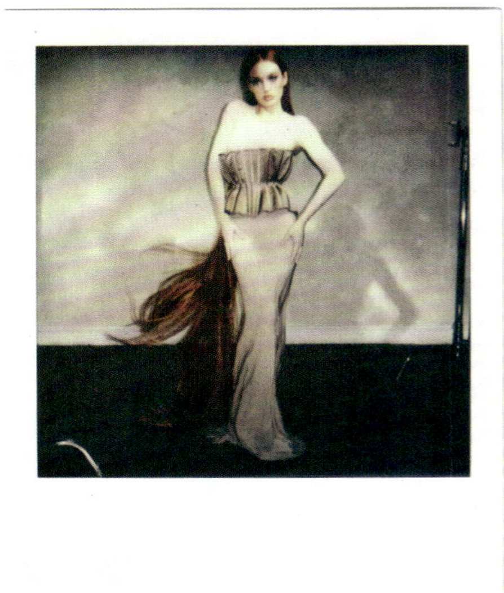

THIS PAGE: Some behind-the-scenes Polaroids from a shoot I did with *Schön! Switzerland* magazine! Always take risks and allow the creative team to work their magic. It can be scary to have yourself portrayed in a way that you haven't experimented with before, but it allows you to find new styles you may fall in love with. OPPOSITE PAGE: This was a fun shoot I did with Tory Burch for the launch of their Animal House collection. It was shot in a bodega in New York City. It was so fun experimenting with poses on top of all the magazines!

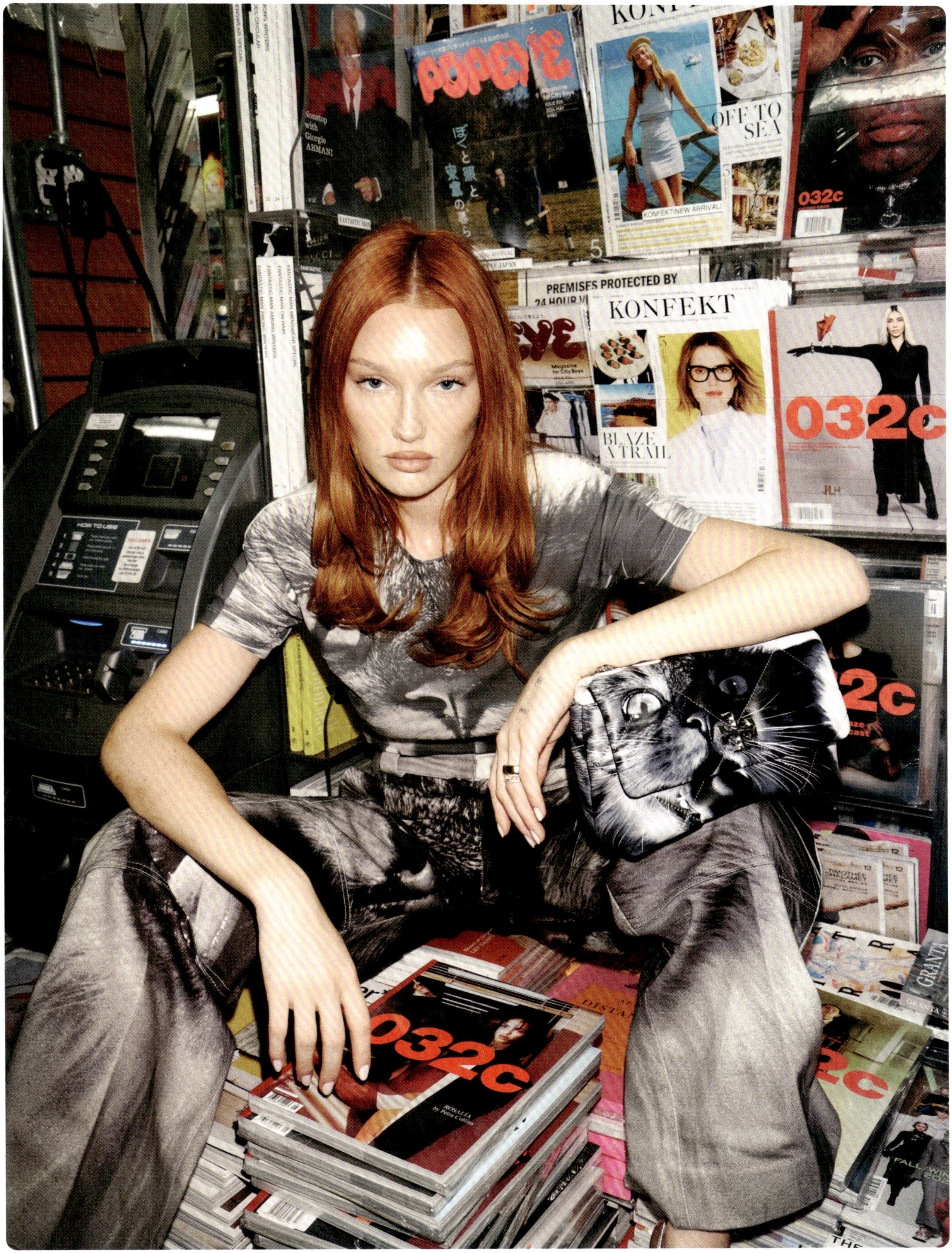
POPEYE
Nonstop with Giorgio ARMANI
KONFEKT
OFF TO SEA
032c
PREMISES PROTECTED BY
KONFEKT
BLAZE A TRAIL
032c
HOW TO USE
032c
ROSALÍA by Petra Collins
GRANTA

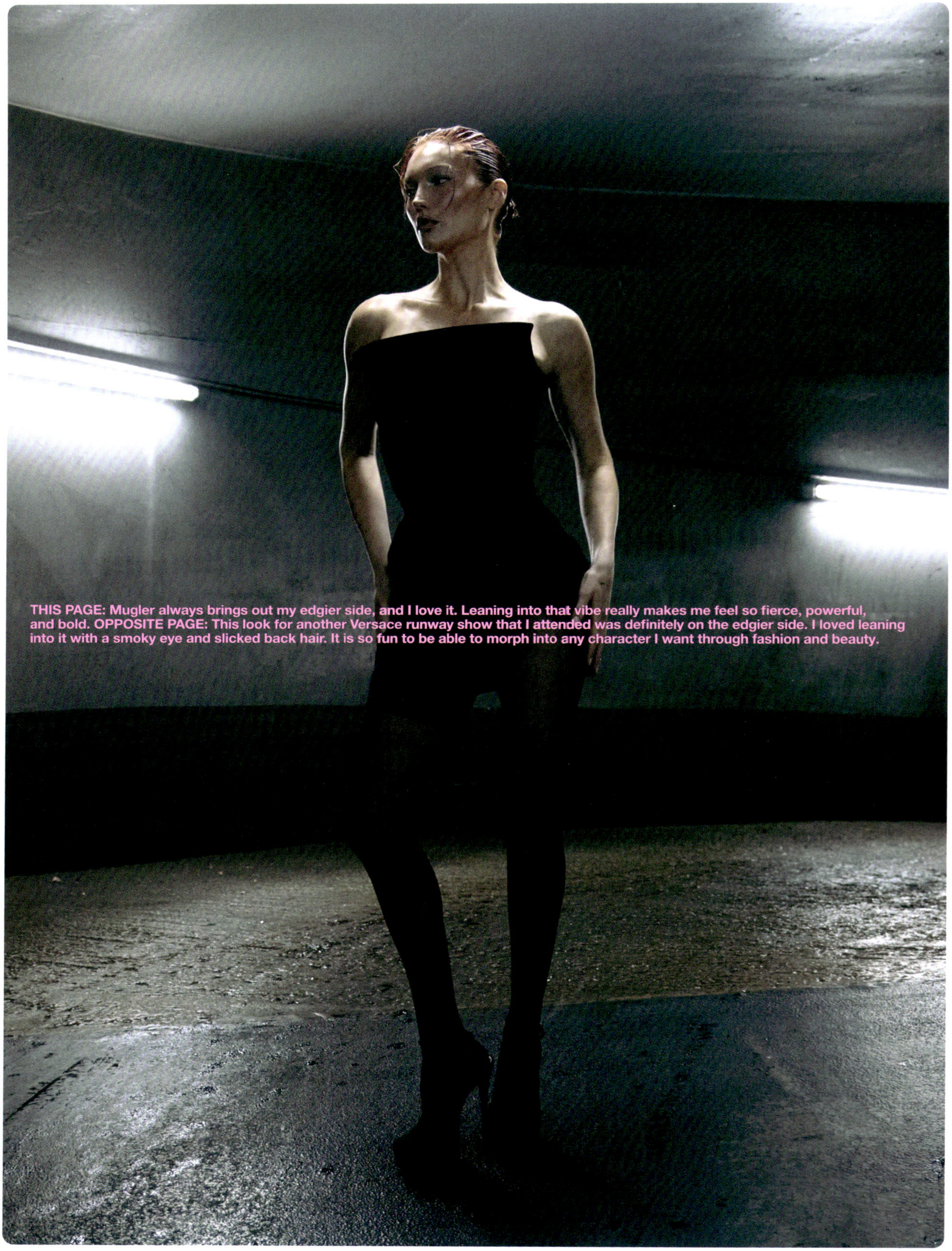

THIS PAGE: Mugler always brings out my edgier side, and I love it. Leaning into that vibe really makes me feel so fierce, powerful, and bold. OPPOSITE PAGE: This look for another Versace runway show that I attended was definitely on the edgier side. I loved leaning into it with a smoky eye and slicked back hair. It is so fun to be able to morph into any character I want through fashion and beauty.

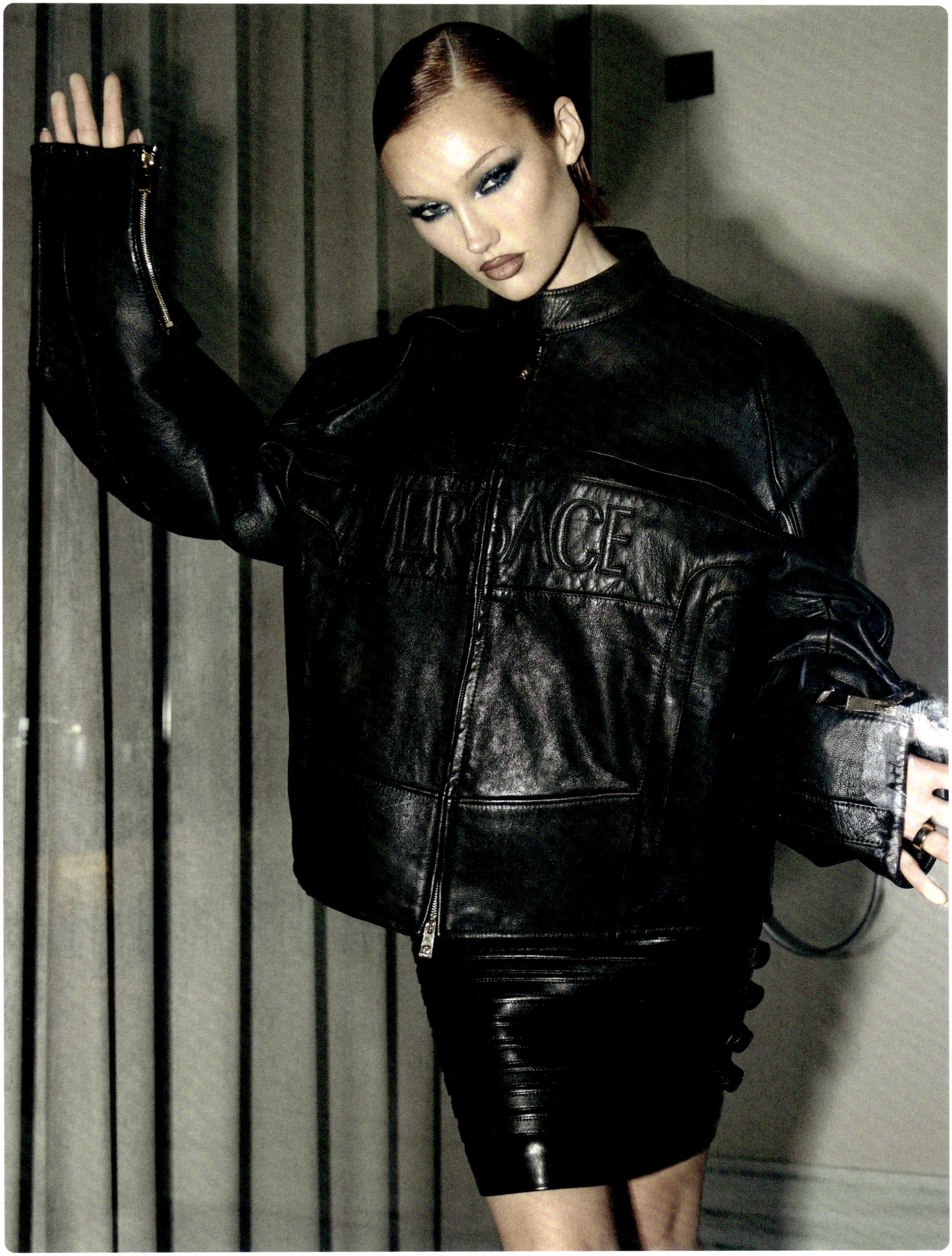

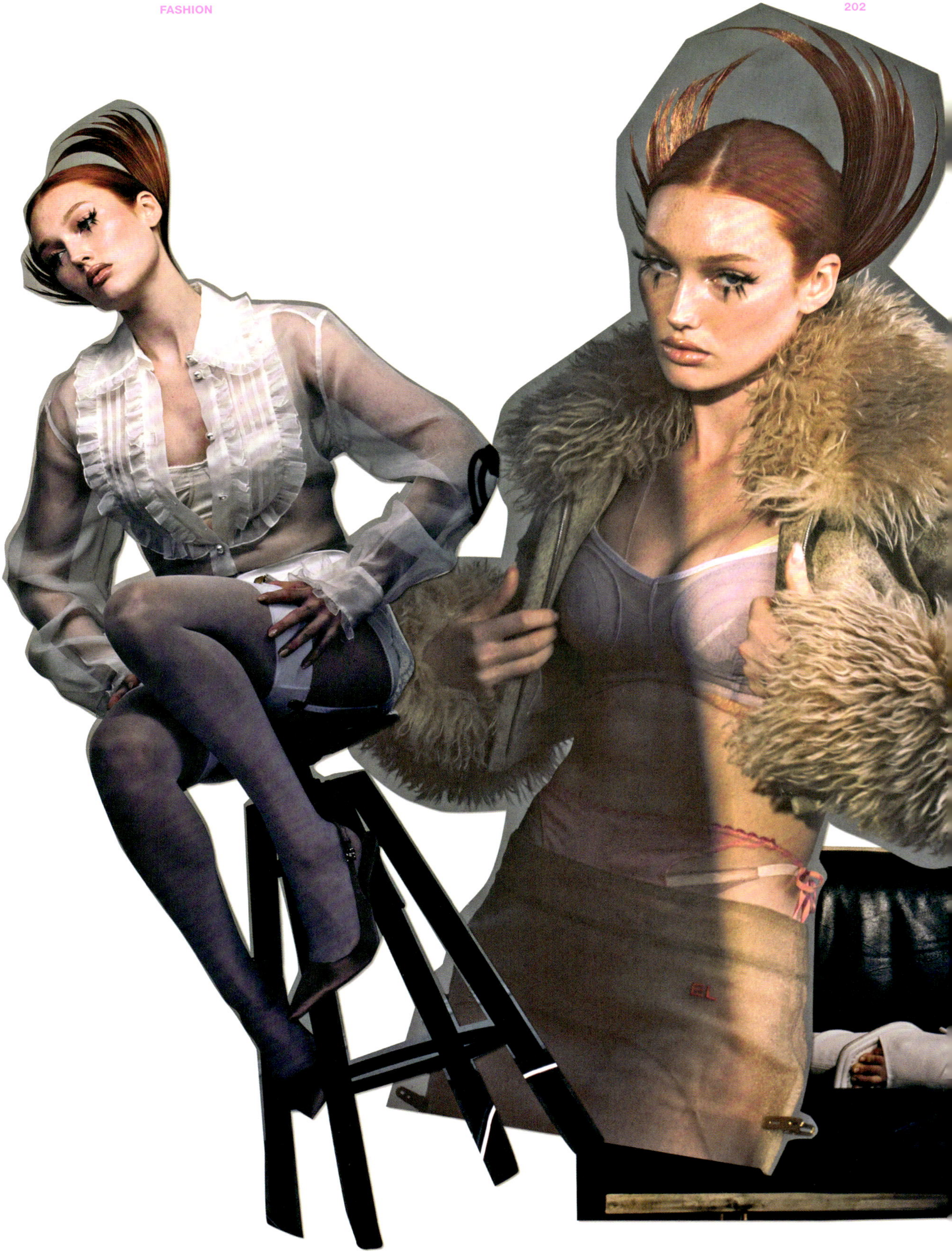

I love being a chameleon and allowing fashion bring me to play a different character for the day. Participating in fun, creative shoots like this really helped to build my confidence in the modeling space as well as allowed me to get comfortable with different poses and expressions.

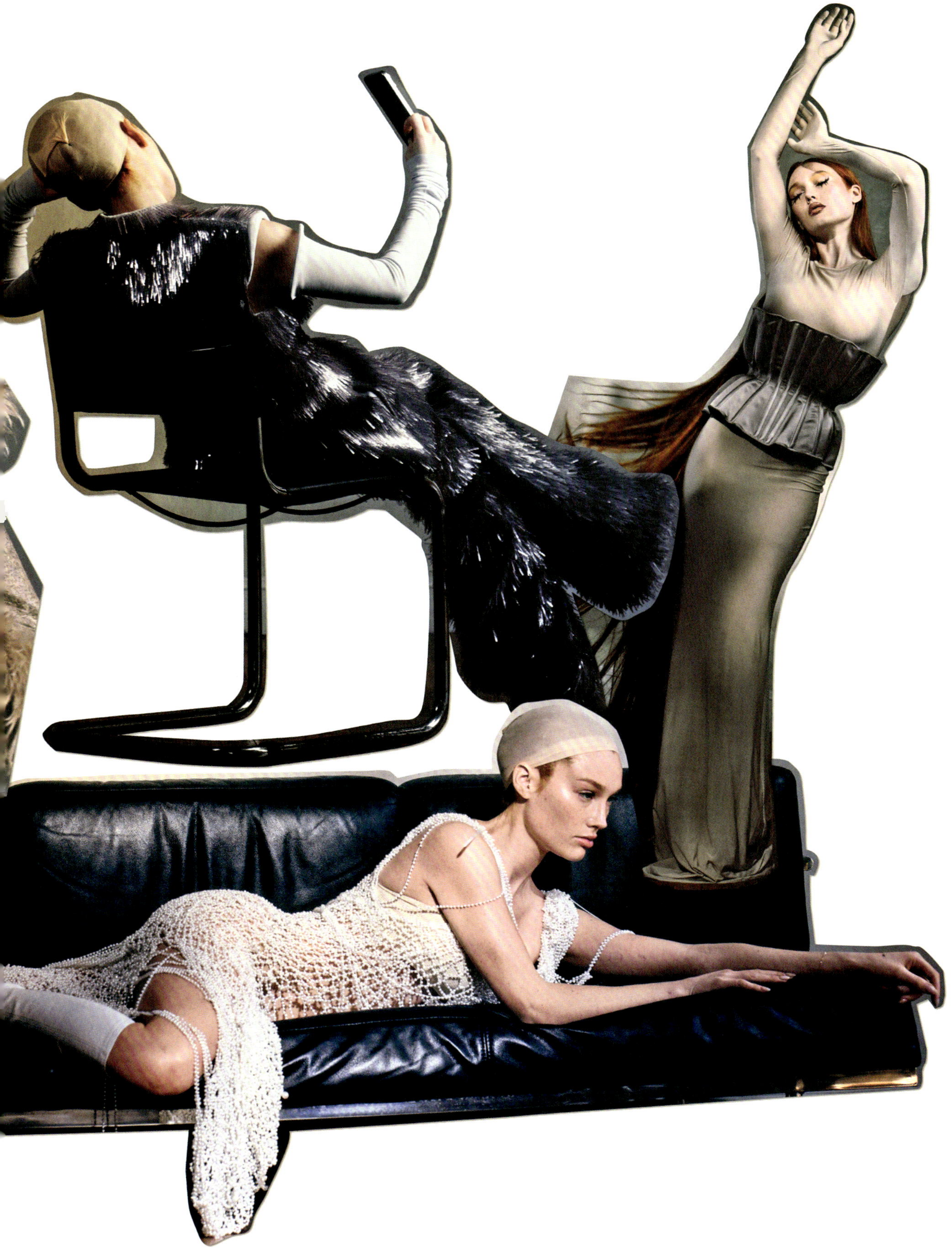

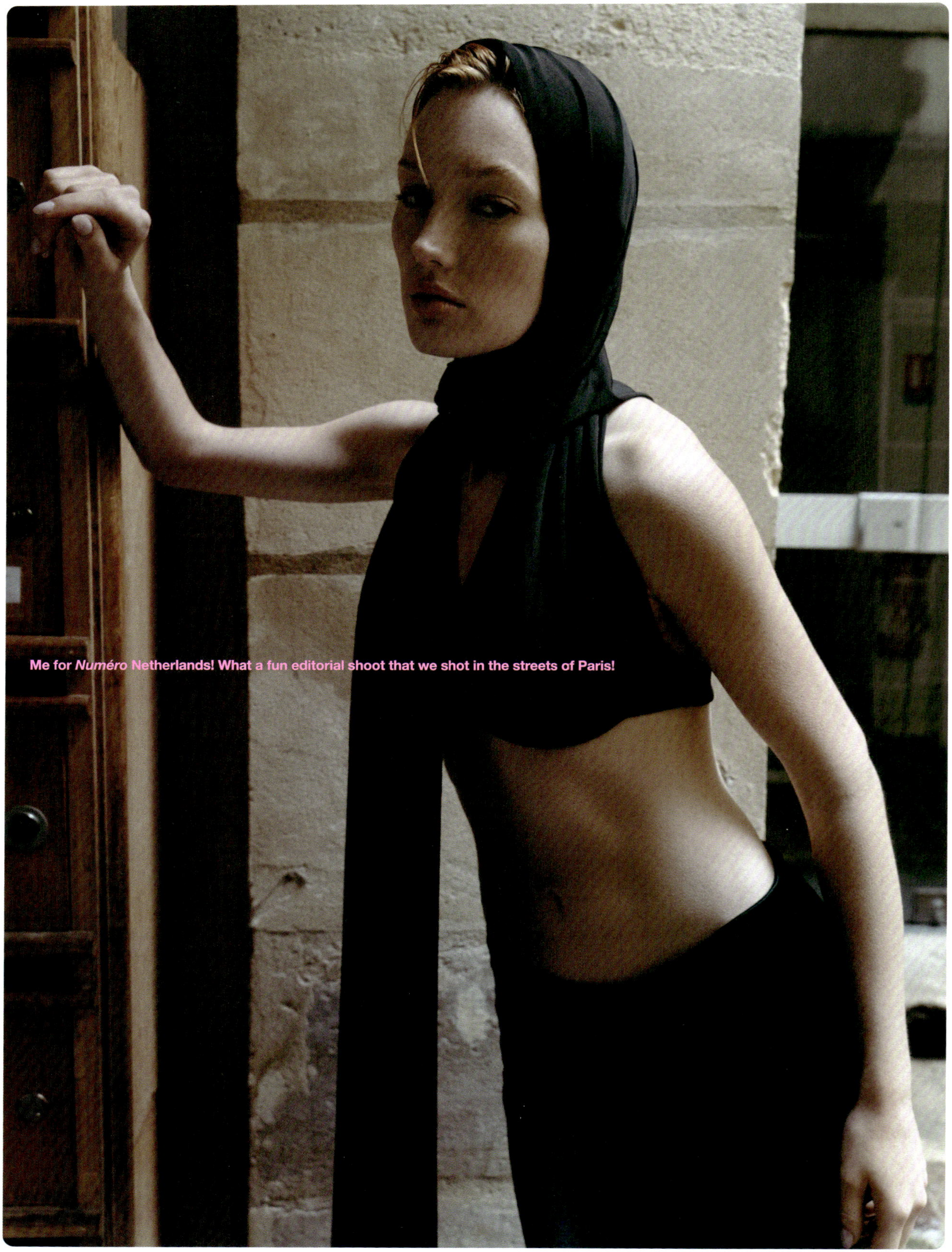

Me for *Numéro* Netherlands! What a fun editorial shoot that we shot in the streets of Paris!

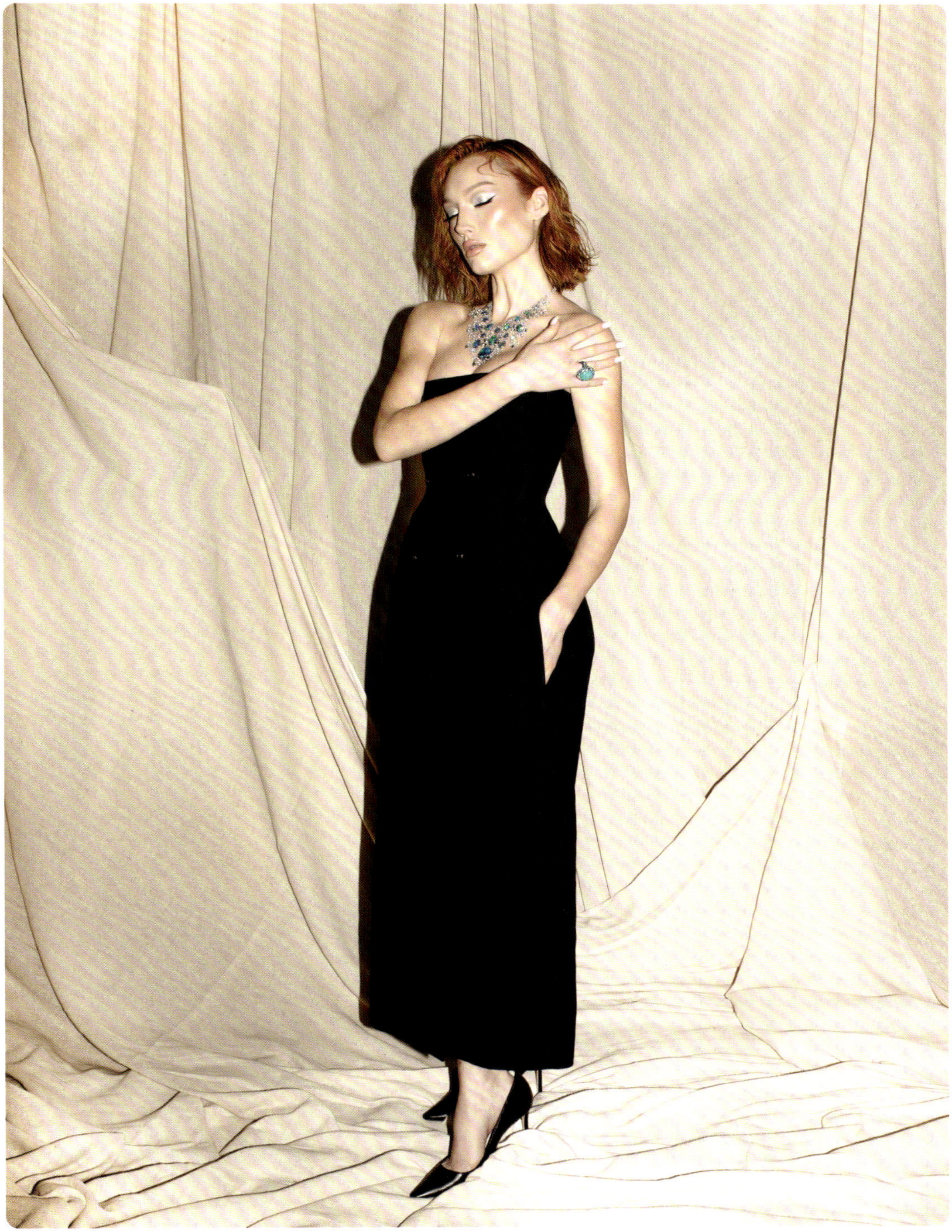

Pre-British Fashion Awards with Charlotte Tilbury! It was so special to join Charlotte for this event, where she was being honored with a Special Recognition Award. She is an icon and someone I look up to. Charlotte's team did my glam, and Chopard dressed me with the most beautiful jewels. The dress was by Stella McCartney!

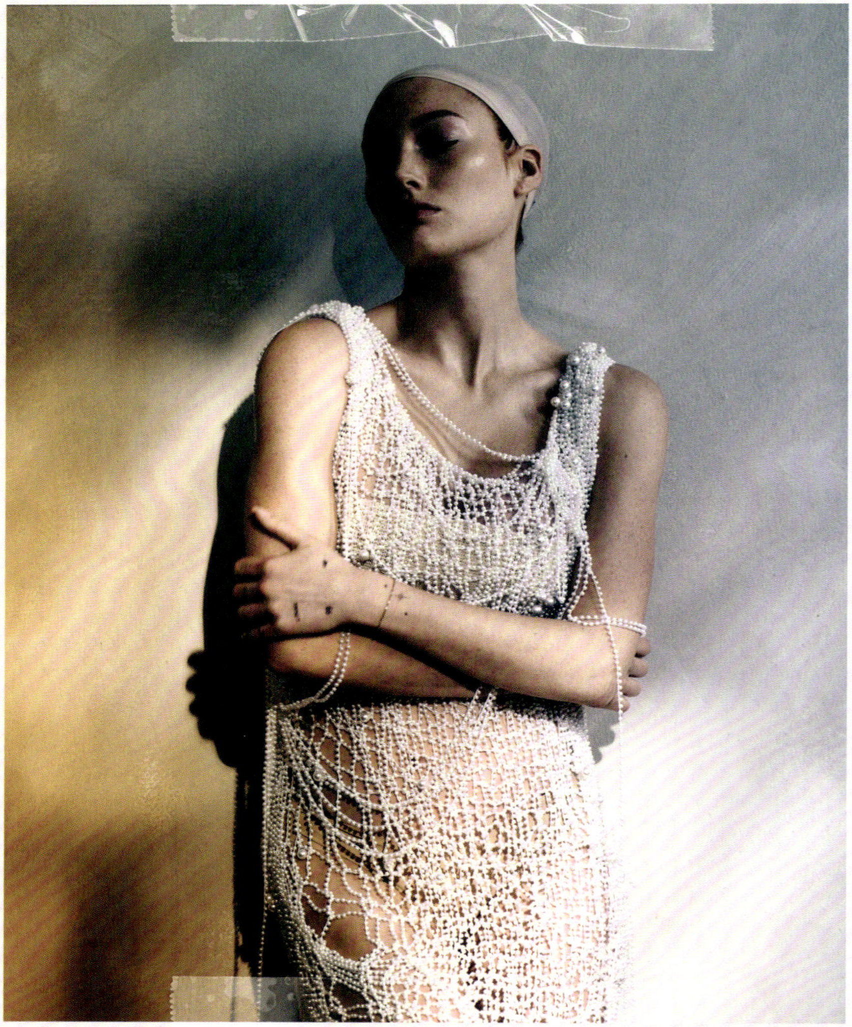

Fashion is such an expressive art, so allowing pieces to speak for themselves is important. I like to lean into whatever mood the clothing is portraying and match that energy. That's when I feel like imagery really comes together best as a whole.

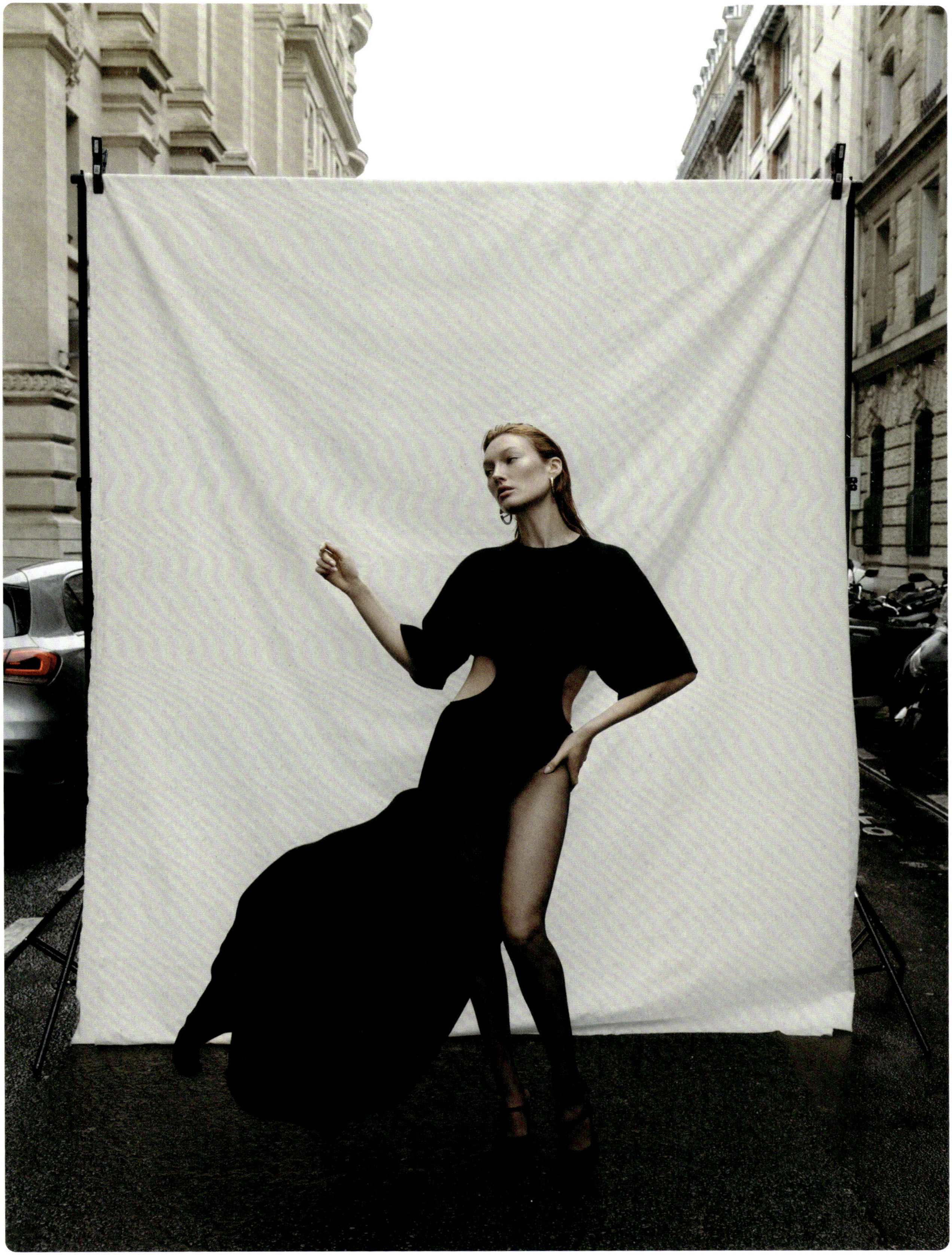

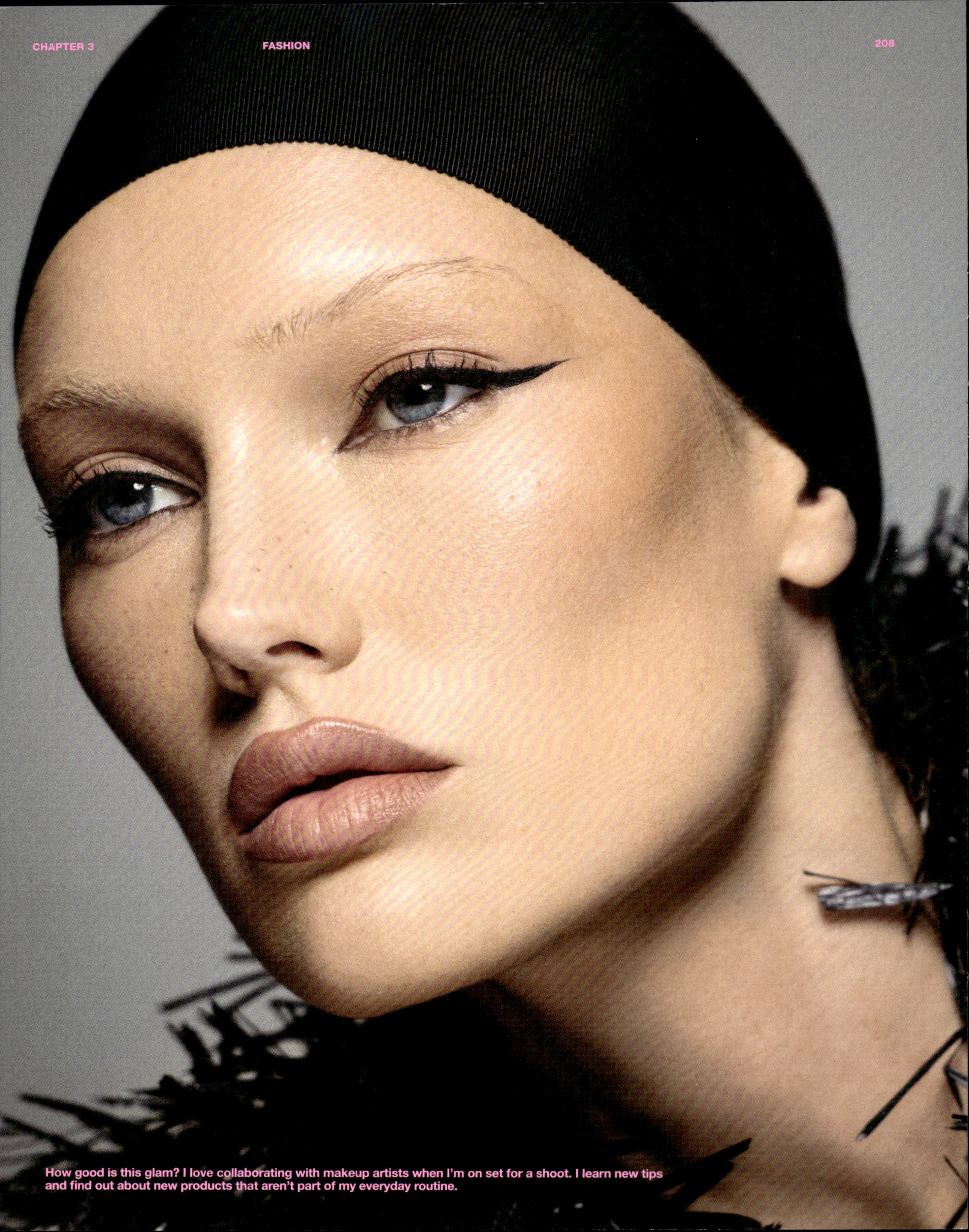

How good is this glam? I love collaborating with makeup artists when I'm on set for a shoot. I learn new tips and find out about new products that aren't part of my everyday routine.

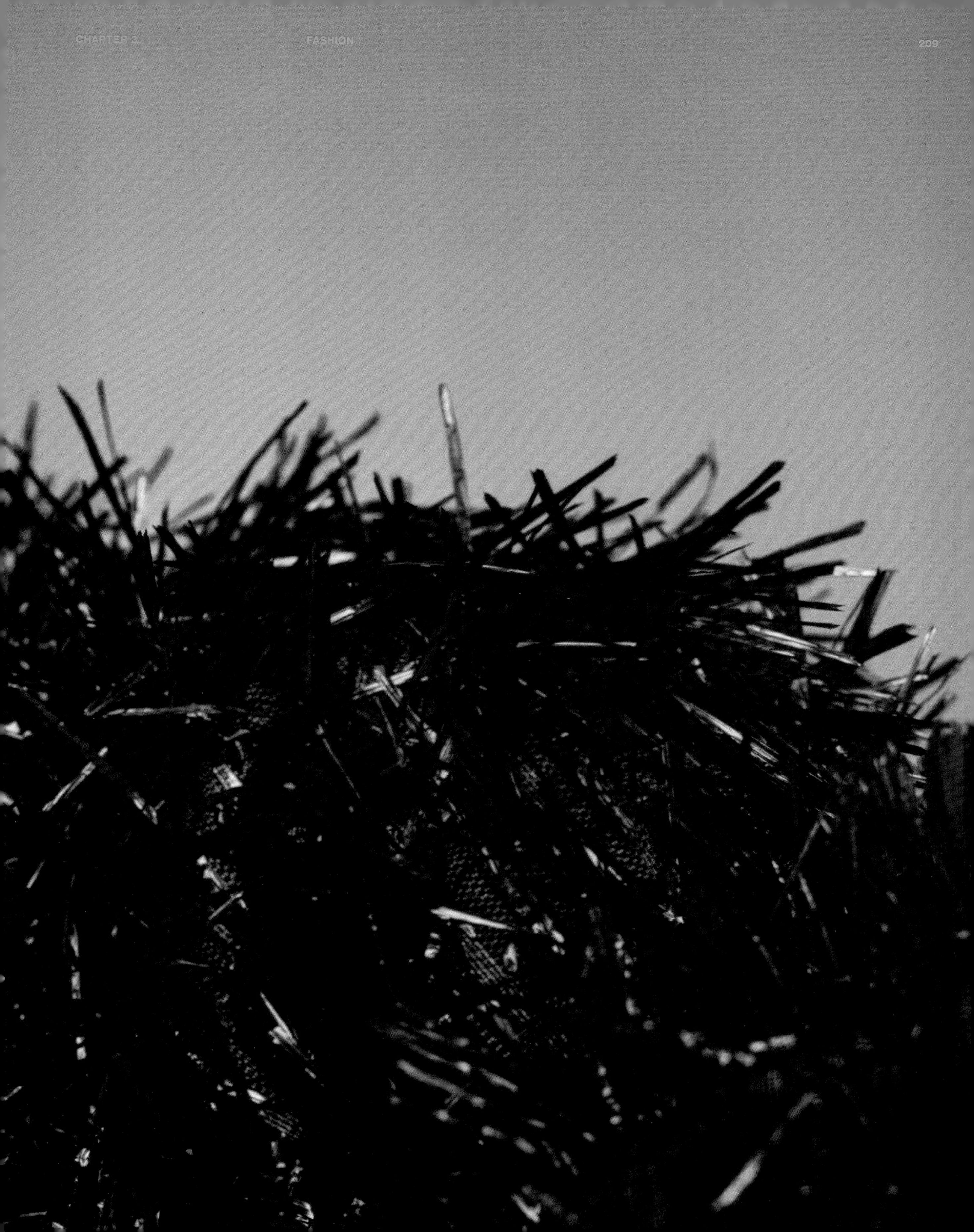

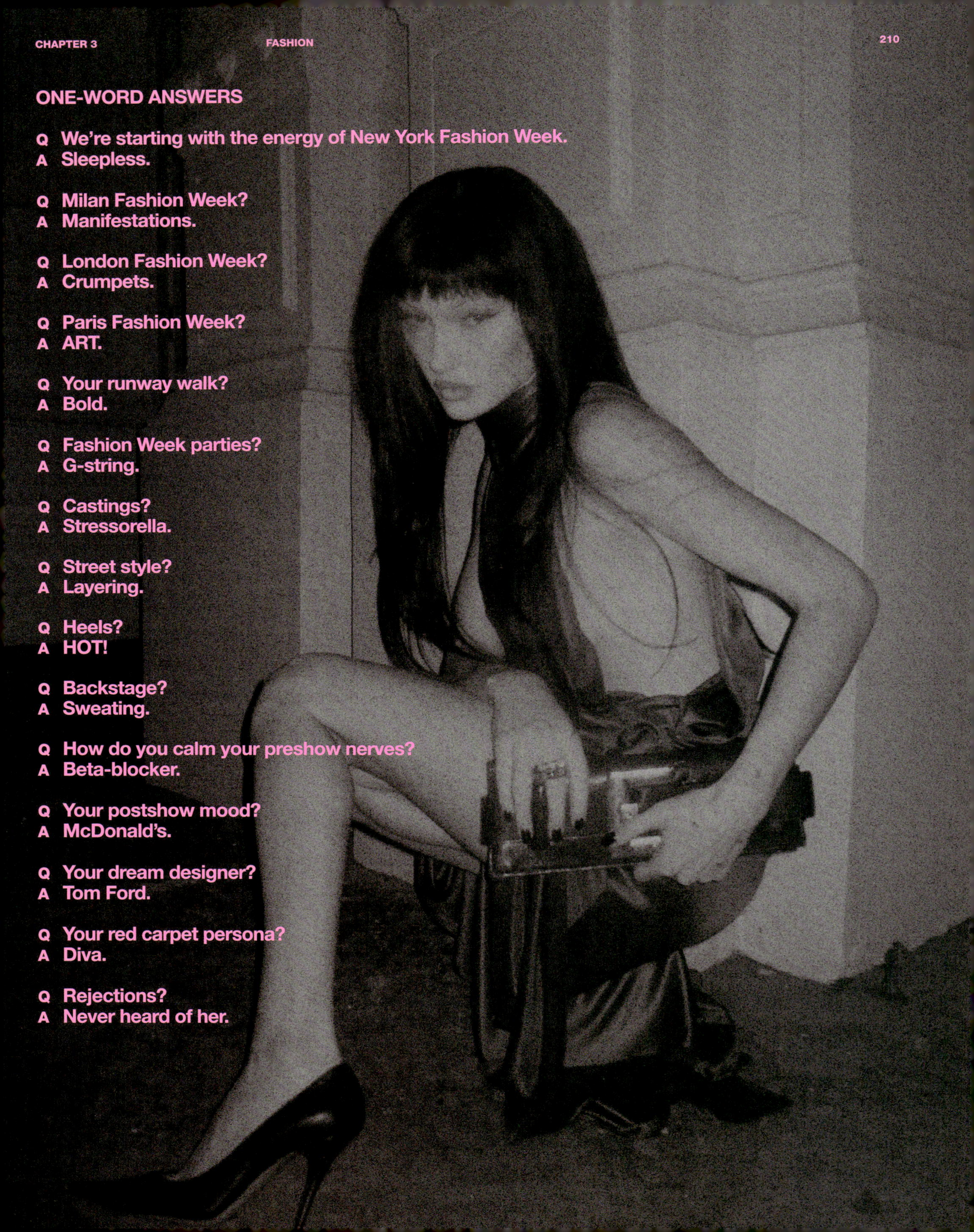

ONE-WORD ANSWERS

Q We're starting with the energy of New York Fashion Week.
A Sleepless.

Q Milan Fashion Week?
A Manifestations.

Q London Fashion Week?
A Crumpets.

Q Paris Fashion Week?
A ART.

Q Your runway walk?
A Bold.

Q Fashion Week parties?
A G-string.

Q Castings?
A Stressorella.

Q Street style?
A Layering.

Q Heels?
A HOT!

Q Backstage?
A Sweating.

Q How do you calm your preshow nerves?
A Beta-blocker.

Q Your postshow mood?
A McDonald's.

Q Your dream designer?
A Tom Ford.

Q Your red carpet persona?
A Diva.

Q Rejections?
A Never heard of her.

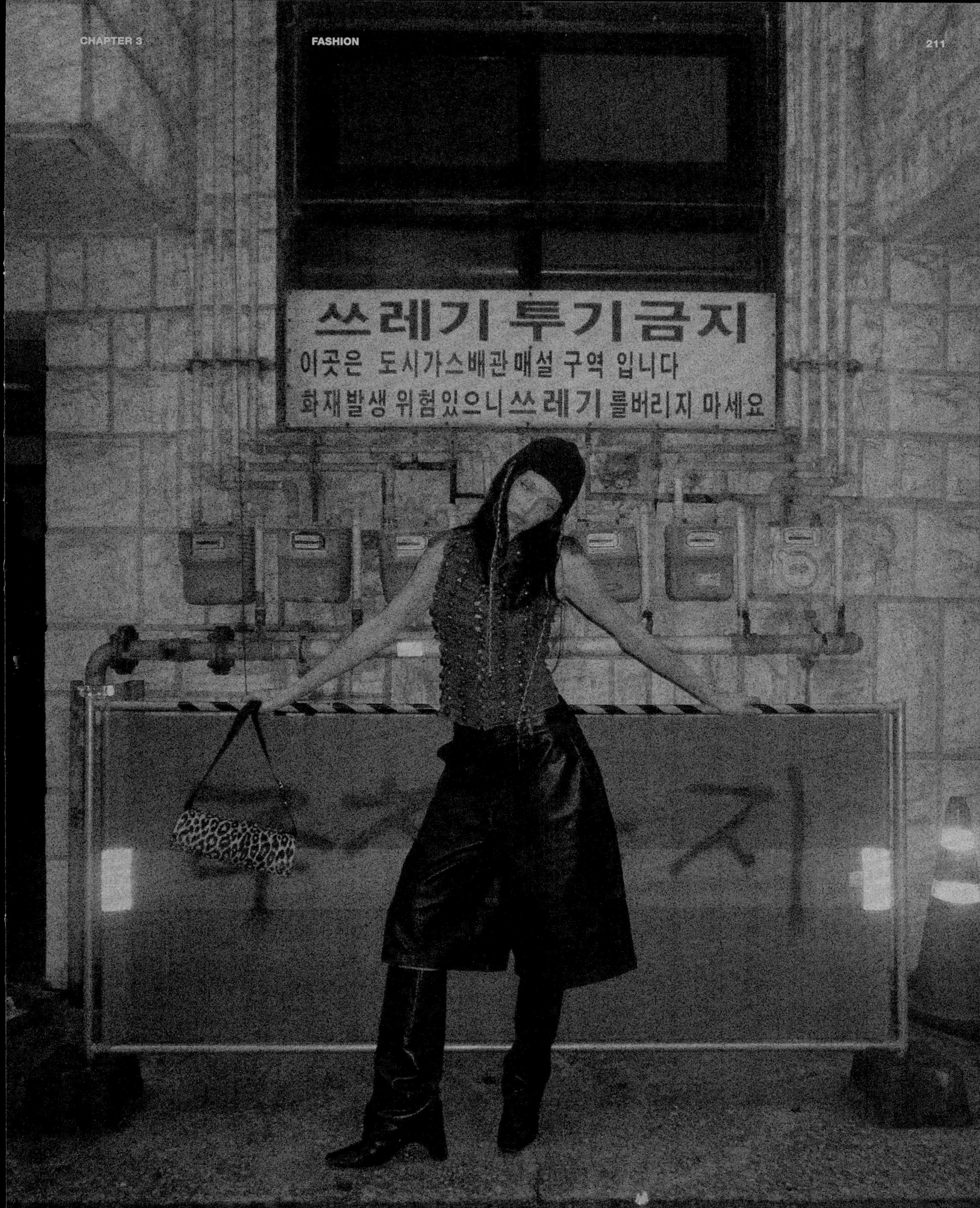
쓰레기 투기금지
이곳은 도시가스배관매설 구역 입니다
화재발생 위험있으니 쓰레기를버리지 마세요

Q Let's talk about your actual debut on the runway, which was for GCDS during Milan Fashion Week in September 2023.

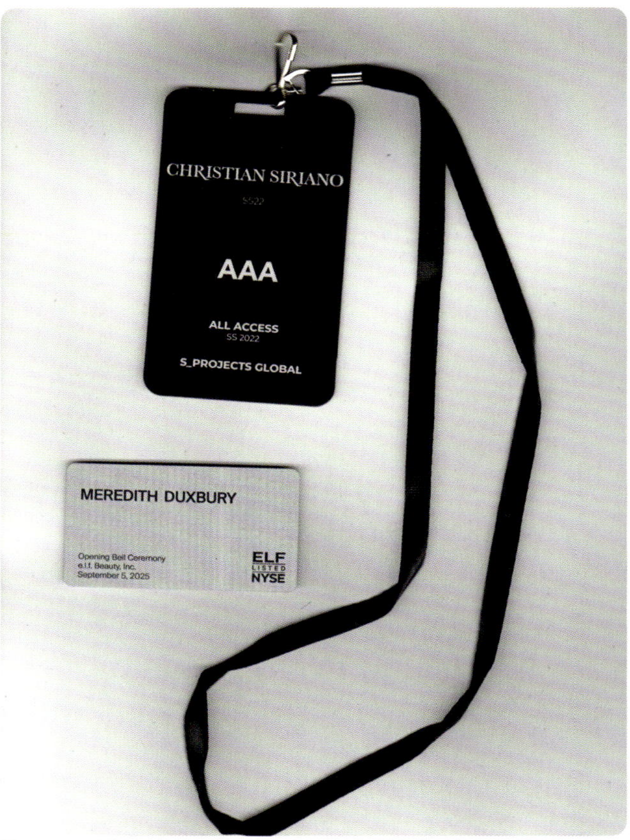

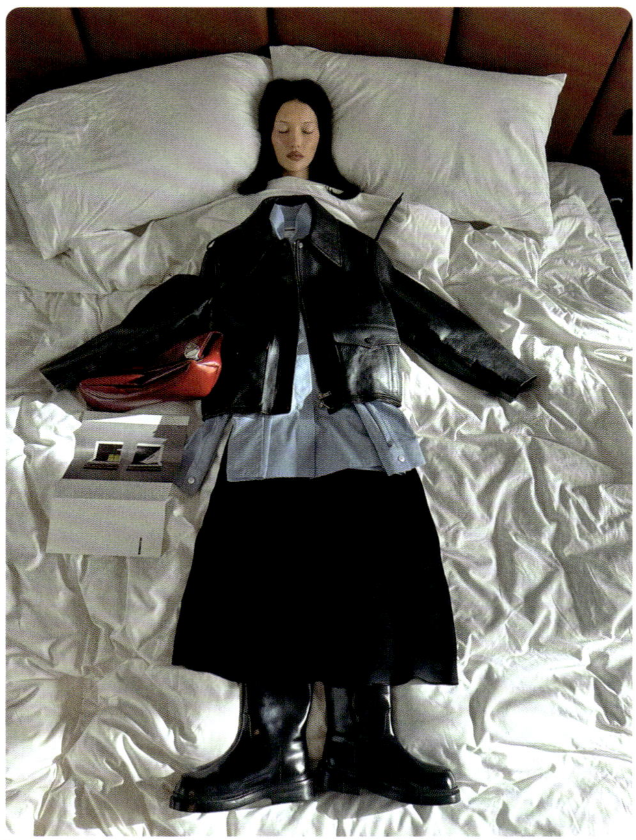

More fun trinkets from shows and events within fashion and beauty that I've attended! Always keep your souvenirs! To the right is the night before the Jil Sander show. I love jumping into fun fashion trends. It's important to have fun in the process of it all!

A I went in for the casting and did my walk for the team. They then started fitting me in different show looks. Giuliano Calza, the creative director, was like, "Whatever you feel comfortable in!" It was so nice to have that as my first runway experience, because ninety-nine percent of the time, you don't have a choice about what's comfortable or not.

Normally, I would leave a casting and be called back to do the fitting, but the design team started tailoring things to my body right away. At that point I thought to myself, "Am I confirmed for the show?!"

Q Who did you call or text when you first got the call?

A My manager and my agent. This has been a dream of ours that we've all been working toward. I dyed my hair red, cut my hair, stripped back the makeup, switched up my style of content...all to try and make this dream of modeling happen. There was a whole strategy, and to feel that all our efforts had finally paid off made me want to call the people who have been working so hard on this with me and just celebrate together.

Q What was the night before the show like for you?

A It was very, very nerve-racking. I have extreme presentation anxiety, and even though I wasn't speaking, I have really bad anxiety in big public-facing things and can get panic attacks. I had to take a beta-blocker that essentially stops the physical effects of panic, before I walked, because I knew I was not going to be able to breathe, and, of course, I wanted to walk my best

The minute that you're standing on the runway, you can see everyone sitting there. When it's your turn to walk, they tap your back and tell you to go. And then you just do it. You have to f***ing do it.

I pretty much blacked out because I had such bright lights in my face. I couldn't see anybody, which was sort of nice because I didn't see all the eyes on me. I just thought about my walk, my posture, and my pace because I had to make sure I kept up so there wouldn't be a large gap between the other models and me.

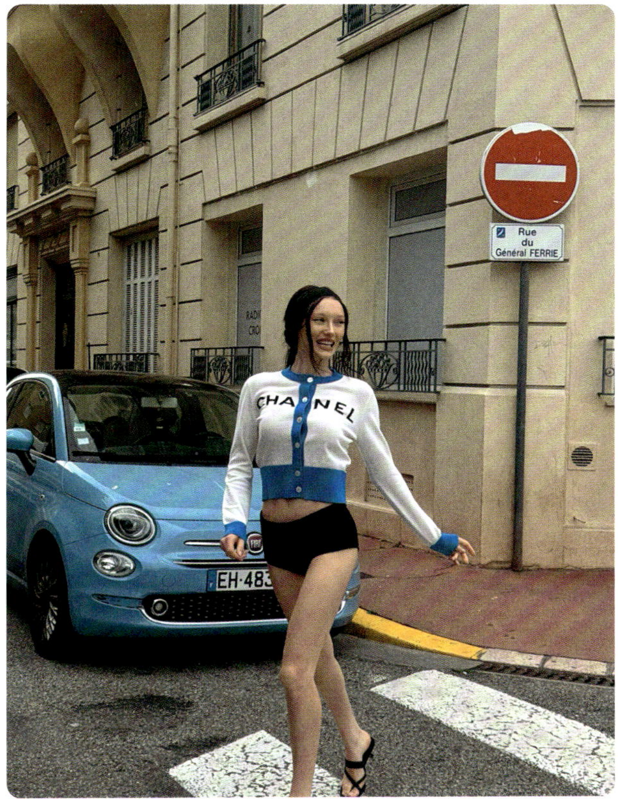

TOP: Chanel and the South of France are always a good combo!
BELOW: rhode always has the best photo booths.

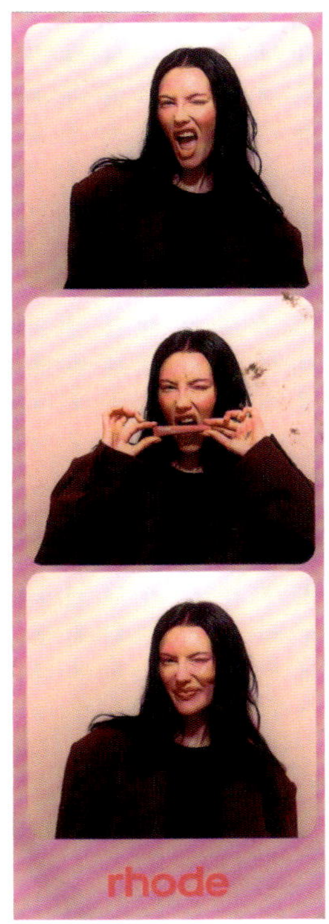

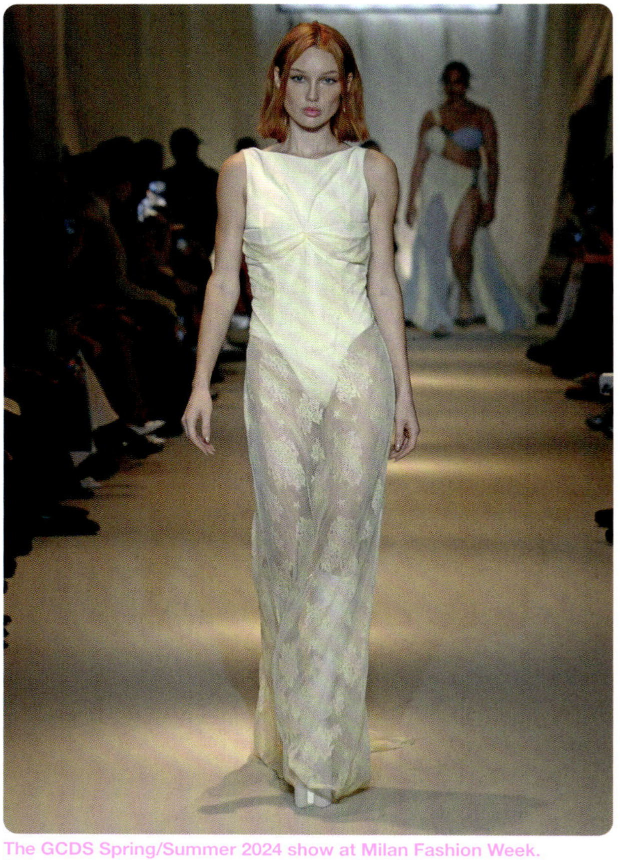

The GCDS Spring/Summer 2024 show at Milan Fashion Week. This was my first-ever runway show for GCDS! I remember being so nervous. I was in eight-inch heels with a lace-train dress.

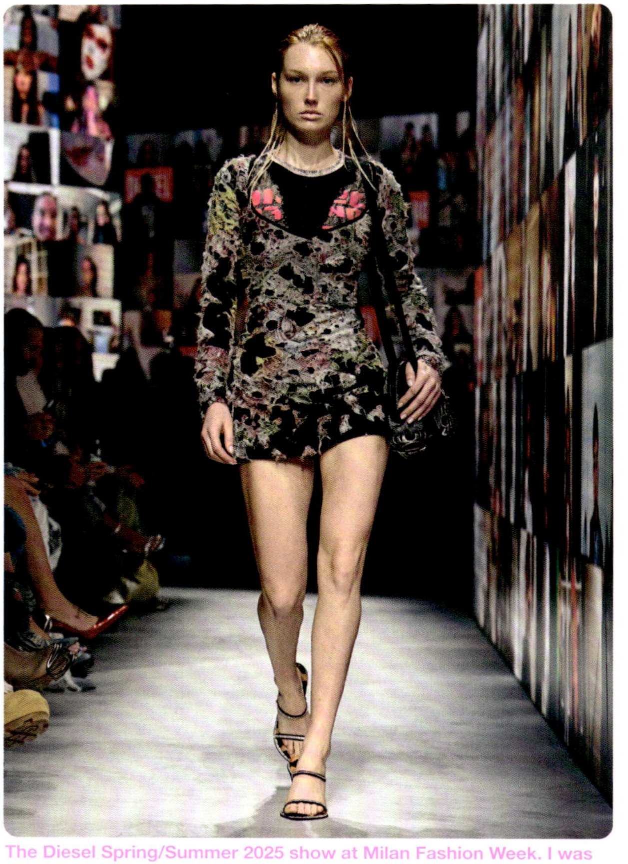

The Diesel Spring/Summer 2025 show at Milan Fashion Week. I was so nervous that my feet were sweating. I had to try my hardest to keep my heels from slipping off on the "runway."

I was listening to the soundtrack and thinking, "When you reach the photographers, that's the picture that is going to end up in *Vogue*, so give your fiercest face."

Q How did you celebrate after the show?

A We went to my favorite pizza restaurant in Milan called Le Specialità and had a bunch of pizzas and chilled. And then I probably called every single person in my family and recited the entire experience fifteen times.

Q Was your experience walking for Diesel the same sort of thing?

A For my second Diesel show, the runway floor was all shredded denim. There was no clear path for the runway, and I had big wedge shoes on that were so wobbly on that type of surface. I was wearing blue contacts, so I couldn't see a thing, and because the contacts covered my entire eyes, I couldn't see where I was walking, lol. It was the most difficult runway I've done, but it was just another challenge I had to overcome!

Q Let's talk about attending shows for a second. Do you remember the very first fashion show that you attended?

A It was Christian Siriano! I was invited to attend through Charlotte Tilbury and her team, who did the makeup backstage for the models. It was amazing to experience—especially after coming out of Covid isolation, when I was sitting in my room every day, doing makeup in my pj's alone.

Q Tell me what was going through your mind when you watched that show. Were you thinking, "I can't believe I'm here?"

A It was exciting just to see everything come to life: the soundtrack, the venue,

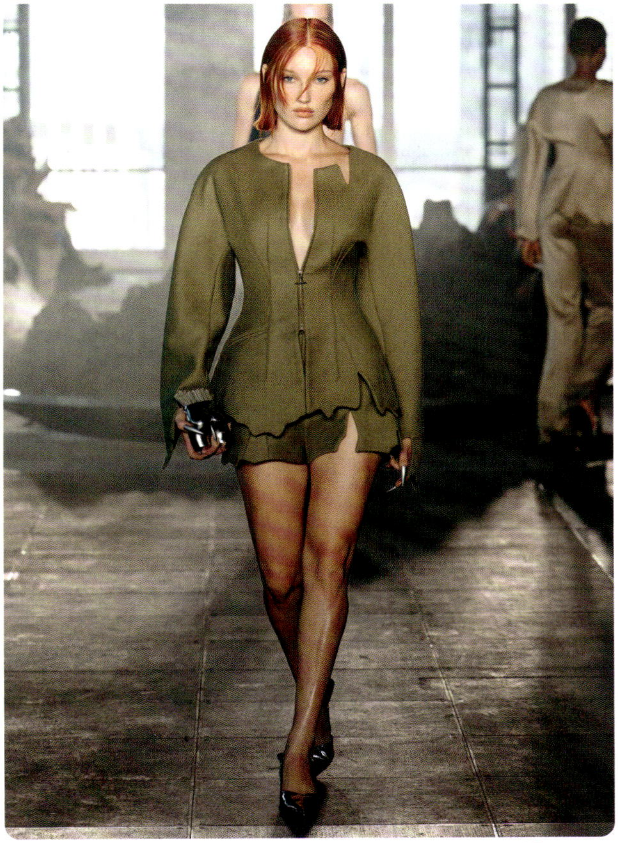

The Grace Ling Spring/Summer 2025 show at New York Fashion Week. Grace Ling has some of the most beautiful designs. I felt like a little Peter Pan in this outfit.

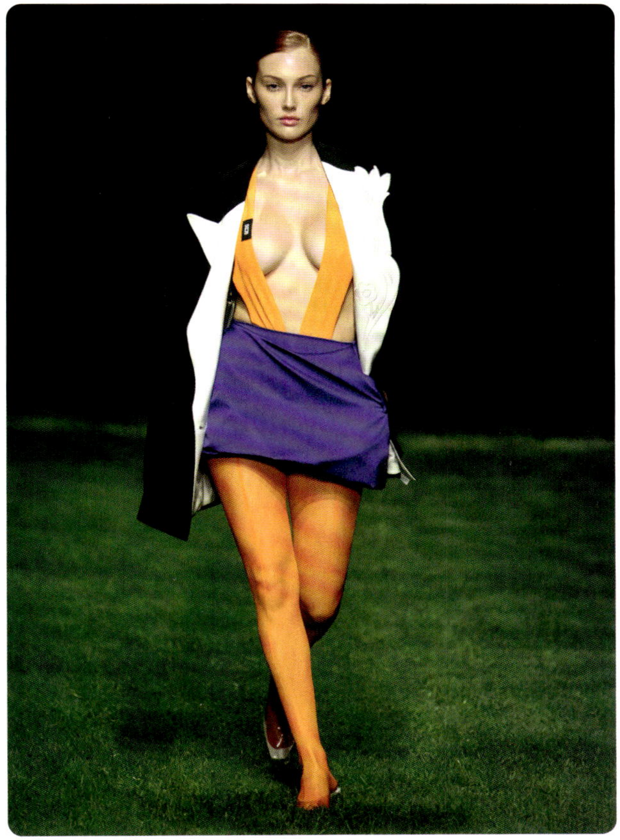

Another GCDS runway show! This one was the GCDS Spring/Summer 2025 show during Milan Fashion Week. How fun is this look! I remember having to tape my feet into my heels lol.

and then the models and the clothes come out. That's also when it sparked my love for modeling and wanting to get back into it.

When I saw the creative director, Glenn Martens, run out at the end, I was in awe that someone had come up with all of this and put their creative ideas into the whole collection. It was very inspiring.

Q You have been to so many fashion shows since. Tell me about a couple of the memorable ones.

A There are so many: Versace, Valentino, Marc Jacobs. Versace is a really fun one for me because it's such an iconic fashion house that can be edgy, fun, yet elevated. That's kind of how I describe my own personal style: edgy and elevated. They also embraced me early into my fashion journey, which I'll always appreciate.

Pat McGrath also does the makeup for the Versace show, so it brings together my two worlds! I love getting to see Pat backstage and admire her amazing work on the models before they go down the runway. She's done my makeup for those shows, too, sending her team beforehand with a look inspired by the show, so that's been a real pinch-me moment.

When attending shows, I always find it special to go into the showrooms, meet the teams, and be dressed by the brand. It's really such an honor. For Mugler Spring/Summer 2026, it was Miguel Castro Freitas's debut show as the new creative director. The collection drew from a lot of archival references. They had a look specifically set aside for me that I loved.

My first Valentino show was very memorable. I loved my outfit. I loved my hair. The collection was beautiful. I think it was the last collection shown by Pierpaolo Piccioli, the creative director at the time.

Q What was working with Pat McGrath like?

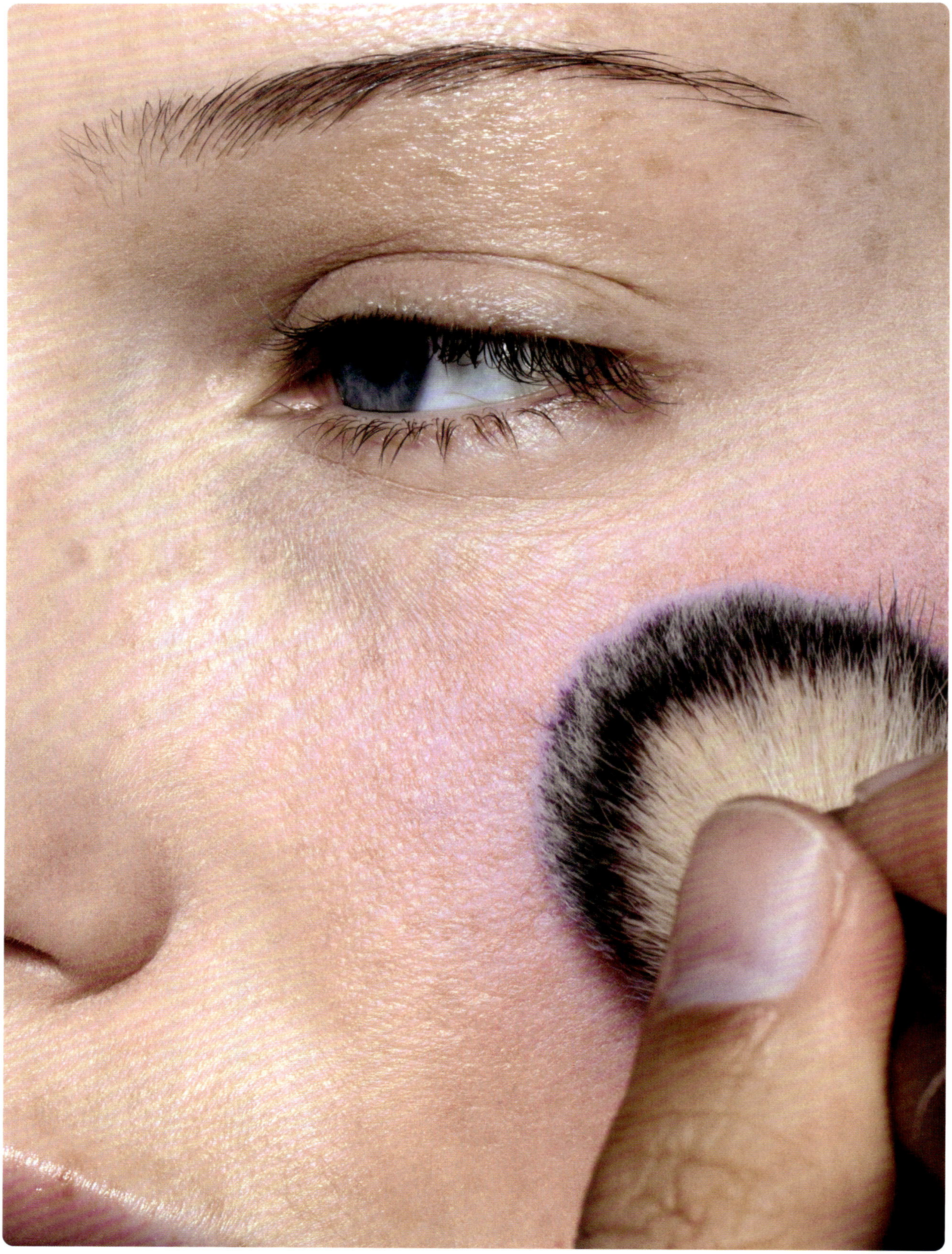

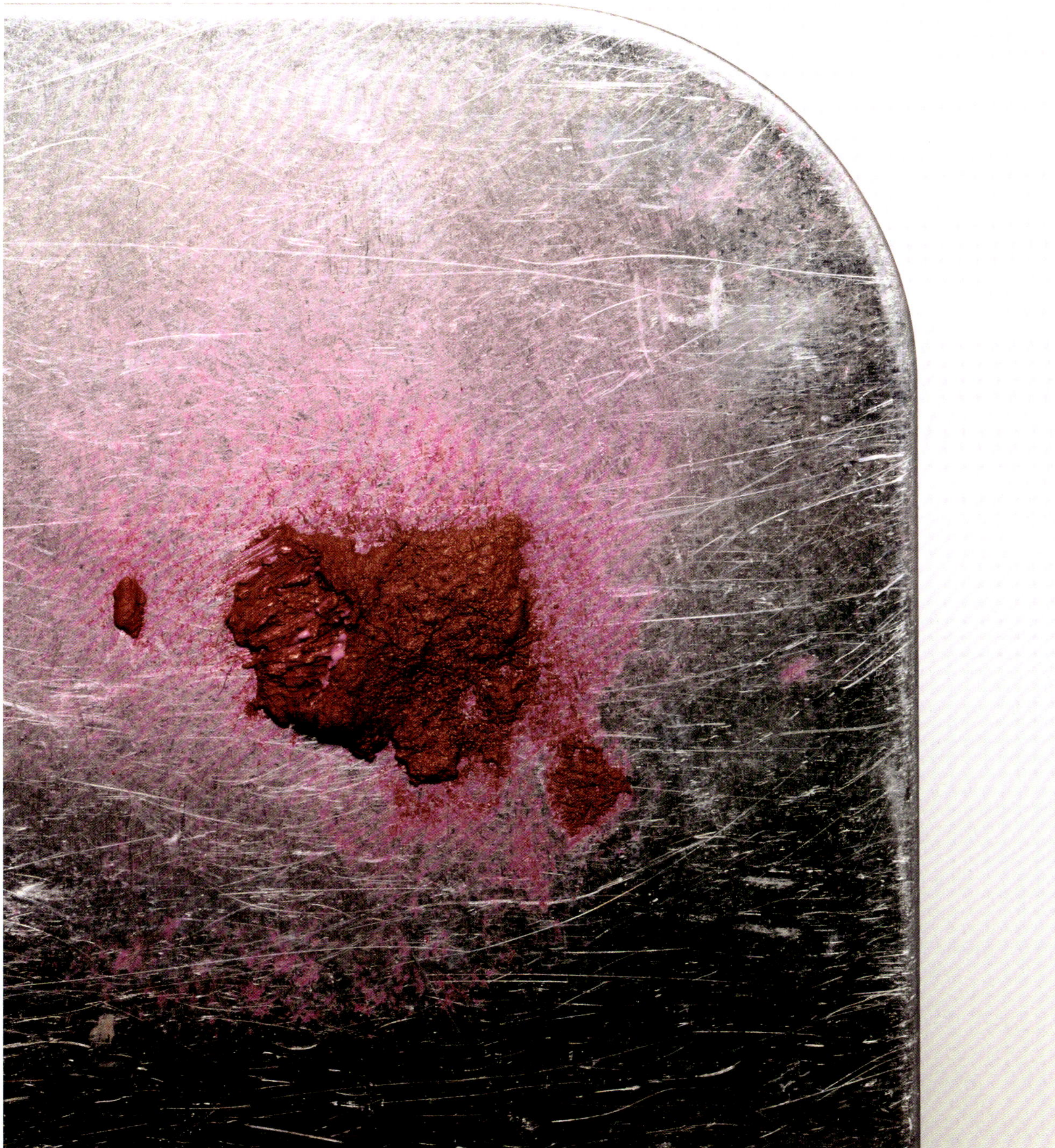

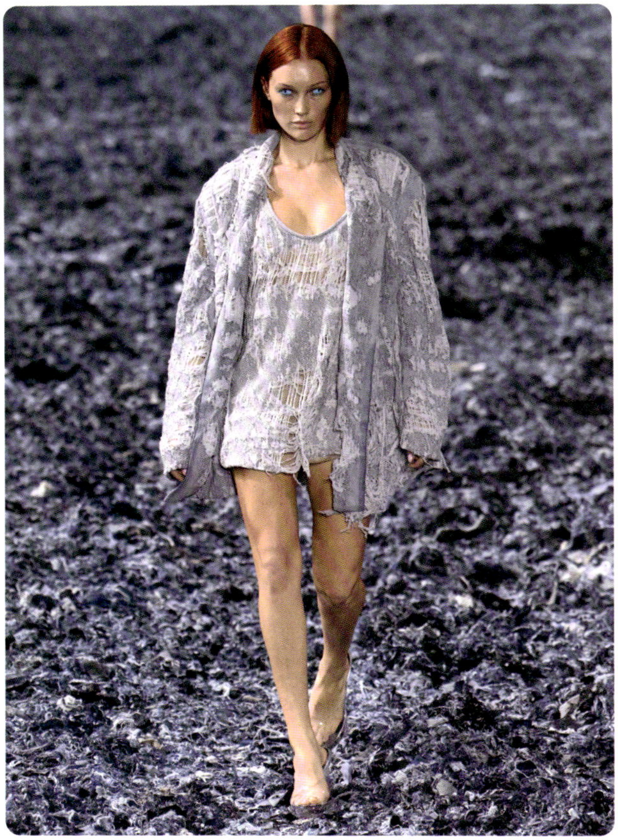

The Diesel Fall/Winter 2024 at Milan Fashion Week. I will say this was one of the most difficult runways I've ever walked. I couldn't see a thing with the colored contacts that they had us wearing, and there wasn't a clear path for the runway because of the ripped denim, so my walk was all from memory of our walkthrough.

A Incredible. First of all, she is the sweetest person ever and has been a mentor to me. She is so creative, and her team is so amazing. Everyone is professional but has fun at the same time. It was nice to see the whole vision come together and have her be a part of it.

Q Tell me about some memorable moments walking on red carpets.

A One of the most memorable was attending the Cannes Film Festival with L'Oréal. Chopard dressed me in beautiful diamonds. I wore a beautiful white gown with a structural waist detail. I loved it.

Q Tell me about your personal style now, because you've talked about its evolution.

A My personal style is elevated, edgy, and chic. Gucci, Chloé, Isabel Marant, Yves Saint Laurent, and Tom Ford really resonate with me. It's nice to have that chic, elevated aspect, but, at the same time, I like to play with color and textures and make it a little undone and messy.

I love the bohemian look. I've also been really inspired by the sixties vibes. It's really fun to bring that type of makeup into the look as well. A little bit of grunginess. I would say that's my personal style.

At first, I was super stripped back, and I really felt that neutrals and very minimal textures were my style because I thought that's what I had to show people for them to see me in a different light. They wanted to see Meredith stripped back, but that's not what I like. This is what I like. And now I feel like I can dress how I want, have my style, and have brands appreciate that—maybe even more so.

Q Is there a collection or a designer whose work has made you rethink your personal style or made you want to try something new?

A I would say Tom Ford has me wanting to try something new because I feel their new collections do a really great job of playing with color in a very elevated way. It resonates with me because I had a really hard time bringing my glam and my color into the fashion industry in a way that was accepted. I feel like Tom Ford brings color in so elegantly, and it inspired me to be able to wear color again!

Q Tell me about a show you are manifesting next, both to walk and then just to attend.

A I would love to walk Miu Miu and attend Saint Laurent.

Q Do you approach fashion the same way that you do makeup, which is kind of a go-big-or-go-home mentality?

A There's a time and place for everything, so if it feels like that fits with the brand's identity and aesthetic, then yes! But there are times when you may want to be more low-key and chill with your look, depending on the event or show as well.

Q Have you ever worn an outfit that was really uncomfortable, but you wore it anyway because it looked good?

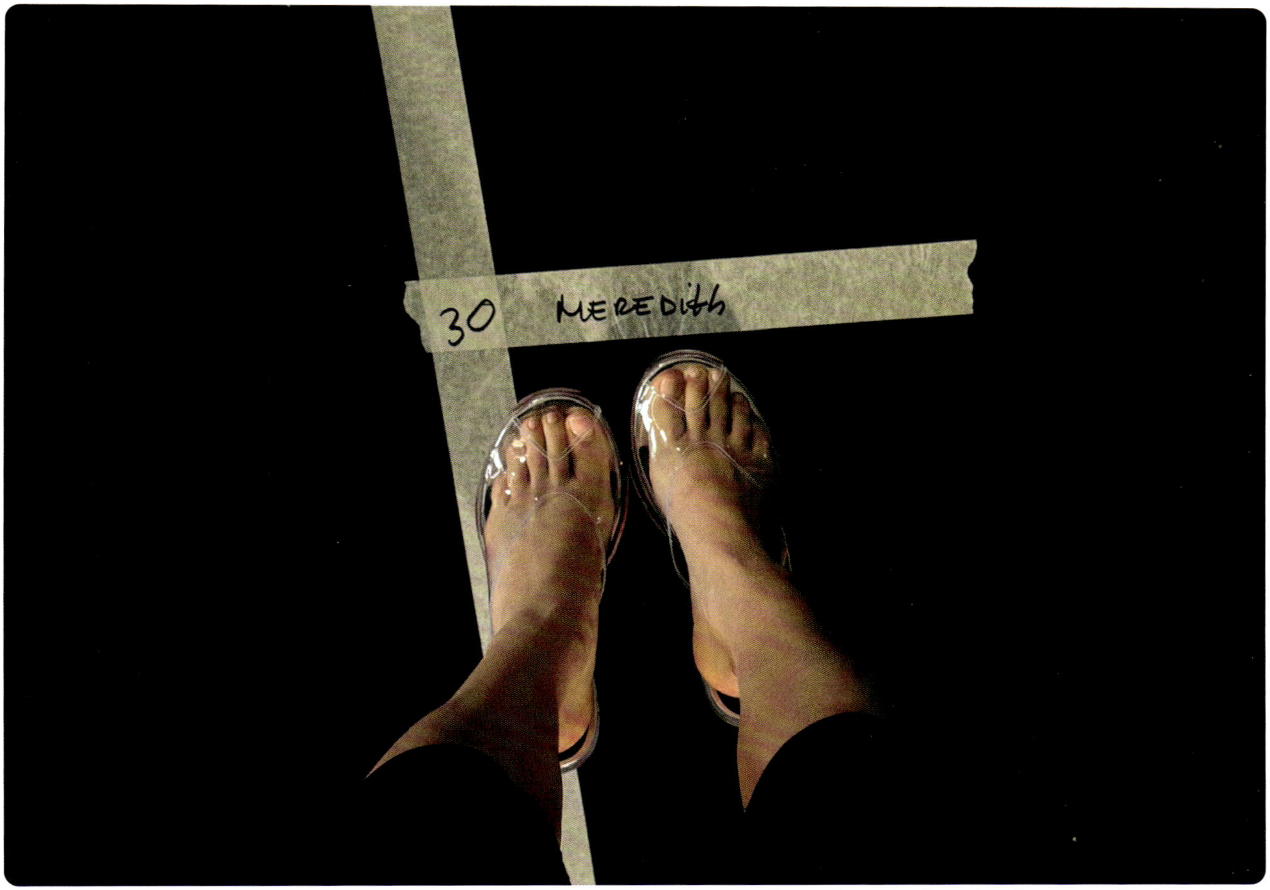

TOP: This is before we did our walk-through for the Diesel runway show. They had us all line up by our look number. I love snapping these quick pics when I'm backstage because it brings me back to the moment and all the emotions I was feeling at the time when I look at them afterward.
BELOW: The backstage board with all the runway models and their corresponding show looks. I was look number 27 for the GCDS runway show that I walked in Milan. My first show ever for GCDS!

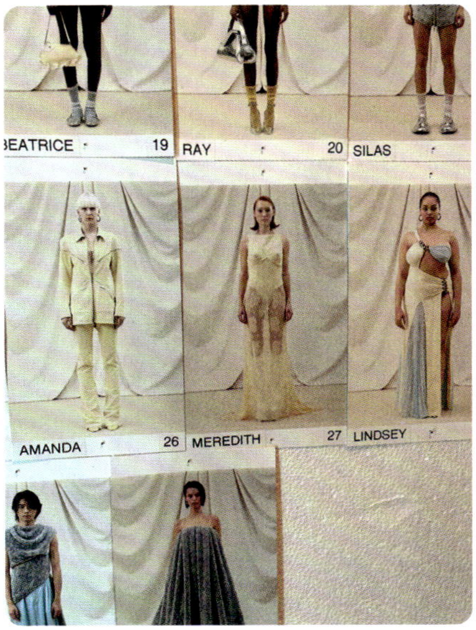

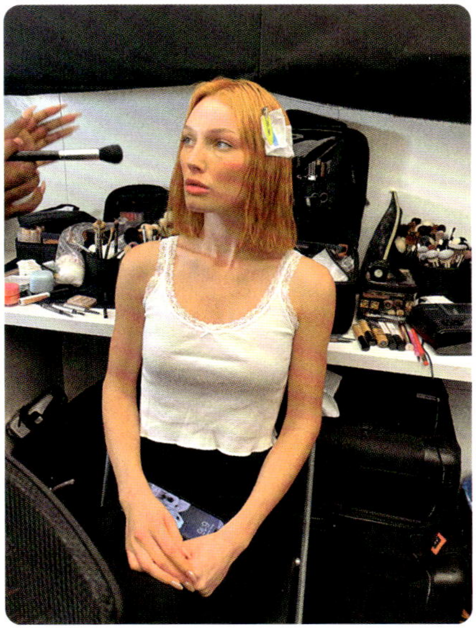

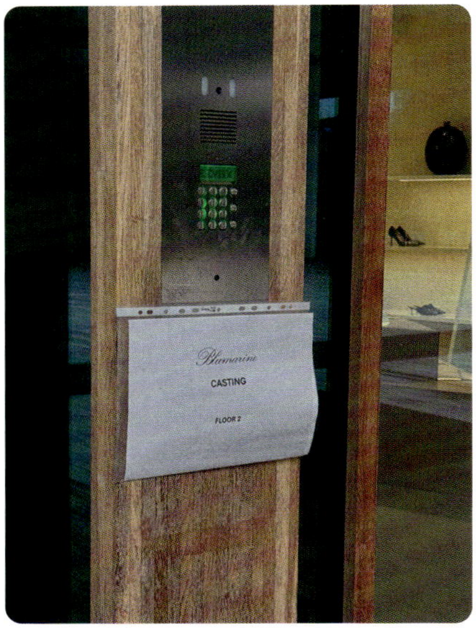
Blumarine
CASTING
FLOOR 2

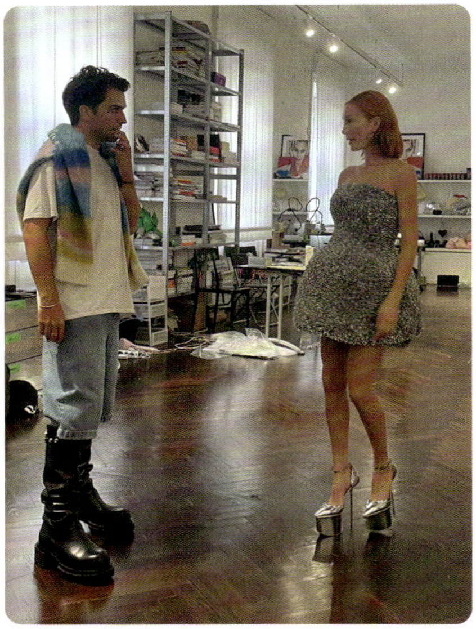

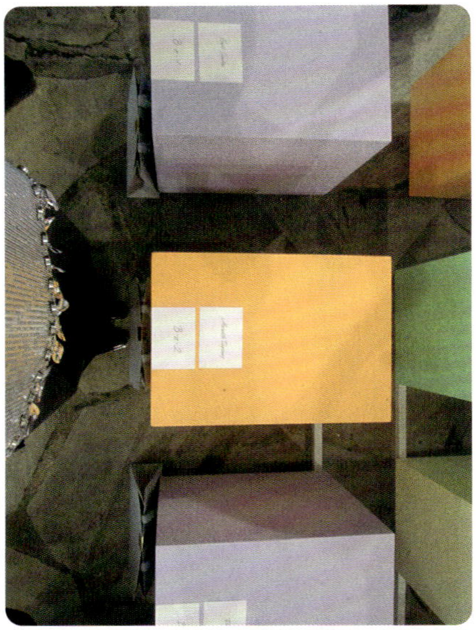

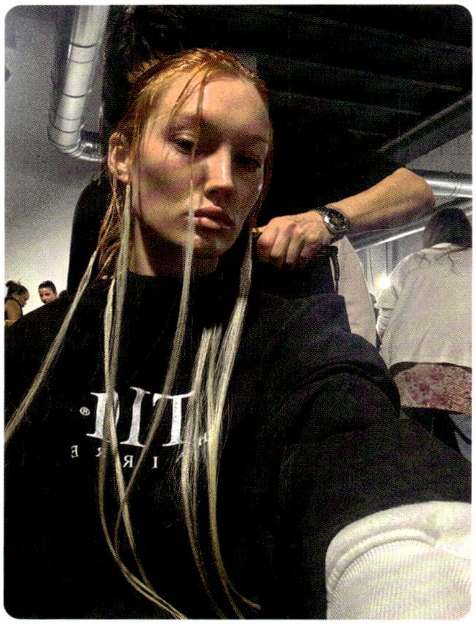

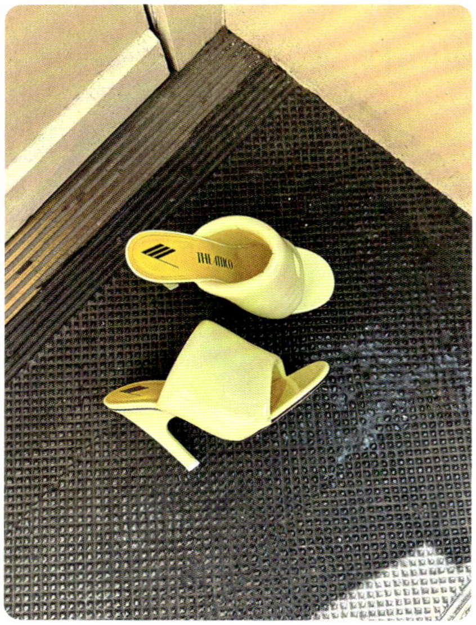

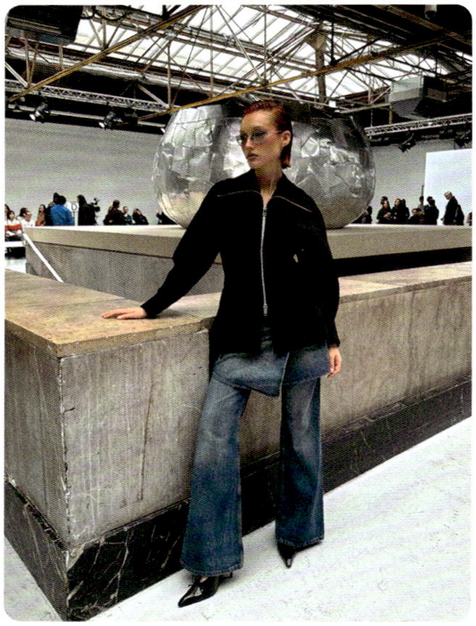

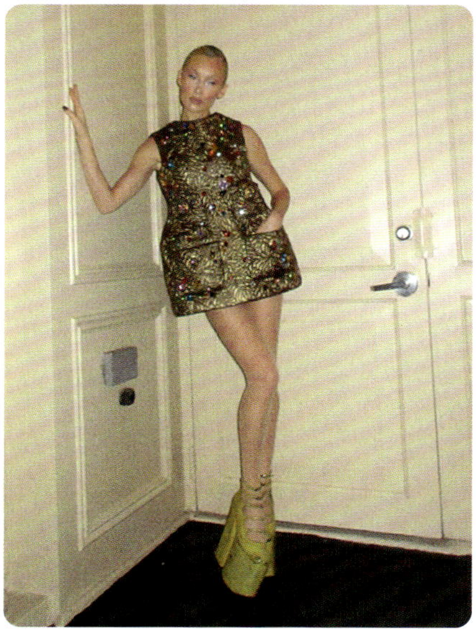

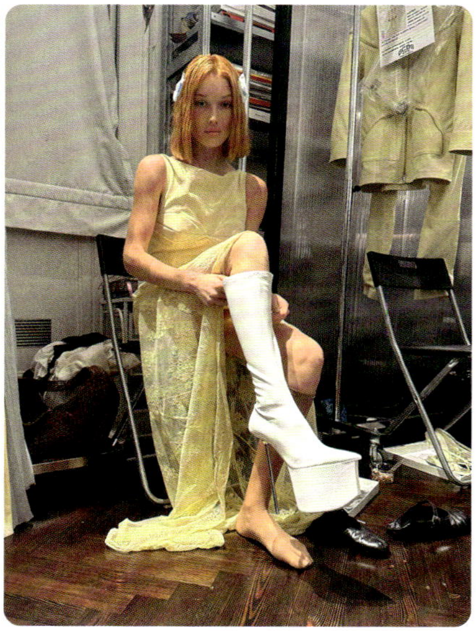

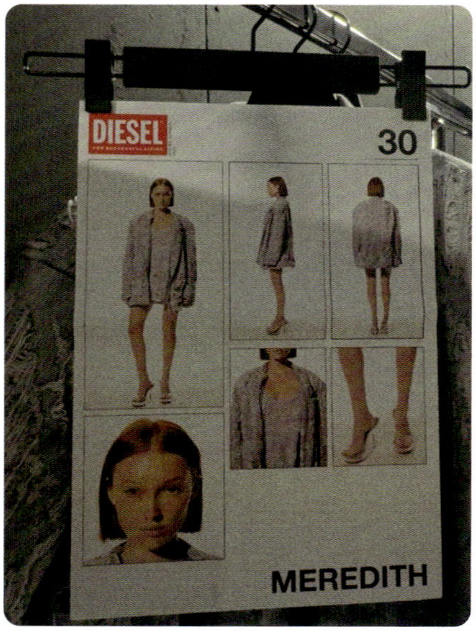
DIESEL
30
MEREDITH

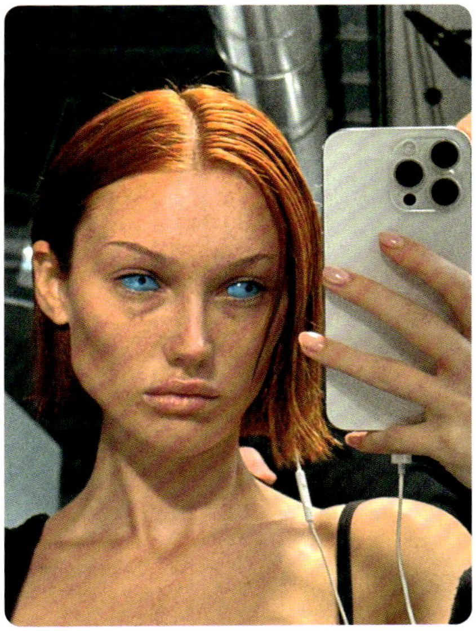

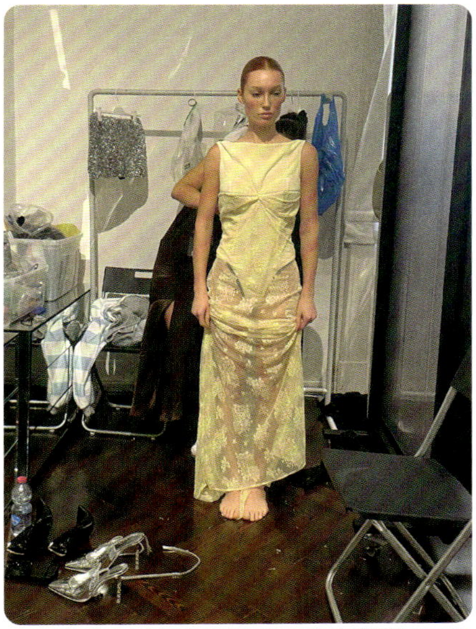

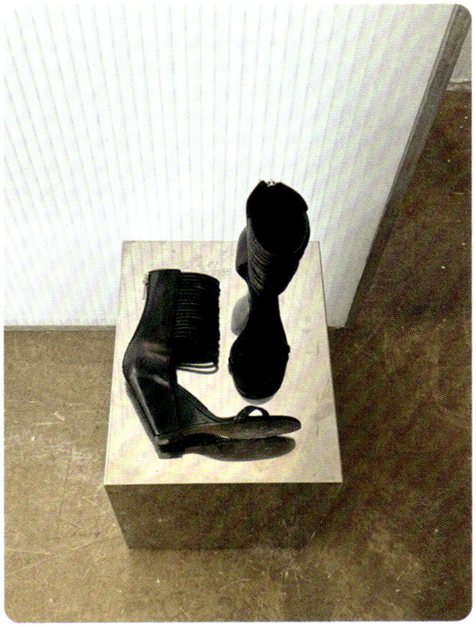

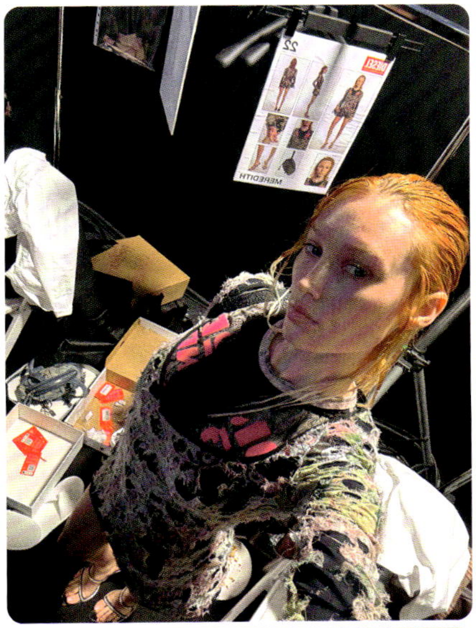

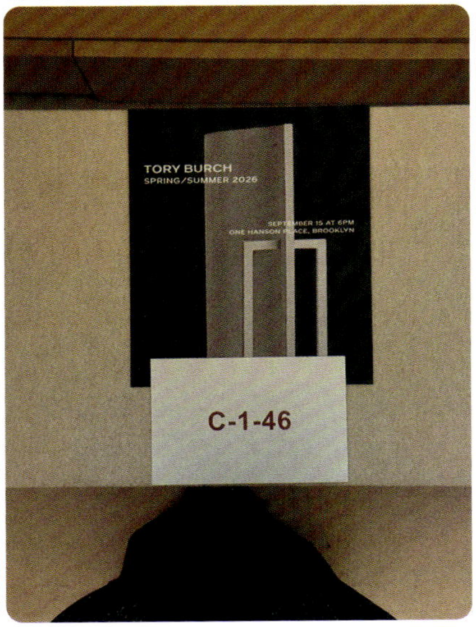
TORY BURCH
SPRING/SUMMER 2026
SEPTEMBER 15 AT 6PM
ONE HANSON PLACE, BROOKLYN
C-1-46

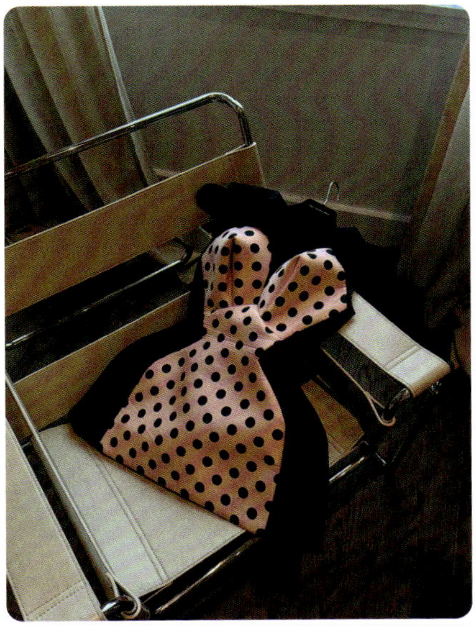

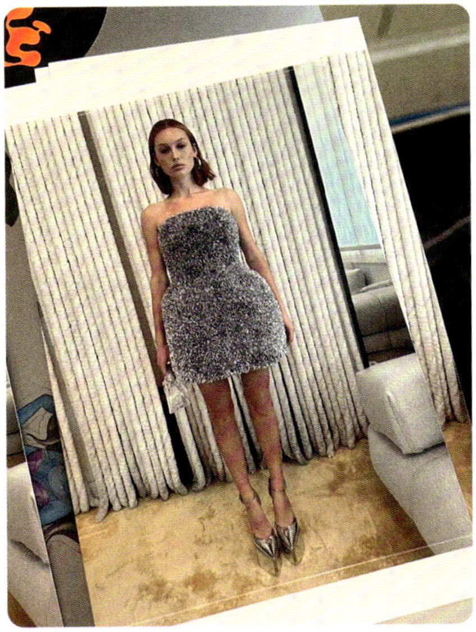

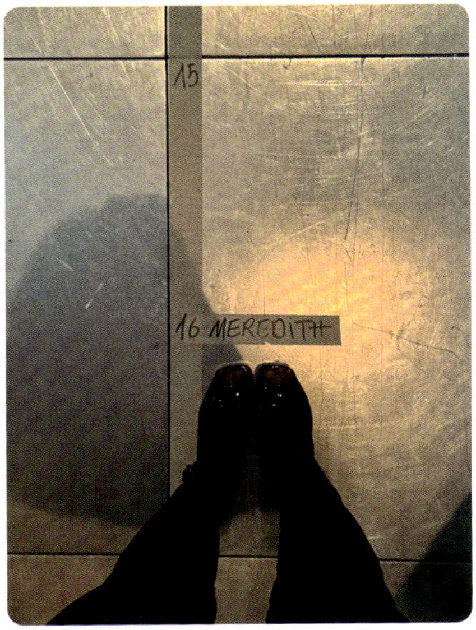
15
16 MEREDITH

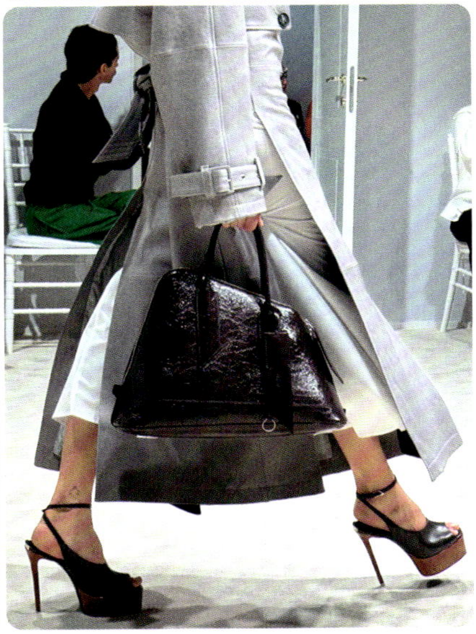

“I THINK IT’S GREAT TO BE A CHAMELEON, BUT IT SHOULD ALWAYS COME BACK TO YOU IN THE END”

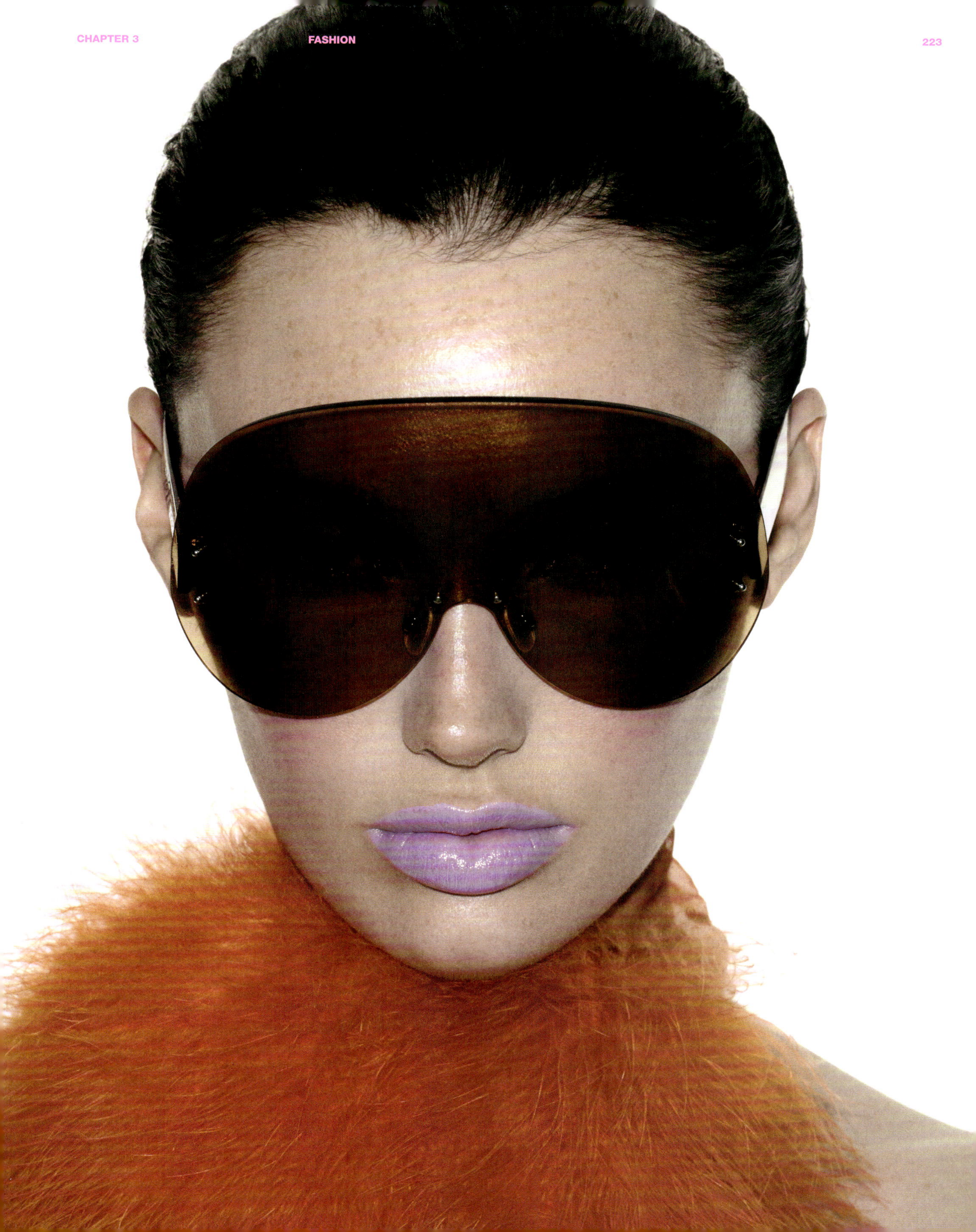

A Of course! I'm so there to have a snatched corset or a shoe two sizes too small if it looks *amazing*. But, for me, comfort comes from how I personally feel about my confidence. I ask myself, "Is this something I would truly wear? Is this something that fits with my personal style and my branding?" If not, I don't want to wear it. I think it's great to be a chameleon, but it should always come back to you in the end.

Q Do you have a name for your current fashion era, or are you still figuring that out?

A Personally, my personal style is always evolving, so I stay away from putting myself in a certain category. But I will say some key words are playful, messy, and colorful!

Q So, how many eras have you had?

A There are too many to count, lol.

Q Are there any eras that you wish hadn't happened, or that you pretend didn't happen?

A I mean, technically, yes, but I will never go back and change anything because it made me who I am today. If I hadn't gone through those eras, maybe I wouldn't have fully explored all my styles and been able to find the one that fits me best now. So, yeah, I look back, and I question why I wore certain things, but it's all part of the process.

Q Who are some other style icons that you look up to?

A Recently, it has been Margot Robbie on her press tour for *Wuthering Heights*. I love how she's playing around with different silhouettes and taking risks within fashion! To me, that's the most inspiring. I like to see someone take a risk and wear something that they wouldn't normally wear!

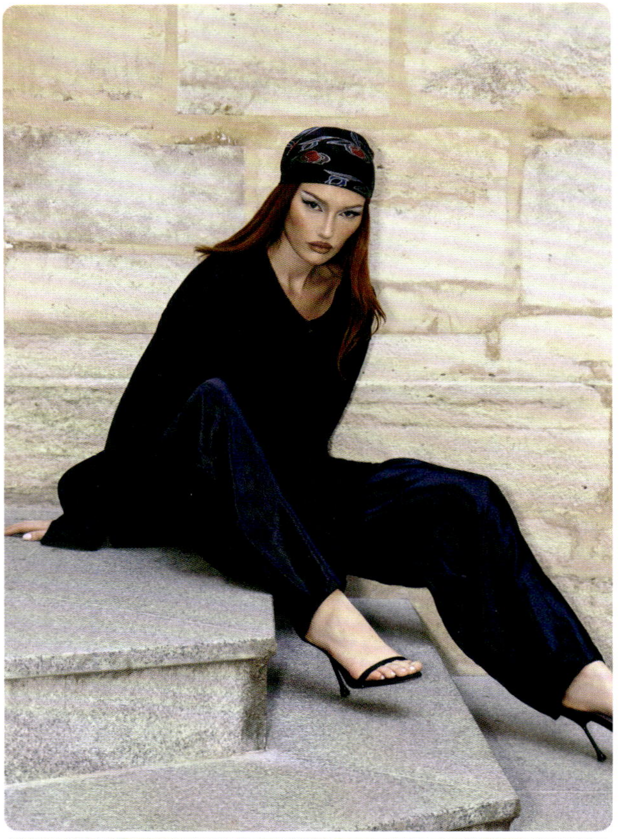

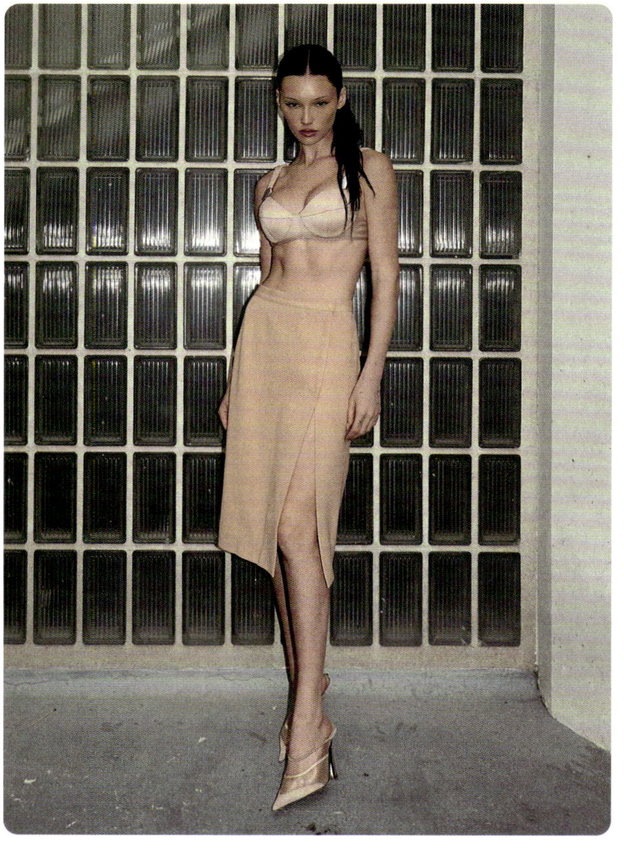

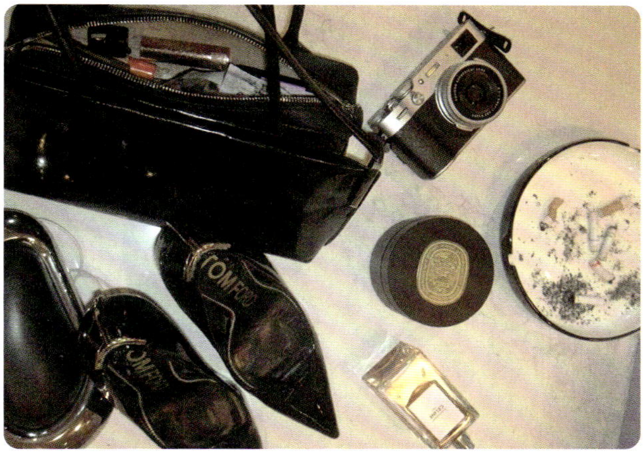

I'm just a girl, lol.

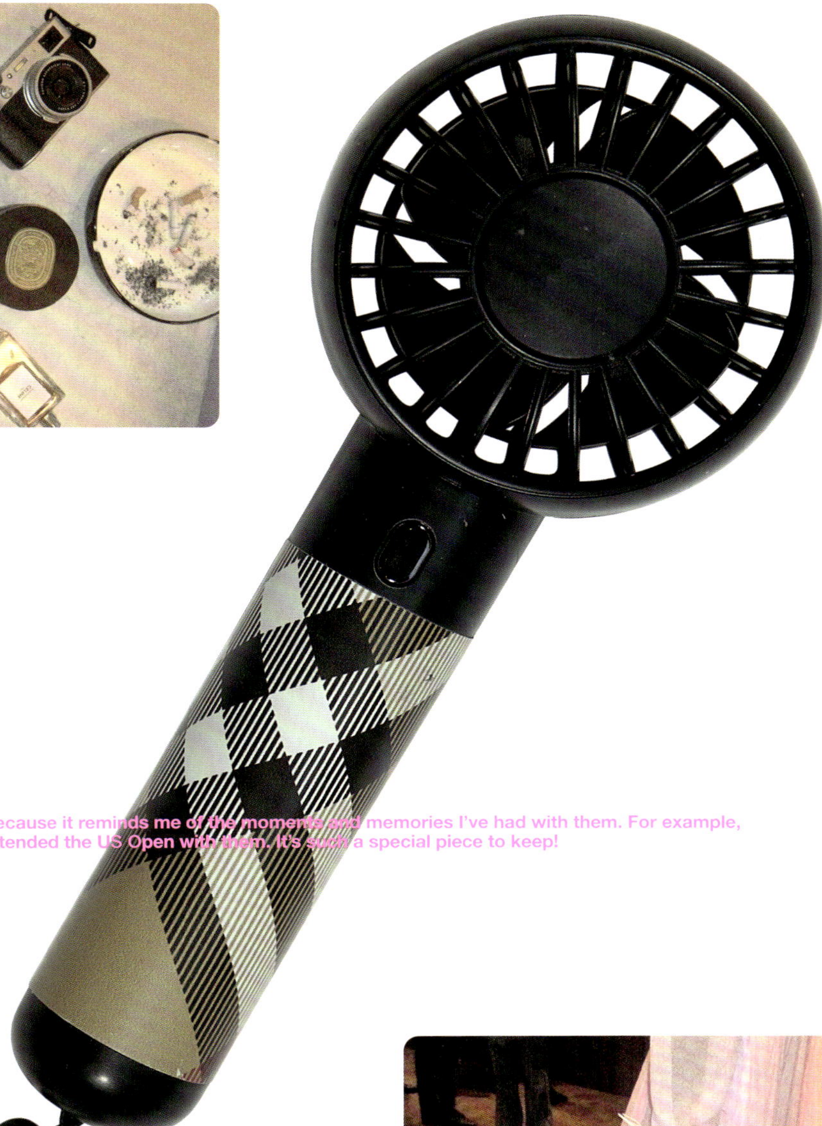

I love keeping special giftings from brands because it reminds me of the moments and memories I've had with them. For example, this Burberry fan was gifted to me before I attended the US Open with them. It's such a special piece to keep!

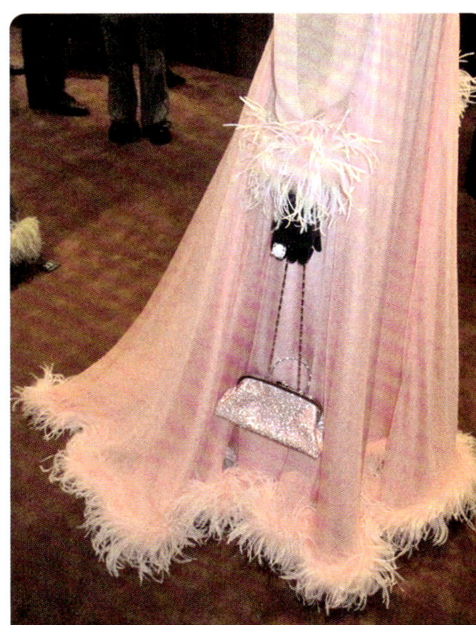

Demna's debut collection for Gucci. Need I say anything else? Iconic!

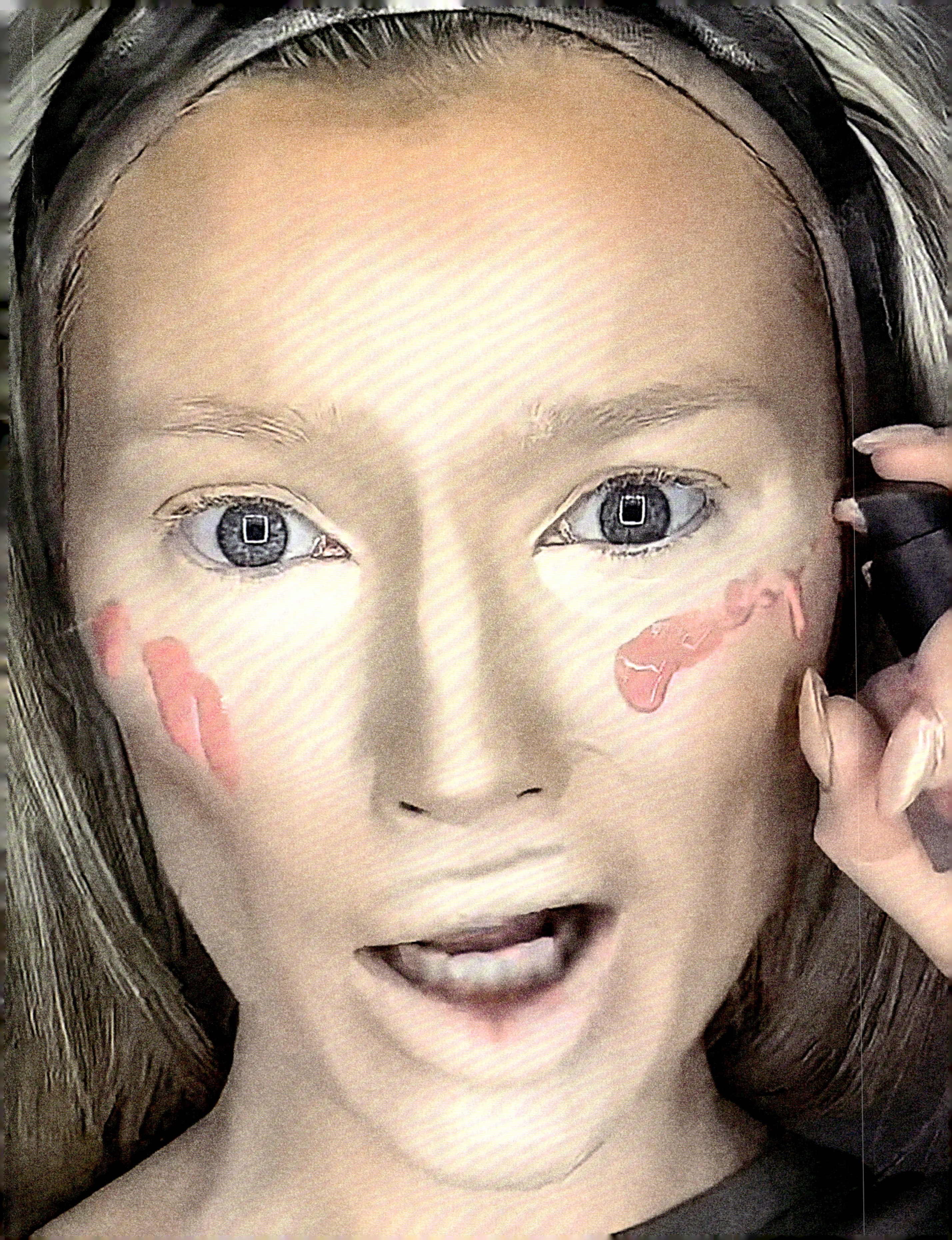

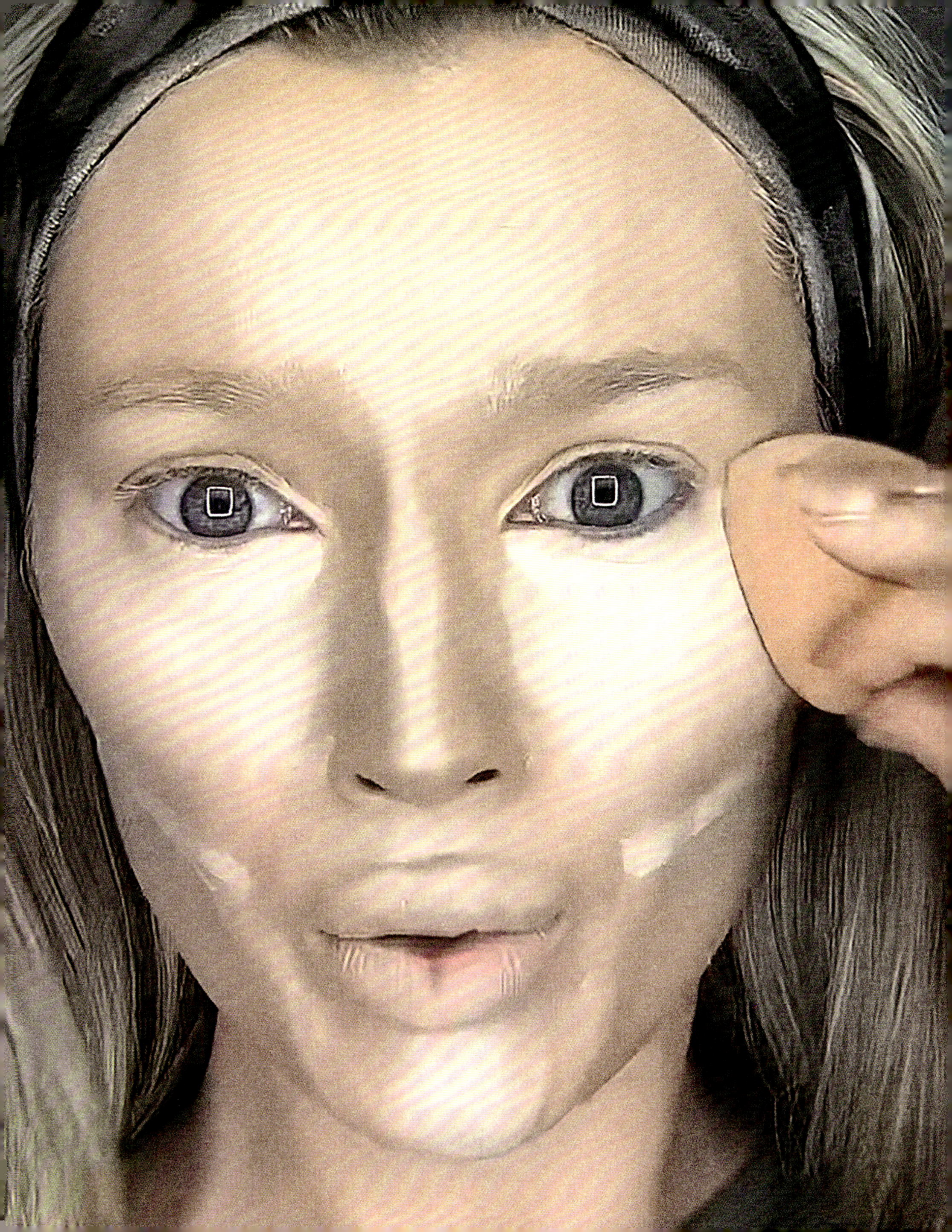

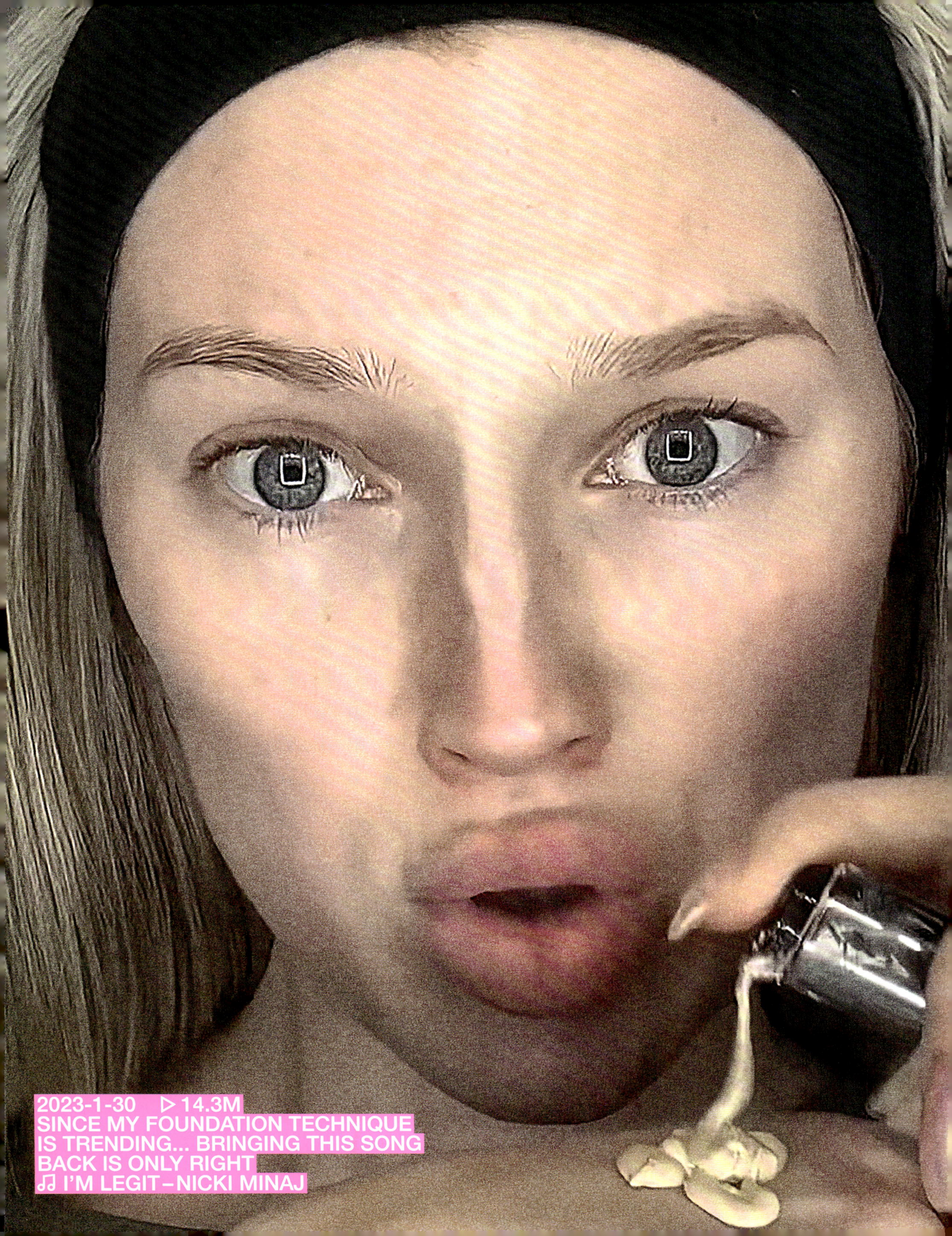
2023-1-30 ▷ 14.3M
SINCE MY FOUNDATION TECHNIQUE
IS TRENDING... BRINGING THIS SONG
BACK IS ONLY RIGHT
♫ I'M LEGIT–NICKI MINAJ

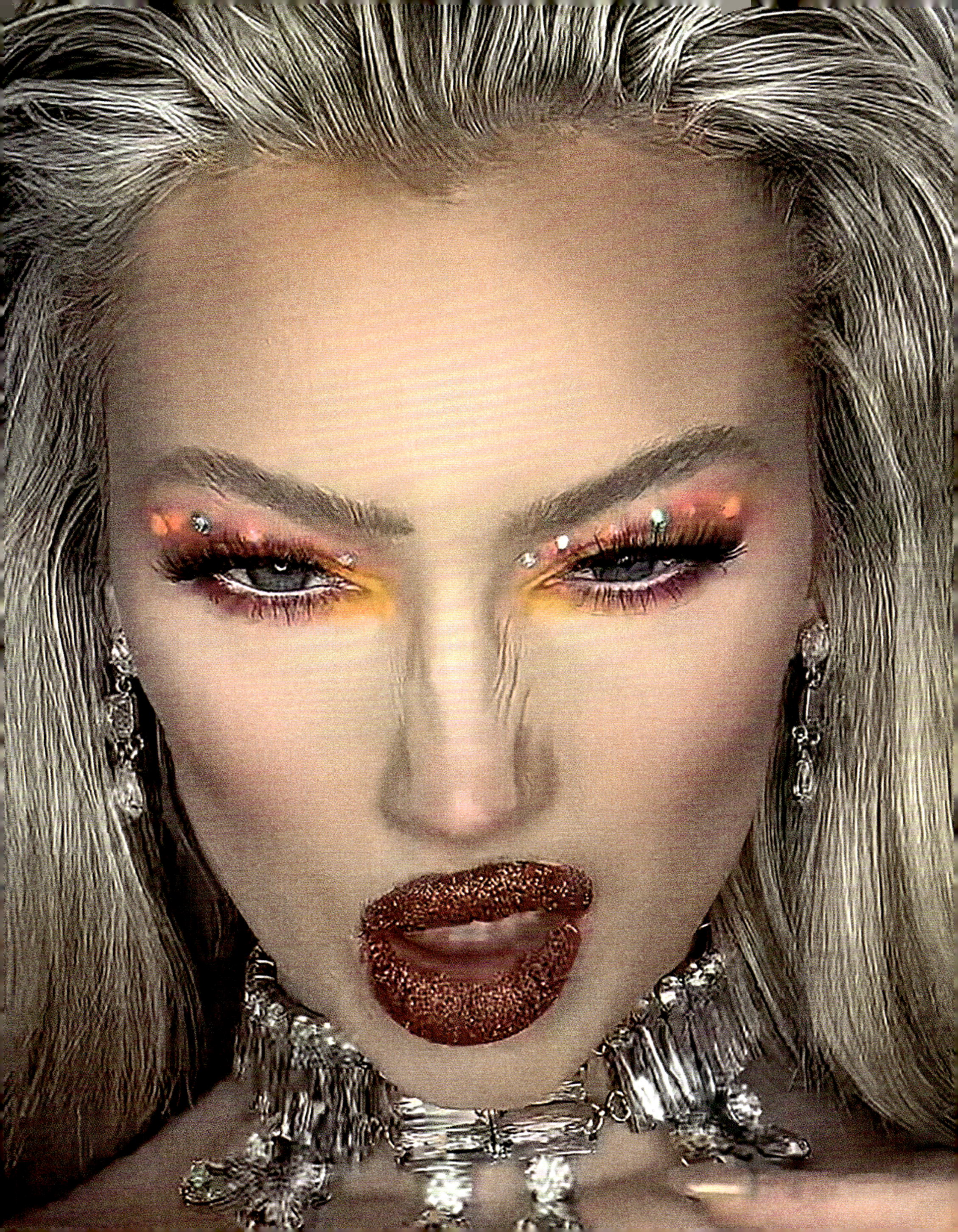

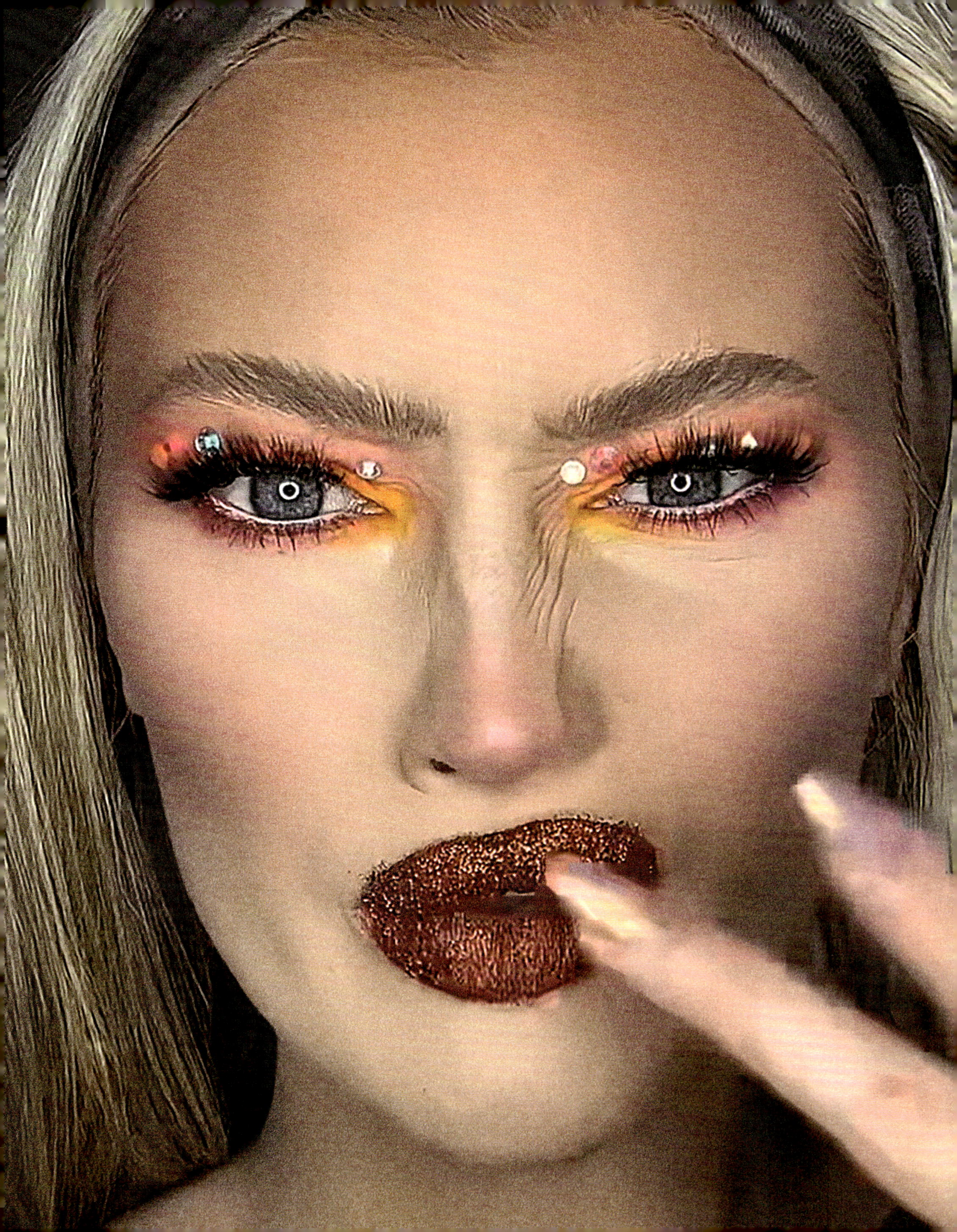

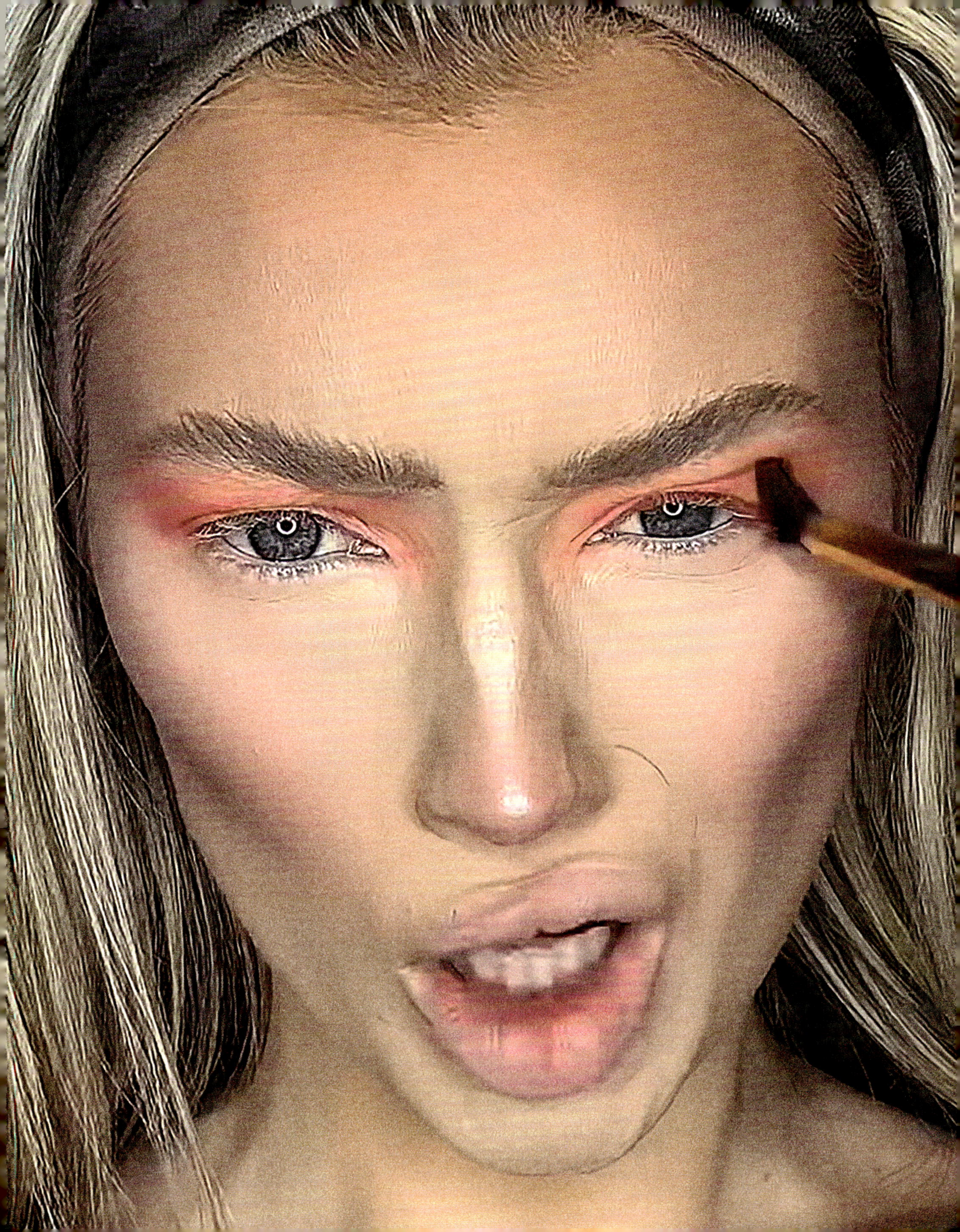

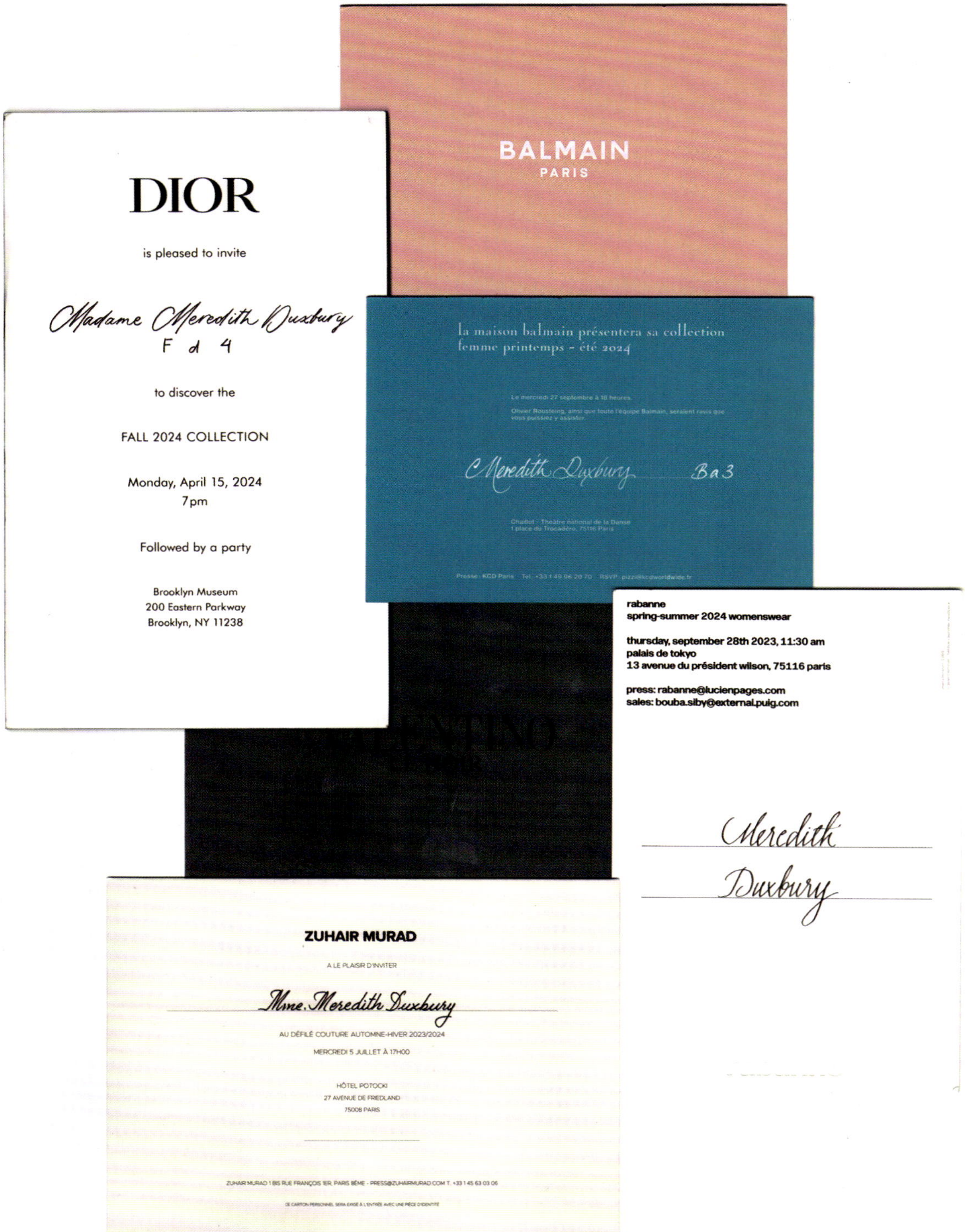
BALMAIN
PARIS
DIOR
is pleased to invite
Madame Meredith Duxbury
F d 4
to discover the
FALL 2024 COLLECTION
Monday, April 15, 2024
7pm
Followed by a party
Brooklyn Museum
200 Eastern Parkway
Brooklyn, NY 11238
la maison balmain présentera sa collection
femme printemps - été 2024
Le mercredi 27 septembre à 18 heures.
Olivier Rousteing, ainsi que toute l'équipe Balmain, seraient ravis que vous puissiez y assister.
Meredith Duxbury Ba 3
Chaillot - Théâtre national de la Danse
1 place du Trocadéro, 75116 Paris
rabanne
spring-summer 2024 womenswear
thursday, september 28th 2023, 11:30 am
palais de tokyo
13 avenue du président wilson, 75116 paris
press: rabanne@lucienpages.com
sales: bouba.siby@external.puig.com
Meredith
Duxbury
ZUHAIR MURAD
A LE PLAISIR D'INVITER
Mme. Meredith Duxbury
AU DÉFILÉ COUTURE AUTOMNE-HIVER 2023/2024
MERCREDI 5 JUILLET À 17H00
HÔTEL POTOCKI
27 AVENUE DE FRIEDLAND
75008 PARIS

I try to keep every show invitation I receive. It's so surreal to me to have such established, well-respected brands send me personal invitations to their runway shows. This industry is so fast-paced that it can often be hard to stop and take a moment to acknowledge all your accomplishments. Looking at these mementos helps me to remind myself of that.

JIL SANDER

Meredith Duxbury A65

SPRING/SUMMER 2026 WOMEN'S AND MEN'S COLLECTION
WEDNESDAY 24 SEPTEMBER 2025 10:30 AM
VIA LUCA BELTRAMI 5, MILANO

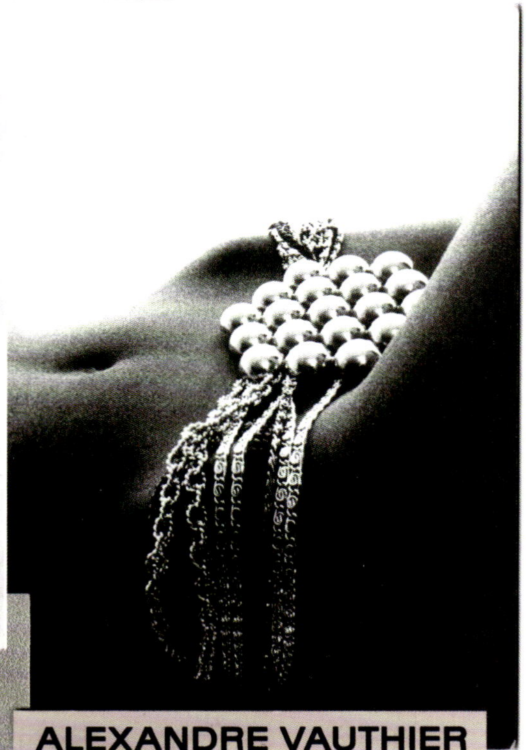

GIORGIO ARMANI

invites

Meredith Duxbury

to celebrate the opening of

ARMANI / MADISON AVENUE

Giorgio Armani Women's
Spring/Summer 2025 Collection
Thursday, October 17th
7 PM Show — 9 PM Party

Park Avenue Armory
643 Park Ave, New York

Black Tie

Seat number
J30

ALEXANDRE VAUTHIER

PRIE : Madame Meredith Duxbury Aa40

D'ASSISTER AU DÉFILÉ

HAUTE COUTURE HIVER 2023

AU PALAIS DE TOKYO

13 AVENUE DU PRÉSIDENT WILSON
75116 PARIS

LE

MARDI 4 JUILLET 2023—16H30

RSVP
ALEXANDREVAUTHIER@BPCM.COM — ALEXANDREVAUTHIER@PRCONSULTINGPARIS.NET
REBECA@ALEXANDREVAUTHIER.COM

MAISON VALENTINO A LE PLAISIR
DE VOUS INVITER A UN DINER POUR CELEBRER LA COLLECTION

VALENTINO
LE NOIR

DIMANCHE 3 MARS 2024
A 20H30

LAURENT
41 AV. GABRIEL, PARIS

#ValentinoLeNoir

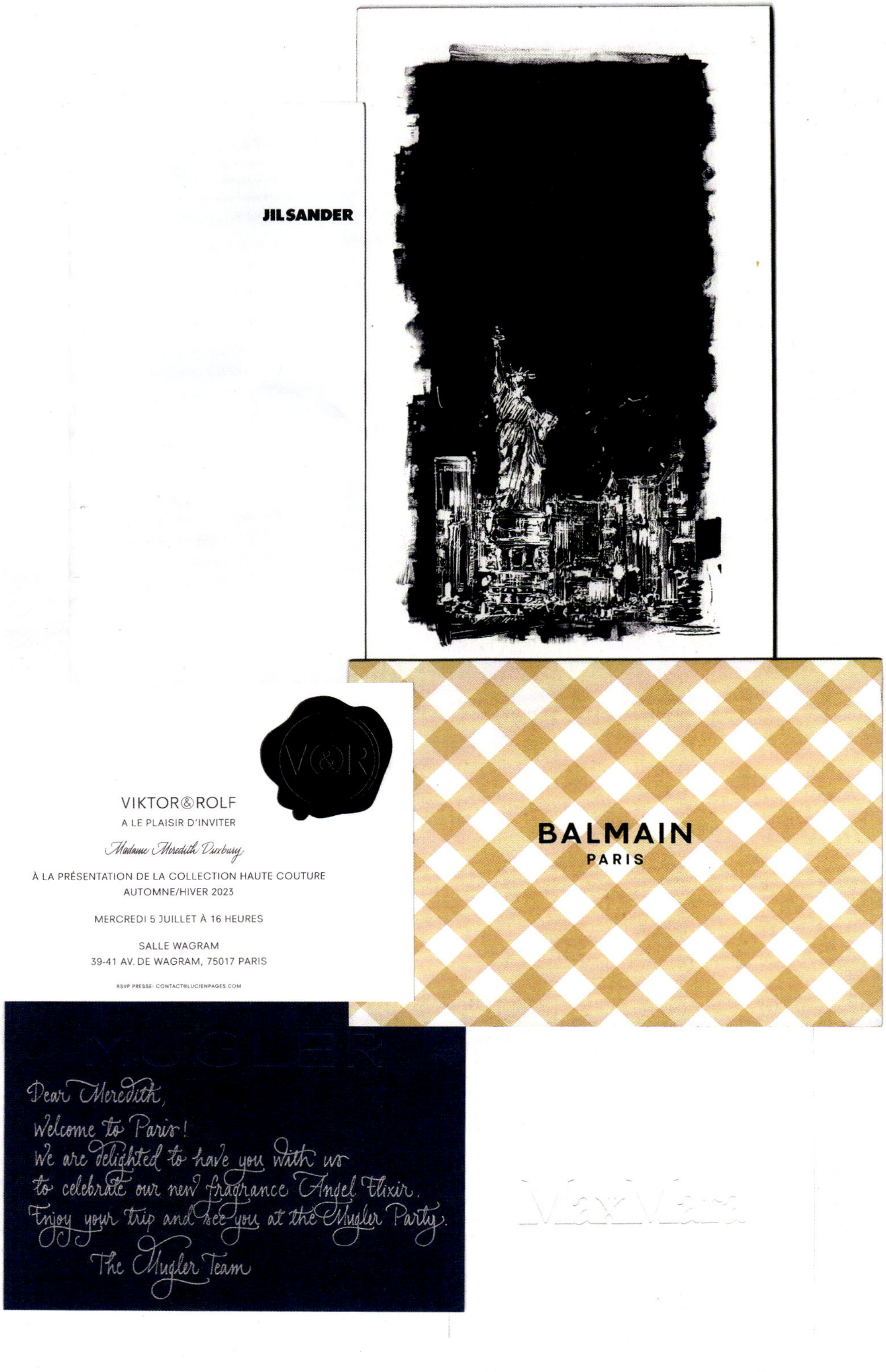
JILSANDER
VIKTOR&ROLF
A LE PLAISIR D'INVITER
Madame Meredith Duxbury
À LA PRÉSENTATION DE LA COLLECTION HAUTE COUTURE
AUTOMNE/HIVER 2023
MERCREDI 5 JUILLET À 16 HEURES
SALLE WAGRAM
39-41 AV. DE WAGRAM, 75017 PARIS
RSVP PRESSE: CONTACT@LUCIENPAGES.COM
BALMAIN
PARIS
Dear Meredith,
Welcome to Paris!
We are delighted to have you with us
to celebrate our new fragrance Angel Elixir.
Enjoy your trip and see you at the Mugler Party.
The Mugler Team
MaxMara

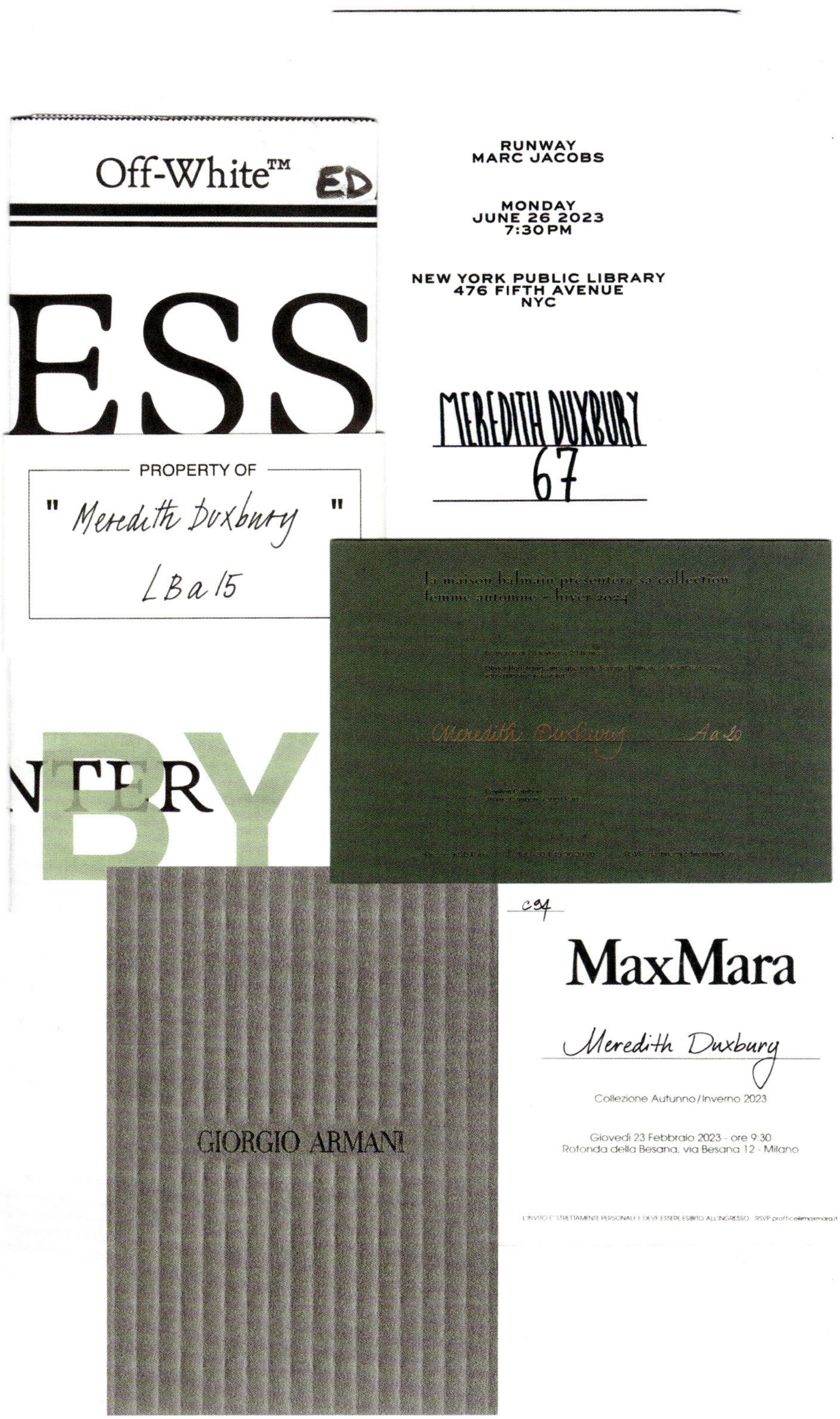
Off-White™
ESS
PROPERTY OF
" Meredith Duxbury "
LBa15
NTER
BY
RUNWAY
MARC JACOBS
MONDAY
JUNE 26 2023
7:30 PM
NEW YORK PUBLIC LIBRARY
476 FIFTH AVENUE
NYC
MEREDITH DUXBURY
67
Meredith Duxbury
MaxMara
Meredith Duxbury
Collezione Autunno/Inverno 2023
Giovedì 23 Febbraio 2023 - ore 9:30
Rotonda della Besana, via Besana 12 - Milano
GIORGIO ARMANI

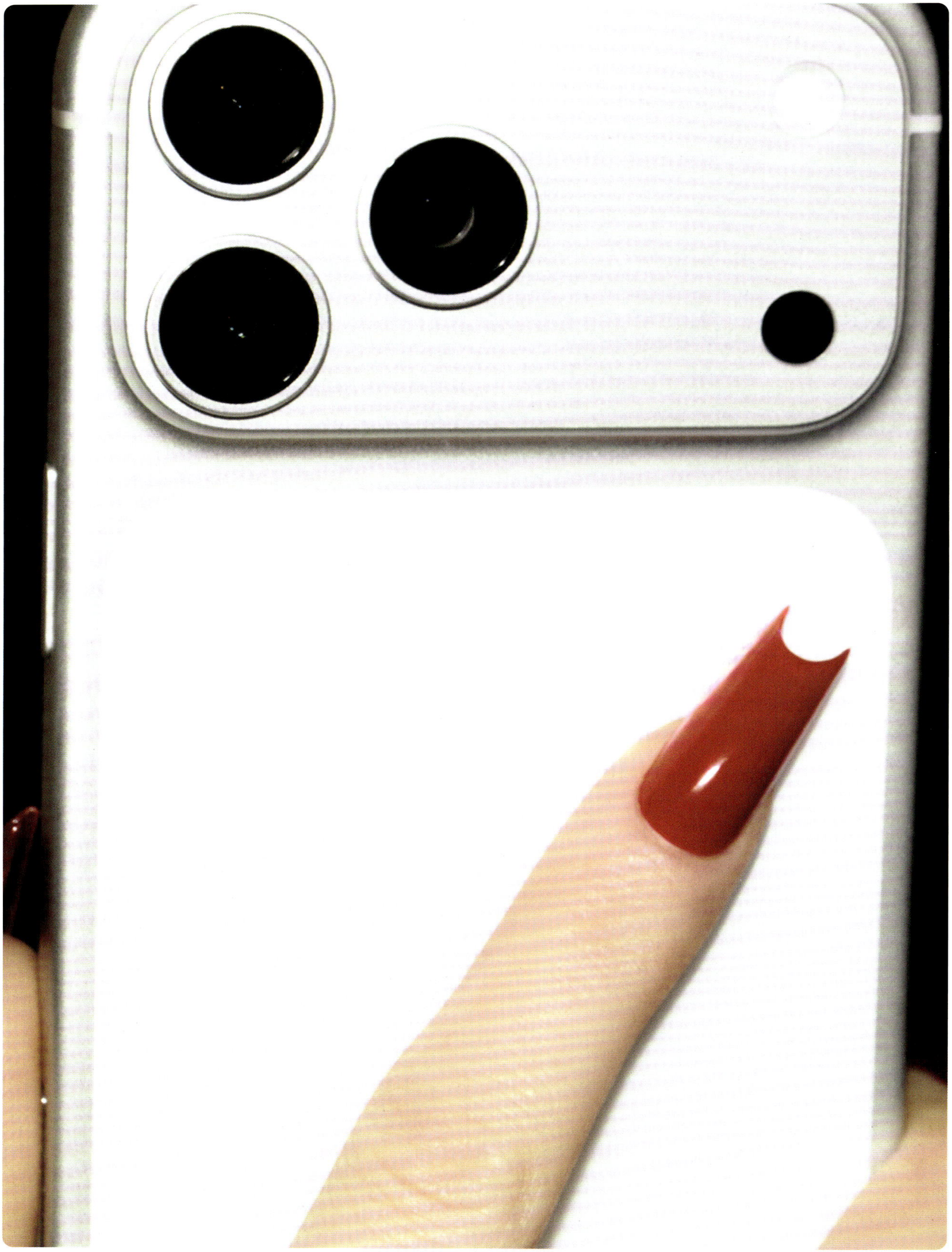

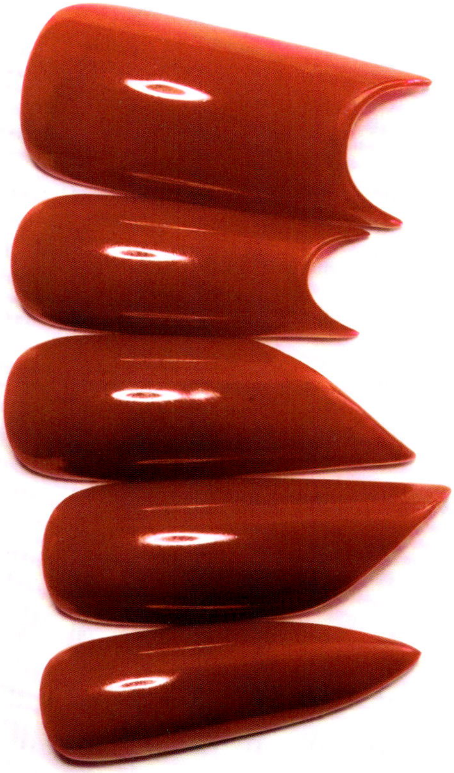

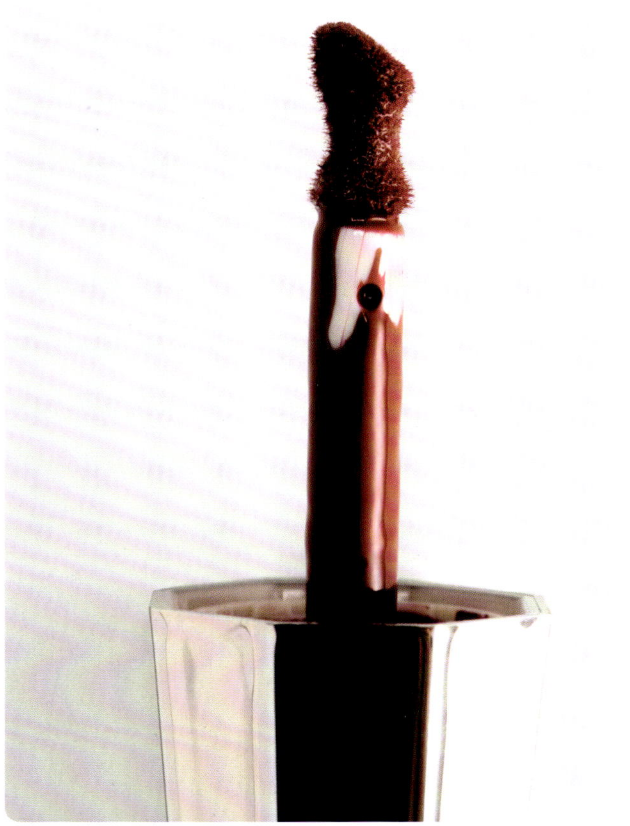

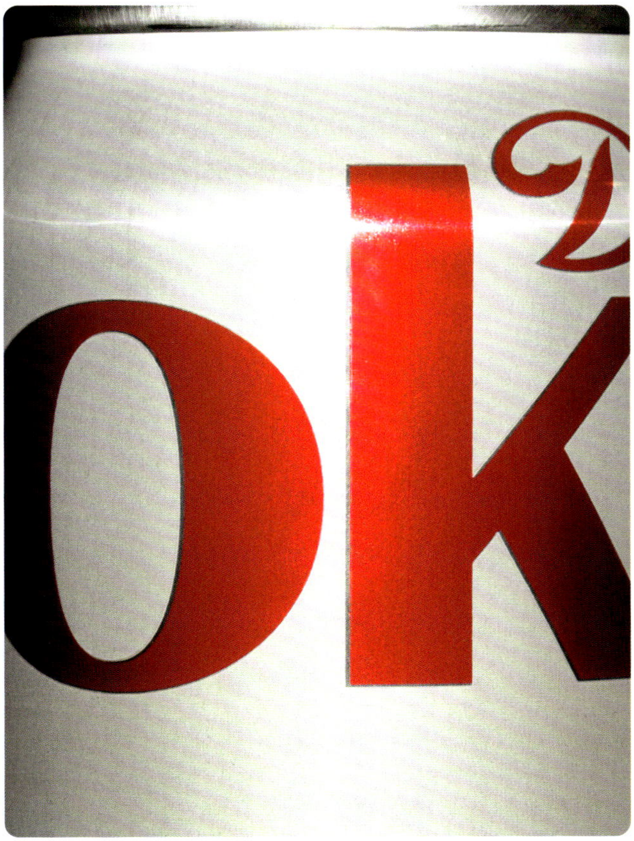

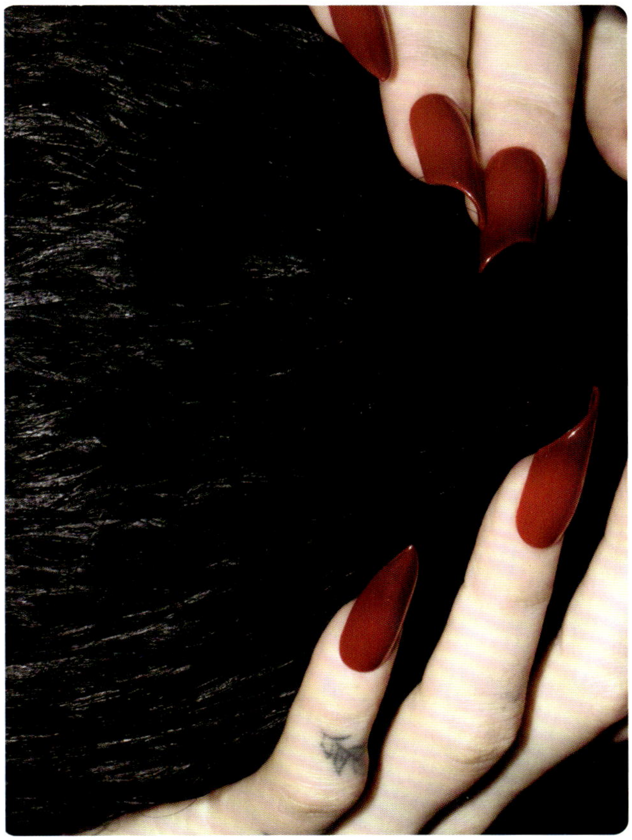

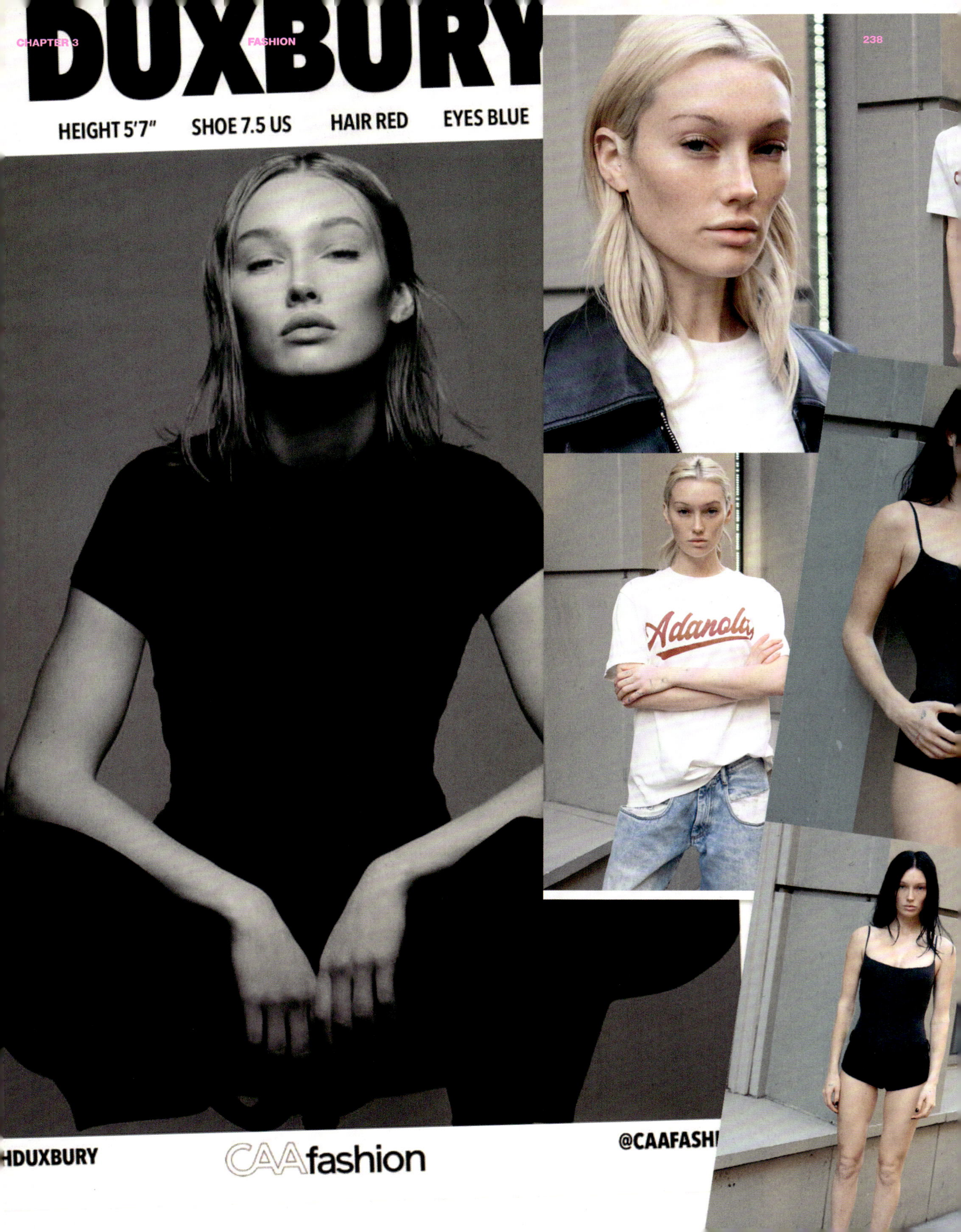
DUXBURY
HEIGHT 5'7" SHOE 7.5 US HAIR RED EYES BLUE
HDUXBURY
CAAfashion
@CAAFASHI
Adanola

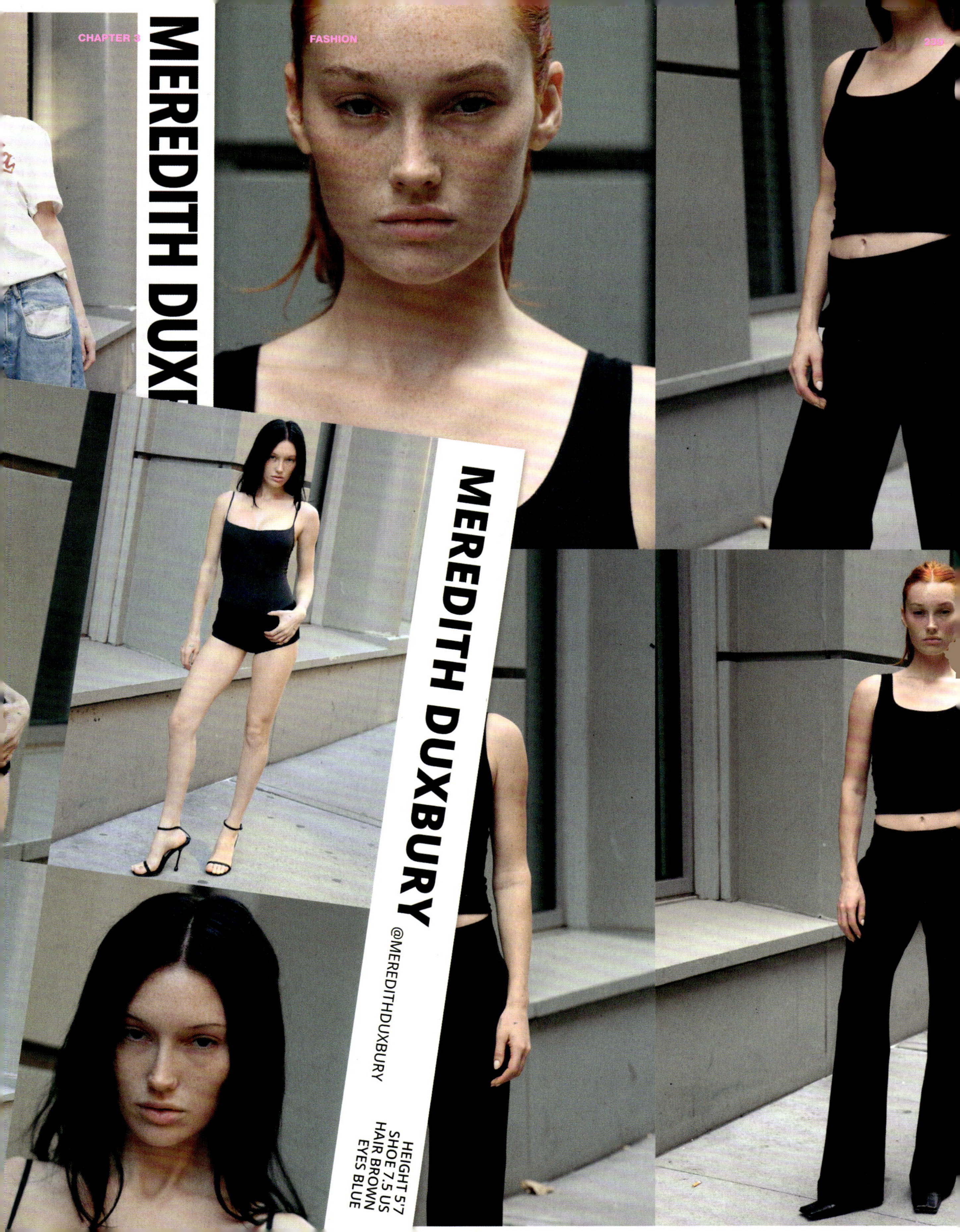
MEREDITH DUXBURY
@MEREDITHDUXBURY
HEIGHT 5'7
SHOE 7.5 US
HAIR BROWN
EYES BLUE

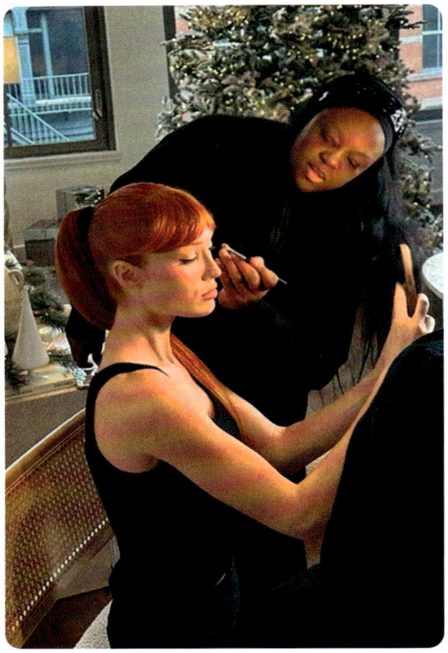

How special is it to have your makeup done by *the* Pat McGrath! I am forever grateful for all the advice and knowledge that she has shared with me. I was getting ready for the CFDA Fashion Awards ceremony here. Pat came over to my apartment and did a look on me. One of my favorite memories to date!

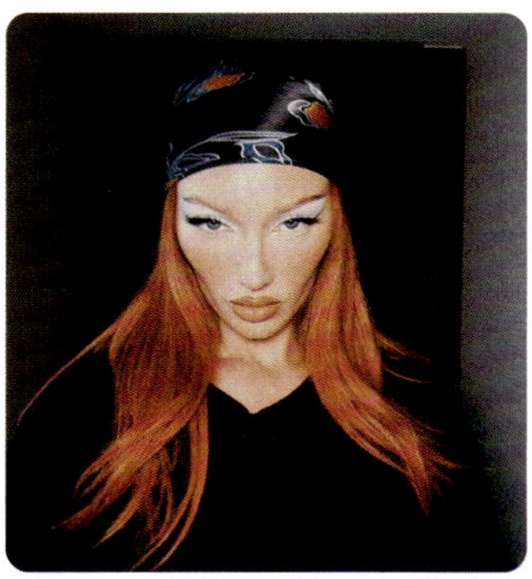

I LOVED this baby-blue eye look a make-up artist did on me for a Giorgio Armani show I attended in Paris, especially with the red hair. It is one of my favorite glams.

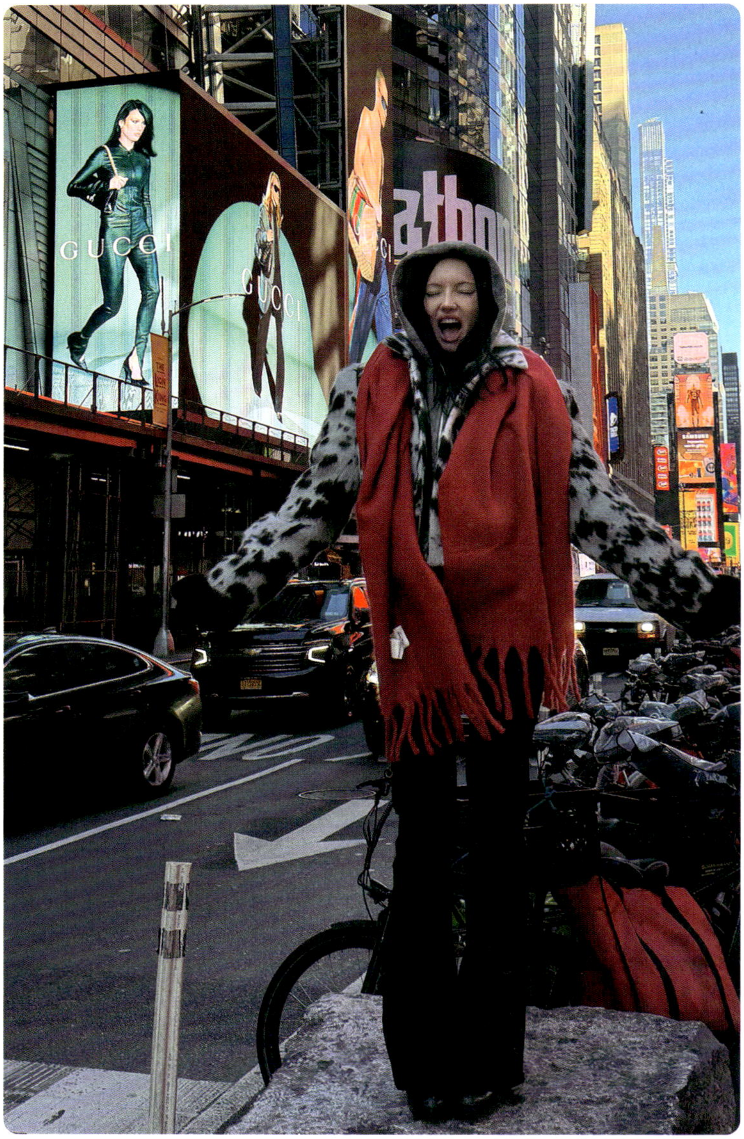

I can't even describe the feeling of seeing myself on a billboard for Gucci in Times Square. I shed so many happy tears. I will never ever forget how lucky I feel to be considered a part of Demna and the rest of the Gucci team's vision.

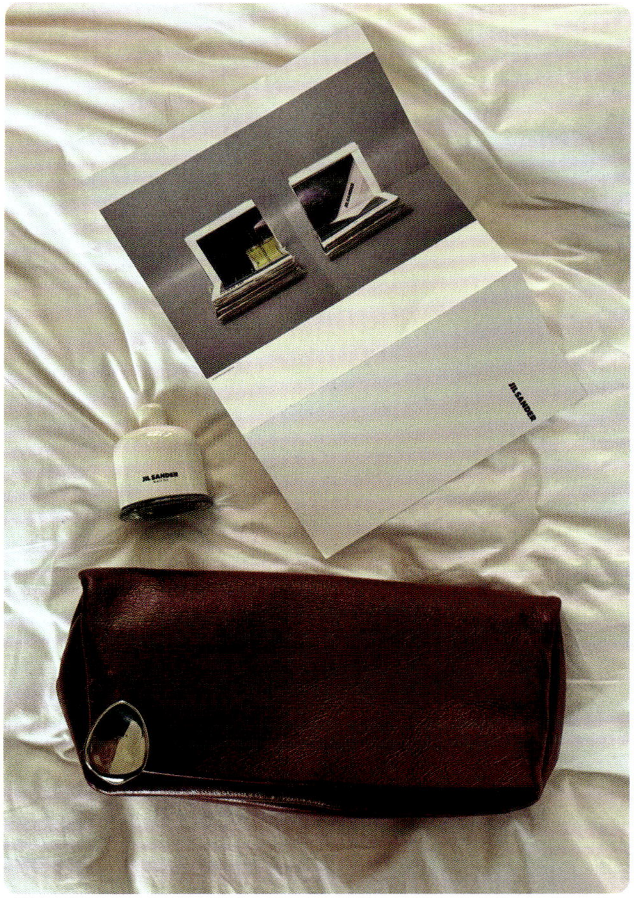

Fashion Week essentials. I always talk about how I use fragrance to remind myself of specific memories and times in my life. I'm always spritzing myself before heading out the door to a show. This is Coffea by Jil Sander. Such a good staple!

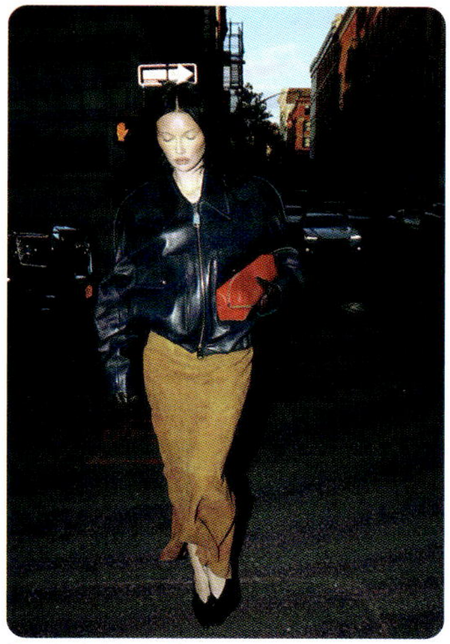

I styled this look myself for the Khaite runway show at New York Fashion Week. I really loved these tones and always get so much inspiration from color when putting a look together.

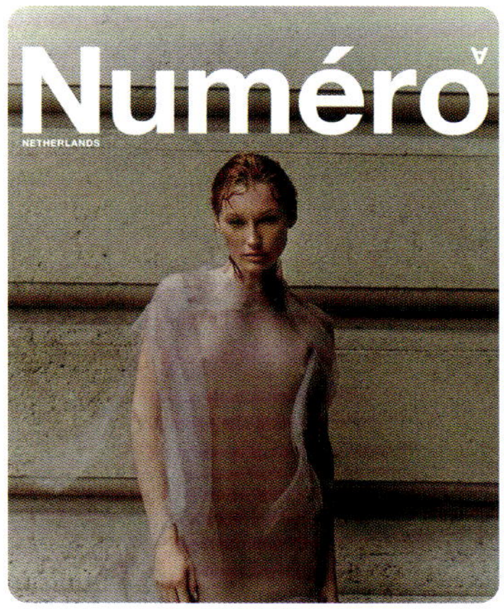

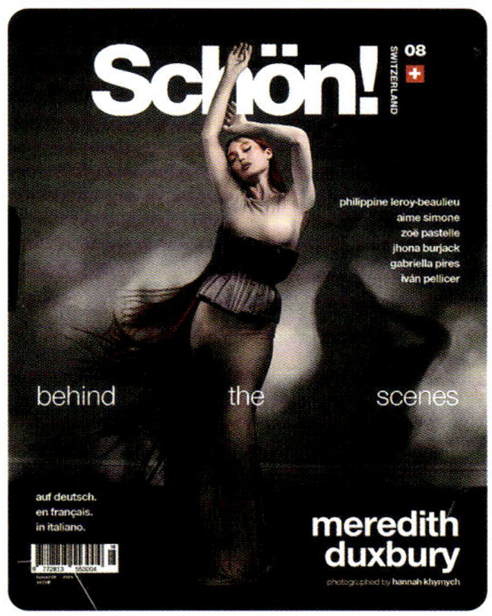

This *Numéro* cover sits on my coffee table. It's one of my faves. My editorial cover with *Schön*! Switzerland. What an accomplishment!

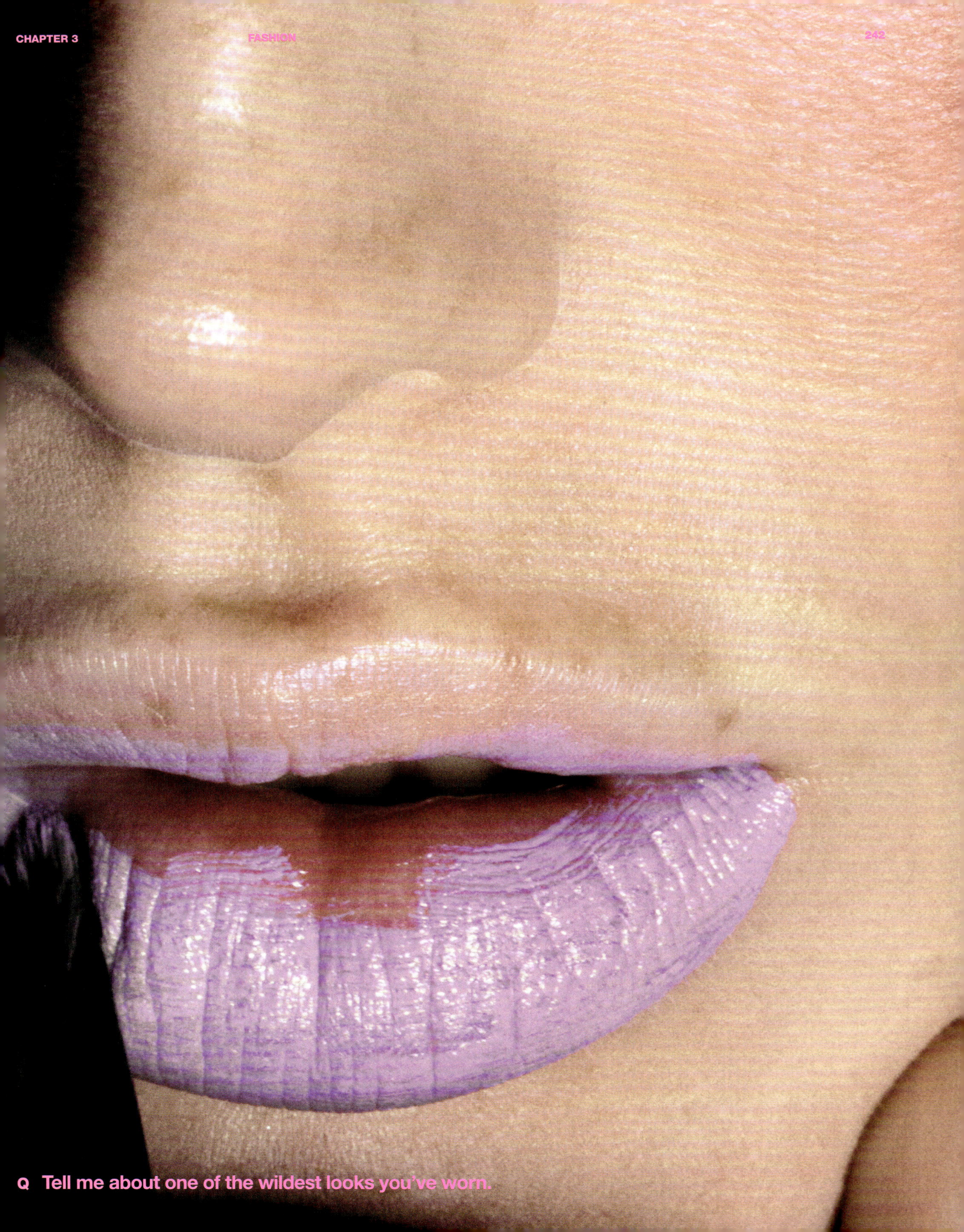

Q Tell me about one of the wildest looks you've worn.

A Probably the wildest was a dress that I wore to an event at the Boom Boom Room during New York Fashion Week in 2023. I don't even know how to describe it. It was a gradient blue-and-red body-hugging dress with an inflatable-looking tube trim that wrapped around my neck and down to my waist. My hair was done up in a huge ponytail braid, and I wore blue eyeshadow and crazy earrings.

Q Have you ever had any wardrobe disasters?

A Name a girl who hasn't had a wardrobe malfunction. One time, a back buckle sewn inside a dress I was wearing broke. I came home at the end of the night alone, and my team had all gone home. I had to figure out how to get a pair of scissors and cut the back of my dress open on my own.

It was couture, and I had to be sewn into my dress in order to wear it. It's actually insane, the things we'll do for fashion.

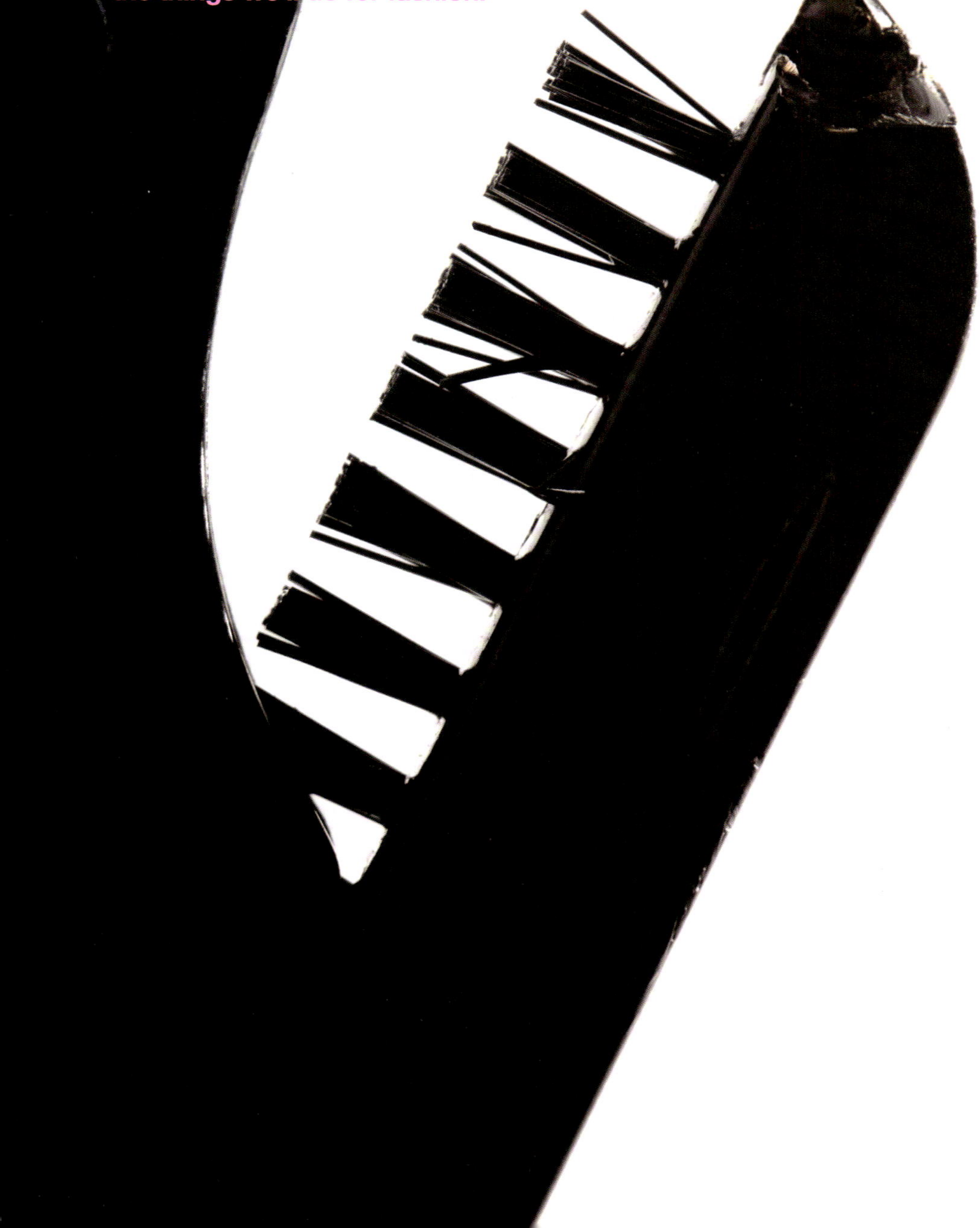

Q What is one trend you will never take part in?

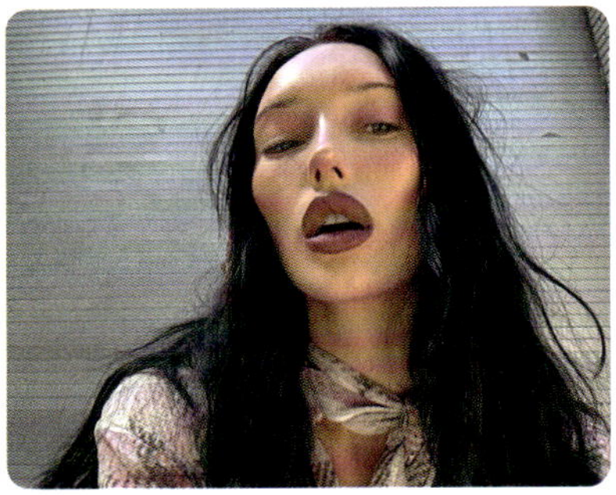

TOP: It's important to switch it up and try new things that you wouldn't normally reach for. In this case above, I tried a burgundy-mauve lip and ended up loving it! If you're ever unsure of your glam, put on an outfit you love that pairs well with your makeup, and I guarantee you'll end up loving it! BELOW: I love a really tailored look and always lean into it when styled in Armani. I remember feeling so good in both of these looks.

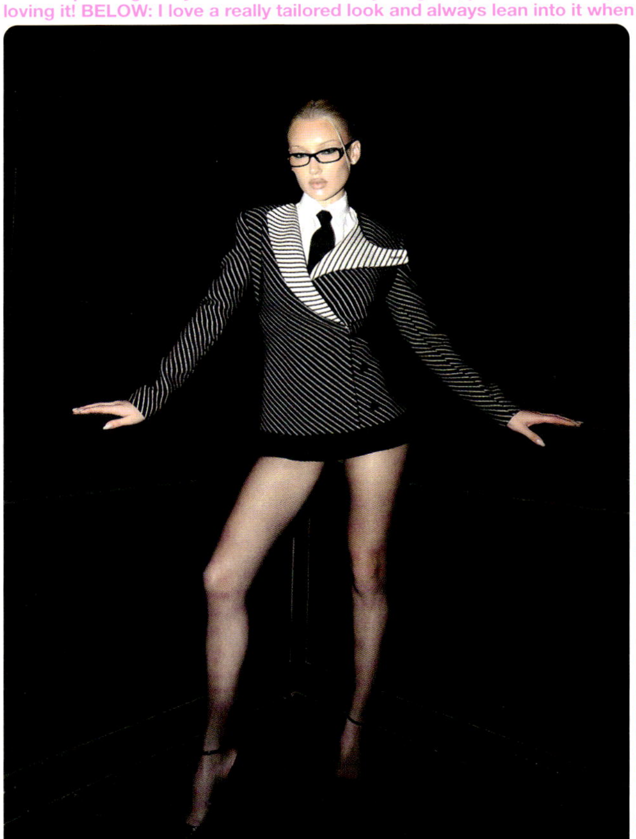

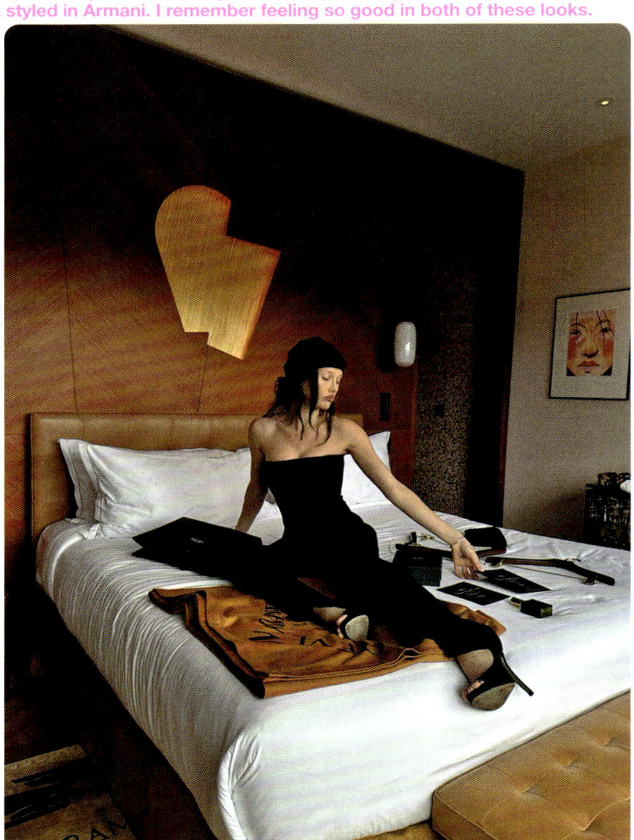

A Honestly, I am so down to try anything. I get adrenaline out of trying something new that's out of my comfort zone. I'm always willing to go for a challenge.

Q What is one trend that you wish would come back, or that you really would like to see take off?

A Napoleon jackets. They're kind of making a comeback, but I think they're supercool. They're very playful, and I think we need more of that in fashion. I got a vintage one in Paris, and I love it.

Q When you imagine your future in fashion—on runways, on red carpets, in editorial shoots—what do you want for yourself? What do you see in that vision?

A I aspire to bring something new and interesting to the fashion industry and bring the fun into it. I want to make people feel good about themselves and challenge them to step outside their comfort zone by exploring different versions of themselves.

I also want to stay true to my personal style and allow myself to absorb different trends and aesthetics, and make a point to always put my personal twist on them. It's so easy to get lost in how I need to portray myself. You can always take inspiration from other people, but being true to yourself is what I always want to carry with me.

Q Is there a dream that you are afraid to say out loud?

A I would love to book a big fashion campaign. There's a billboard I walk by every day to get my matcha in SoHo, and I always look at it and manifest that it will me be up there one day. I would love to book Gucci, Miu Miu, or Saint Laurent and do a huge show. (I'm here a week after writing this, and I got booked to walk the Gucci runway show!!!!! Eeeekkkk! See...keep manifesting, you can and will make it happen!) I would love to go to the Met Gala and do the red carpet there.

I know that's insane, but it's good to strive for big goals. Whenever people tell me something is unrealistic, I know I'm on the right path.

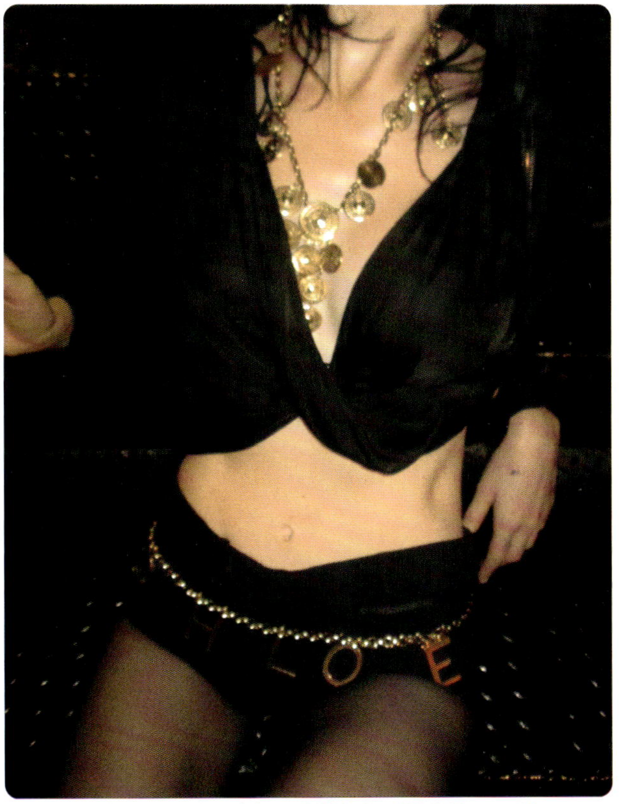

I styled this look for a fun night out! Chloé and Saint Laurent have some of the most beautiful accessories and jewelry. I always find myself drawn to them.

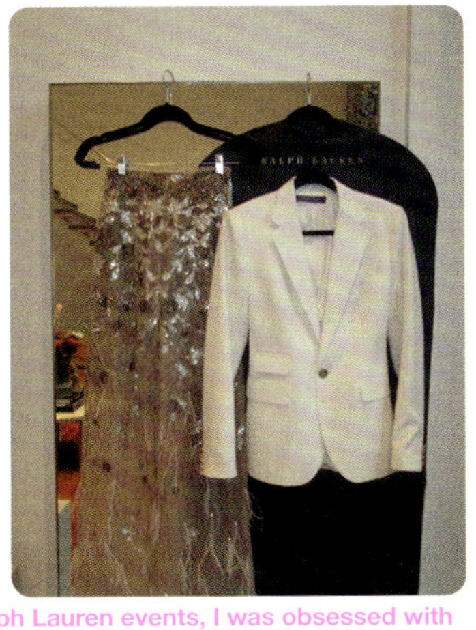

My look for one of my first Ralph Lauren events, I was obsessed with this look! They dressed me in the most fun beaded, embroidered sheer pants with a crisp, tailored white blazer. 10/10.

GET UNREADY WITH ME

4

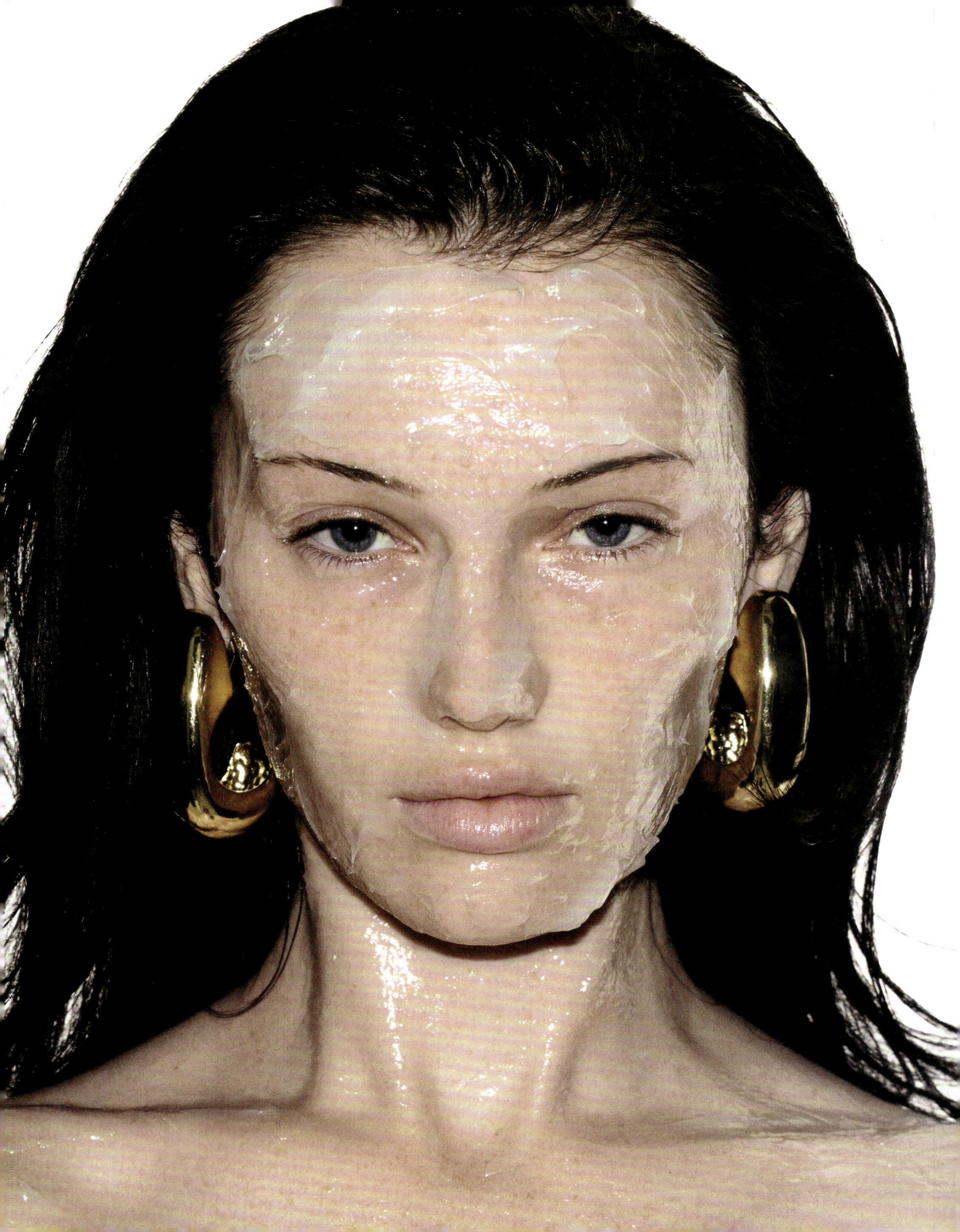

To me, getting unready is about saying goodbye to whatever stress, expectations, and pressures I've built up or held onto for the day. Removing my makeup has never been about just cleaning my face. It's peeling back the layers I've needed throughout the day to show up for the world.

Glam is fun, but taking it off is how I return to my truest version. Getting unready is a time to check in with myself and be vulnerable. Sometimes, you can feel scared to let go and allow yourself to feel your truest emotions, but when you allow yourself to indulge in yourself, you may find that it becomes your favorite part of the day.

There's a version of me that only exists at night. She's the girl who doesn't need to pose or keep her posture perfect. She's just a girl in her bed with her dogs, scrolling, laughing at a meme, or overthinking a conversation from earlier. She compares herself to others, she feels pressure, and she worries she's not doing enough, but she is also the girl who learns to forgive herself.

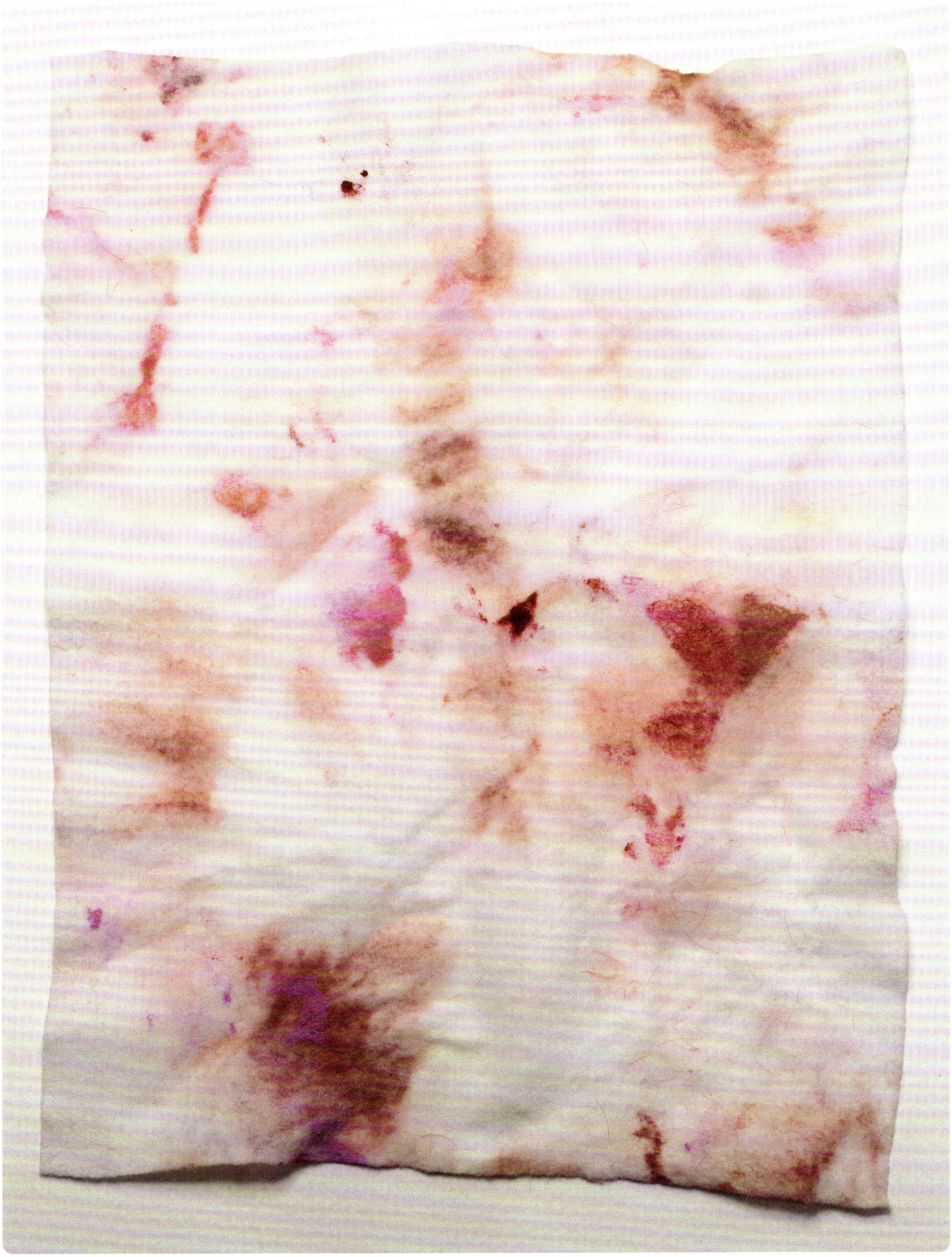

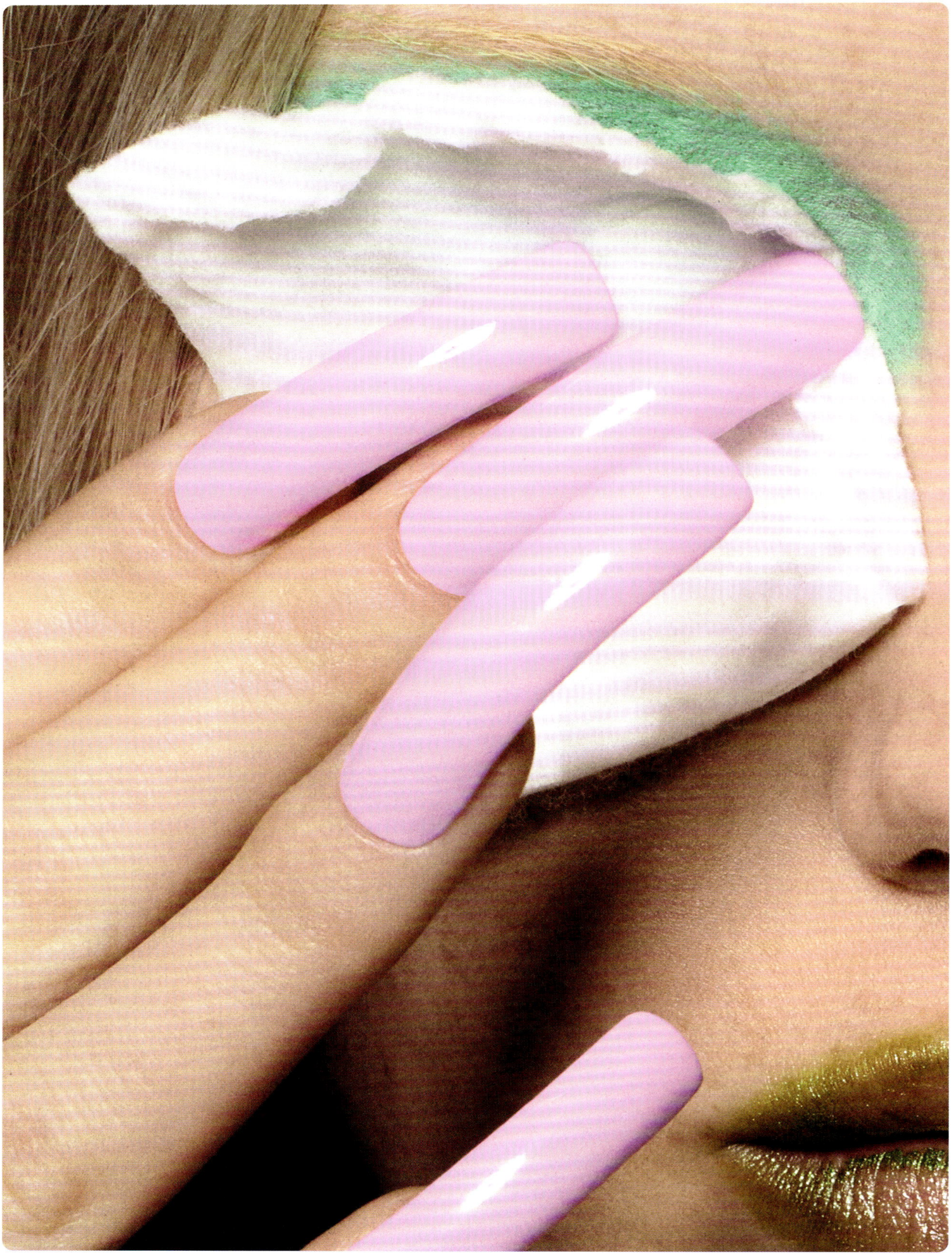

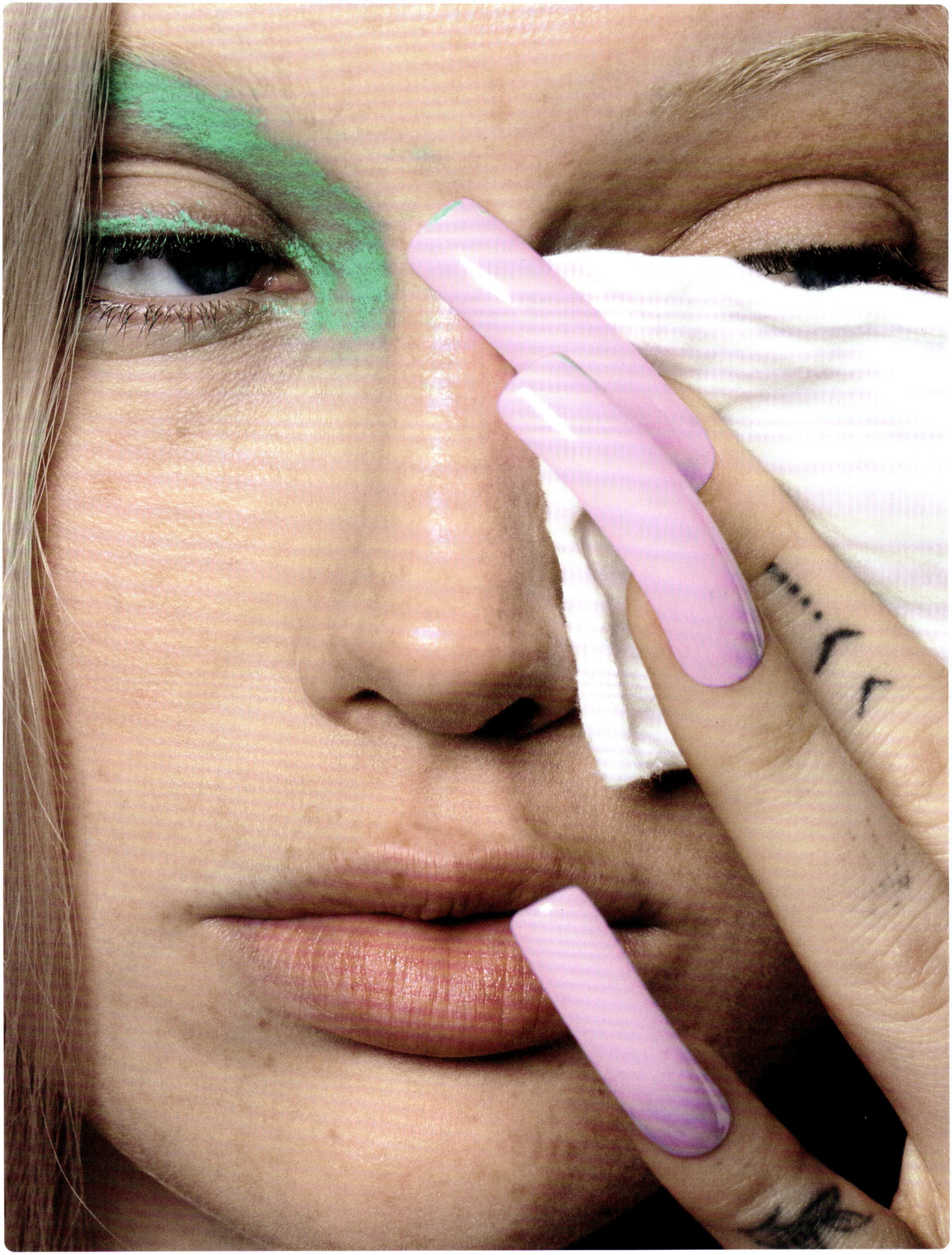

Q What does removing your glam symbolize to you?

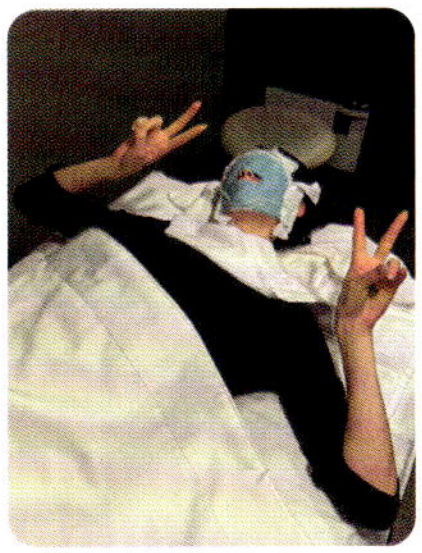
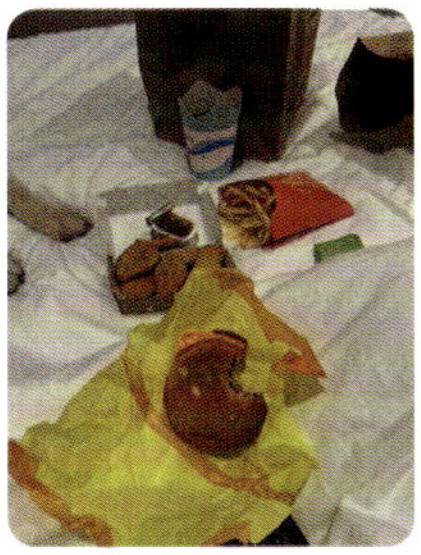
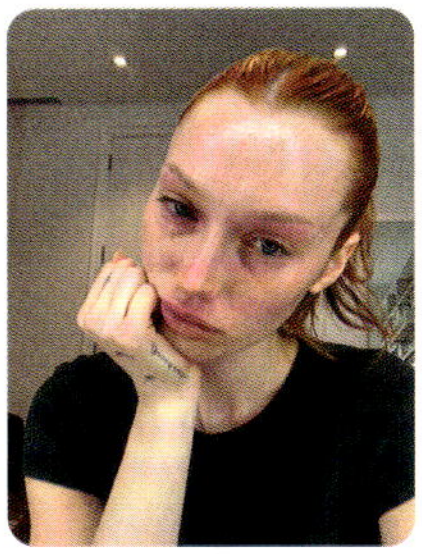

TOP: Life is all about balance. Take the time to get a facial, order your favorite fast food, or have a good cry. Listen to what your body needs and don't feel guilty about taking time out to give it that! BELOW: Skincare is such a huge part of my life, not just for the health of my skin but for my mental health as well. Something about carving out time for yourself and nourishing your body. I find face masks to be one of the best ways to reset and slow down my mind.

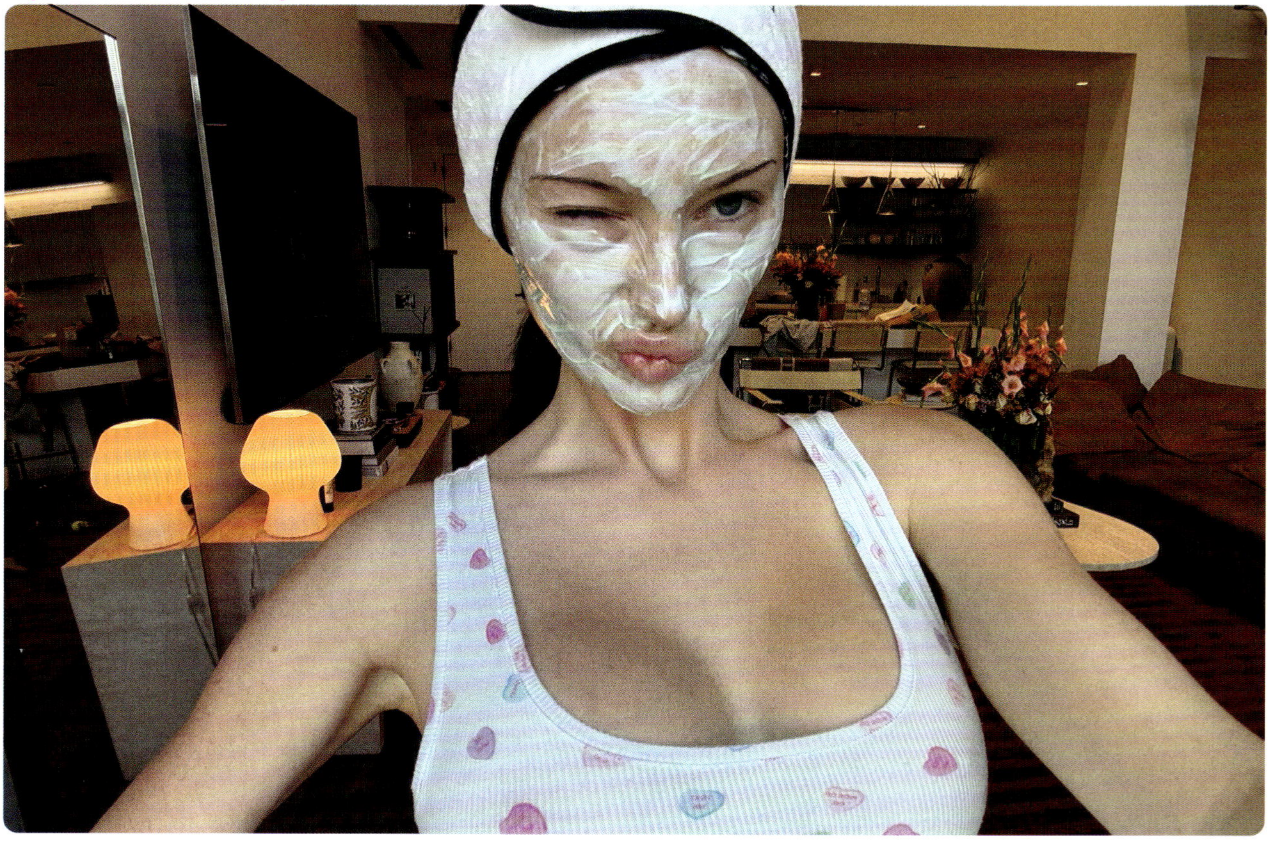

A Removing glam for me symbolizes coming back to myself and who I truly am. It's fun to be experimental and play around, but it's important to recognize yourself for your truest version.

Q When you take everything off, what part of you becomes louder?

A The way I care for myself becomes a bigger priority. It's easy to feel confident when we have makeup on, but when the makeup comes off, that's when we need to show ourselves the most love.

Q Do you ever feel more confident with your glam off?

A Yes! There is something so special about embracing your natural skin—I'm all about embracing your raw features and what makes you unique.

Q Has taking your makeup off taught you anything about who you are as a person, not as a creator?

A It's taught me that I am more sensitive than I am perceived to be. I can be vulnerable, and self-care has taught me to embrace that rather than see it as a bad thing. It's taught me to slow down and work on mindfulness and being present. It's easy to forget to care for yourself.

Q Is there a version of you that only exists at night that no one gets to see?

A We are truly the most comfortable with ourselves when we're alone. When you're alone at night, and your makeup is off, and you're just in your bed by yourself, watching your movie or vegging out, you're not worrying about other people's thoughts or opinions about you.

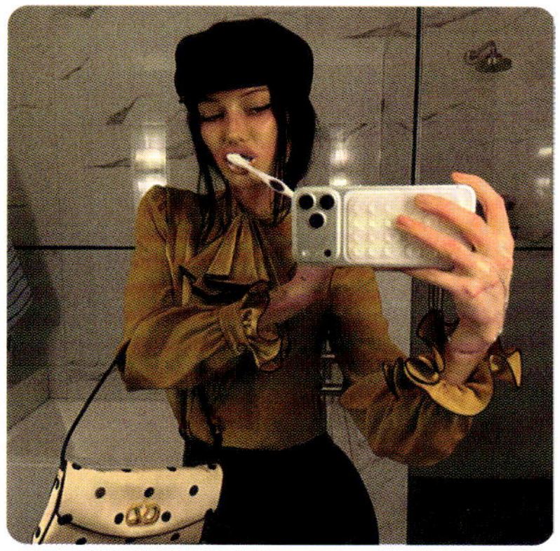

TOP: Even after a long night out, it's so important to take care of yourself and do your nighttime routine! BELOW: My dogs, Pancake and Crumpet, play a huge role in the way I unwind. I love spending time with them and cuddling them after a long day. Animals bring me so much peace, so taking the time to be mindful and slow down with my puppies is very important to me.

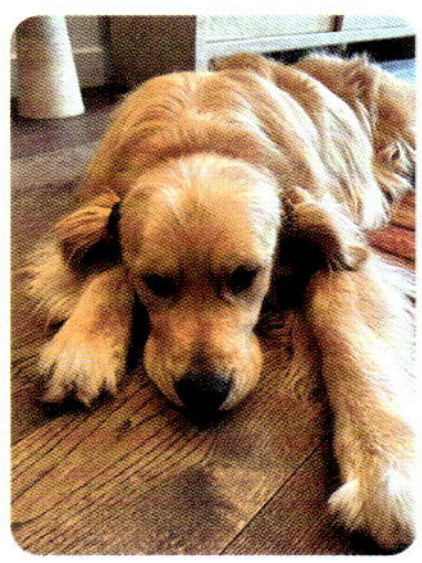

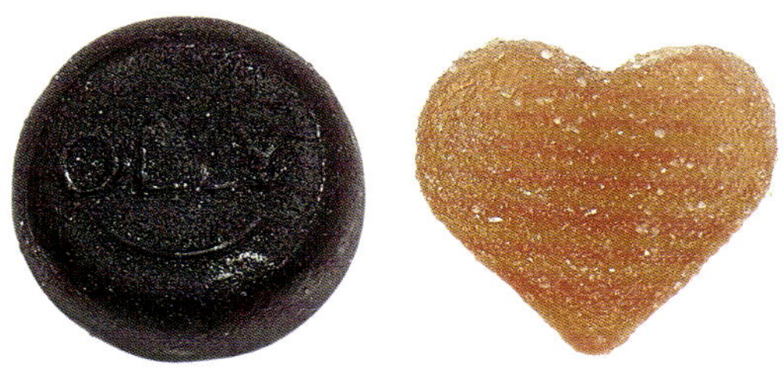

My two daily gummies: Vegamour GRO Biotin Gummies for Hair Wellness and OLLY Extra Strength Melatonin Sleep Gummies.

"I'VE TRA
FOR JUS
REALLY
WORKE

DED
'BOSSY'
T
IAVING A
STRONG
THIC"

Q When everything is quiet, what thoughts get the loudest? Is there something in your head that is talking to you?

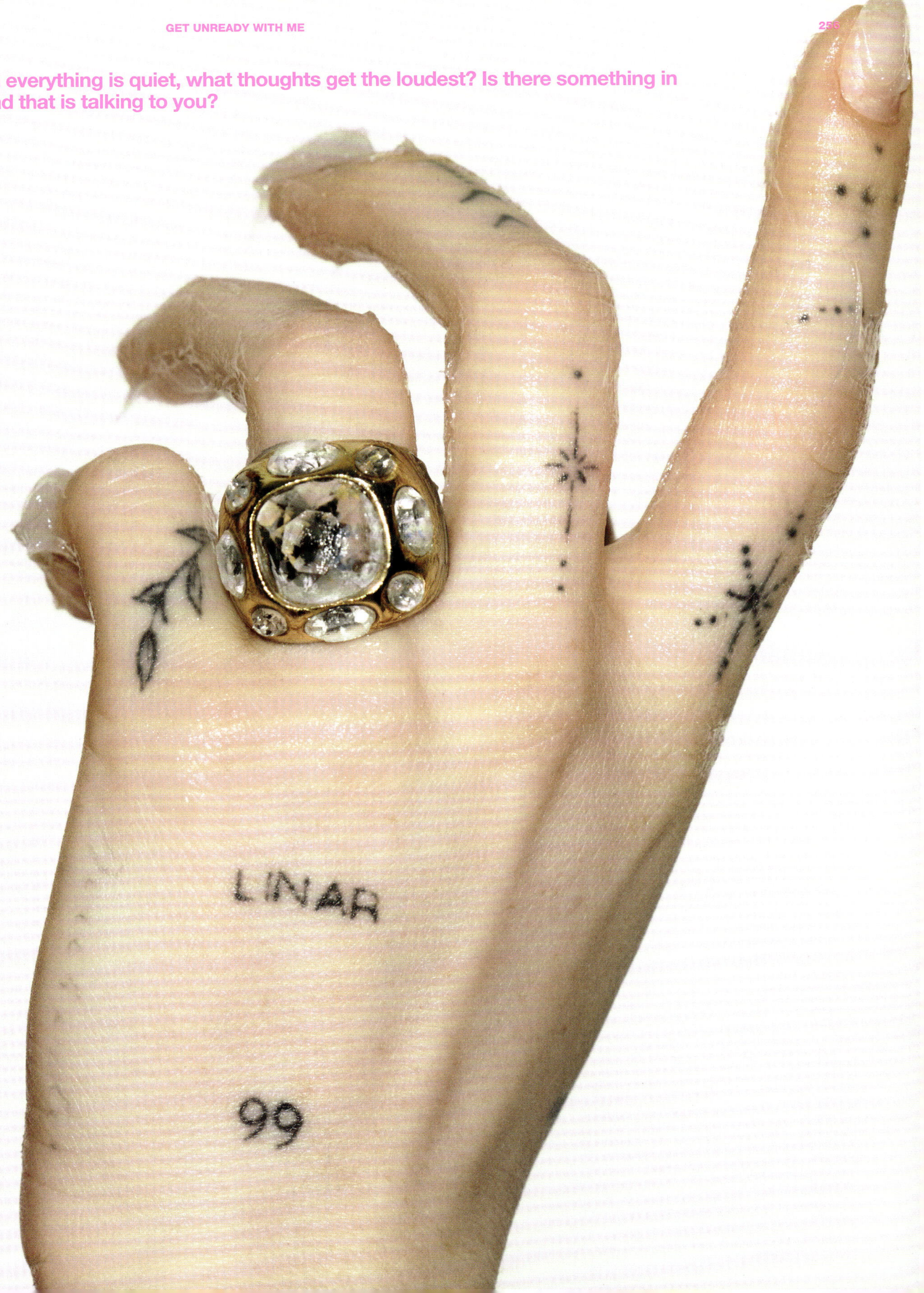

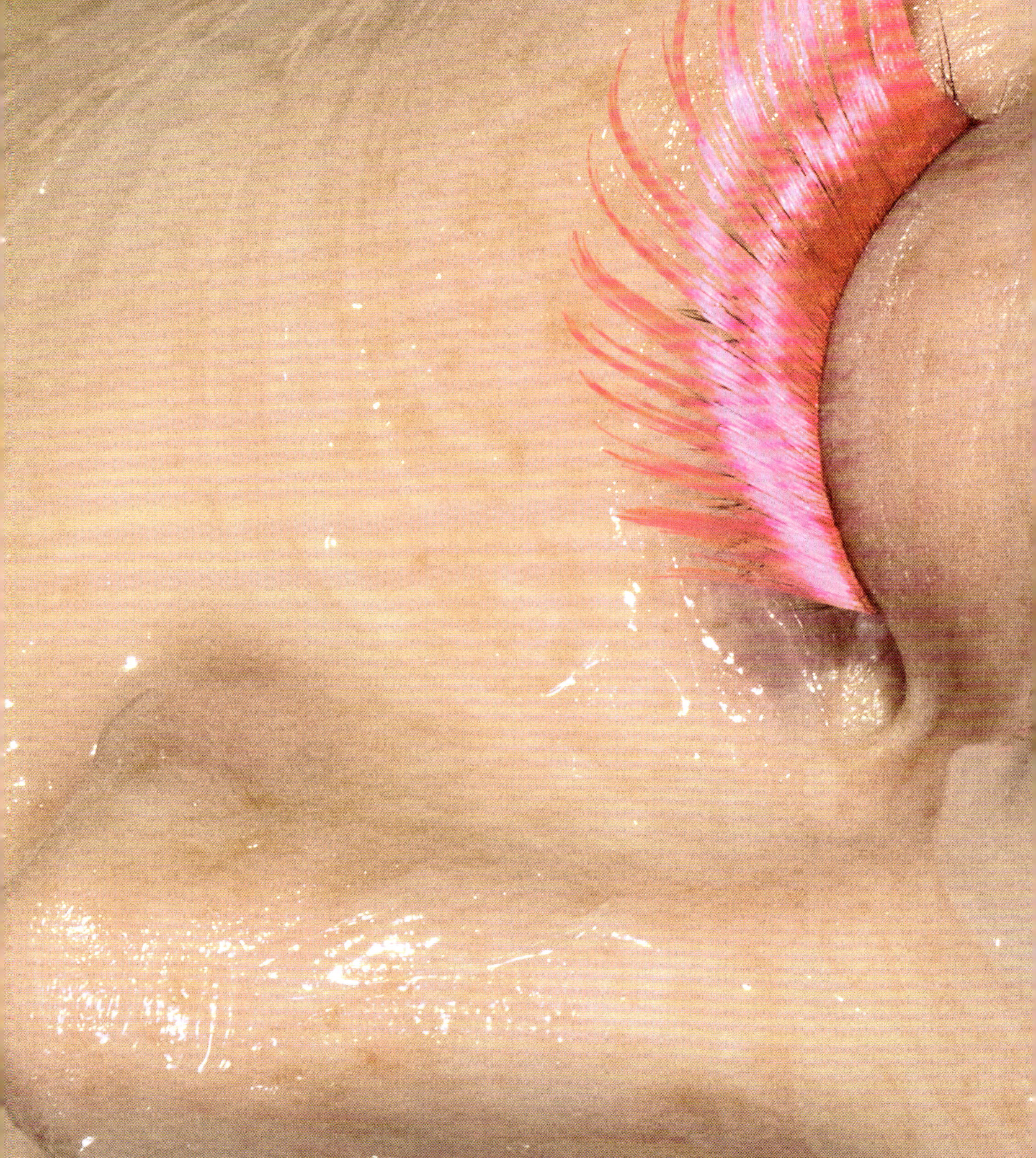

A Societal pressures, for sure!! And the need to feel like I need to accomplish everything at once. I reflect a lot in silence, and it's easy to get lost in your mind. But again, this is when you need to be the most honest with yourself and know you're enough and doing your best.

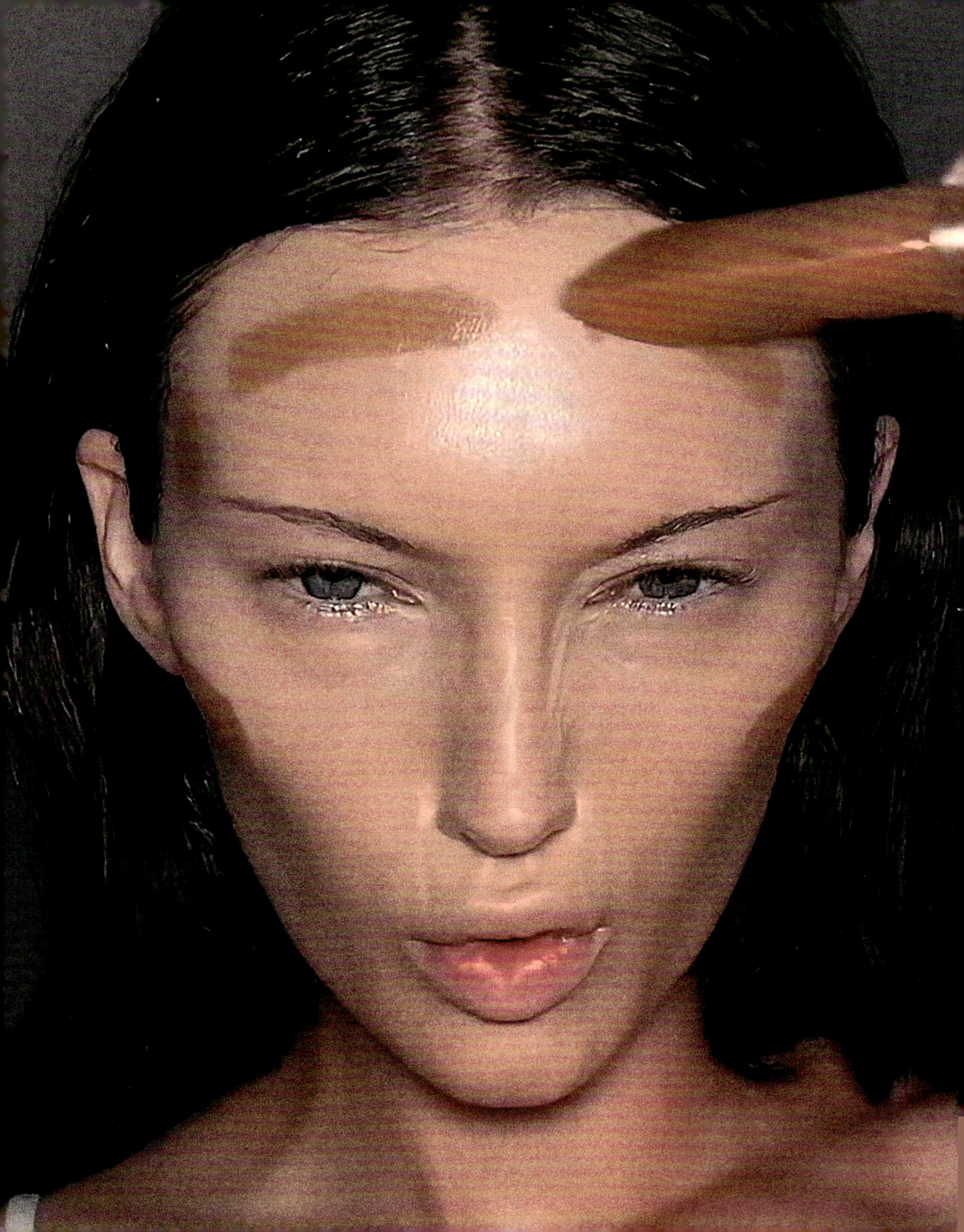

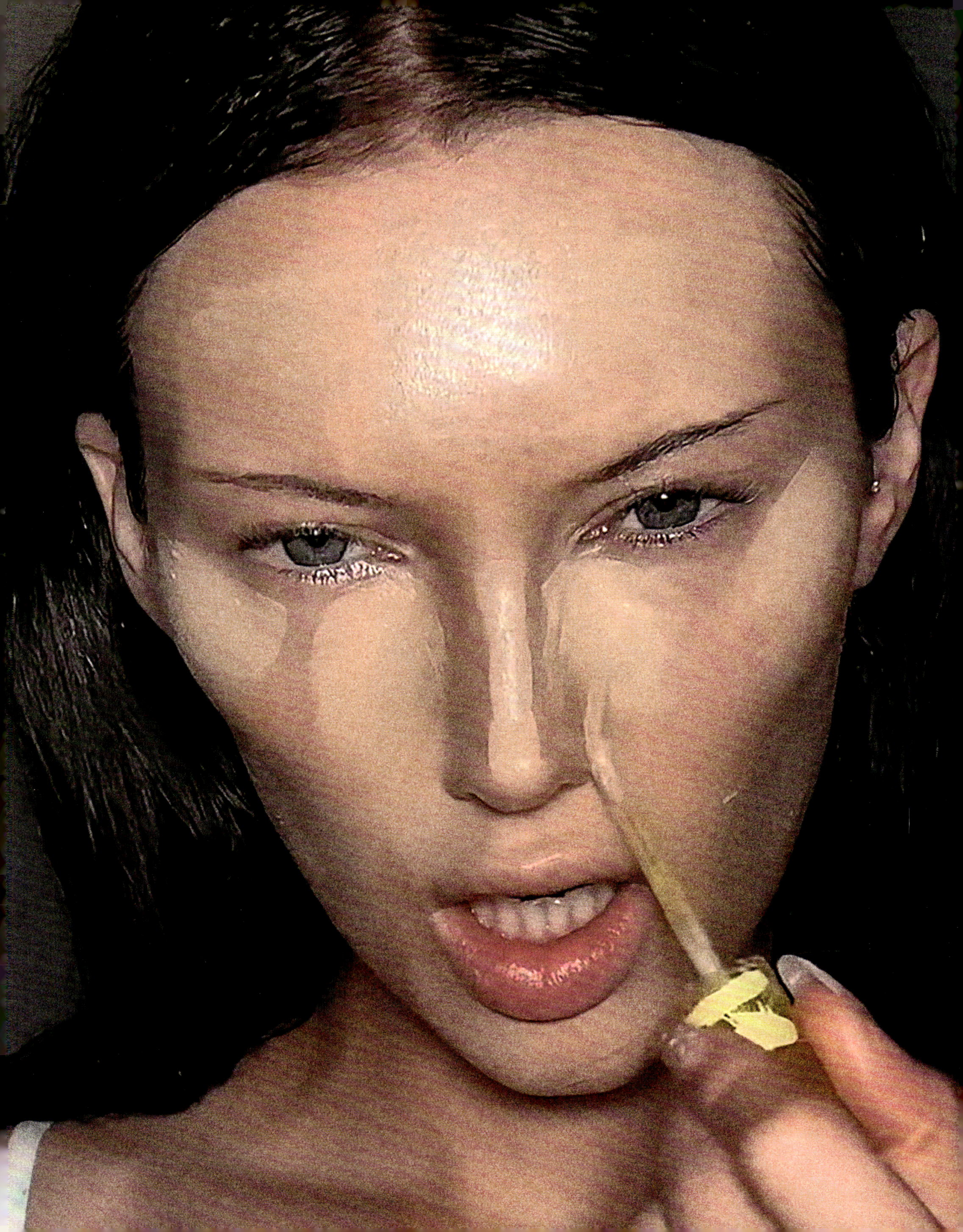

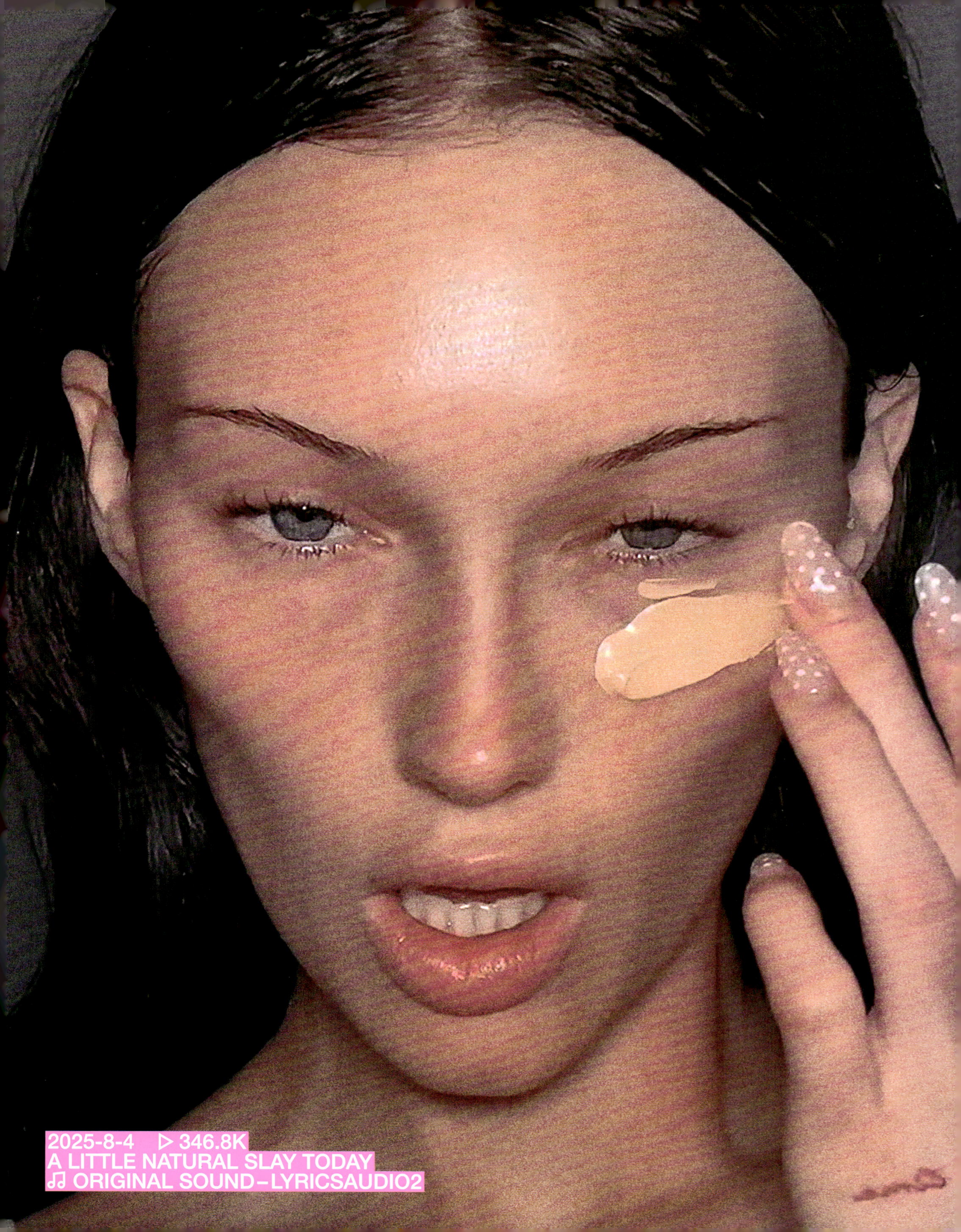
2025-8-4 ▷ 346.8K
A LITTLE NATURAL SLAY TODAY
♫ ORIGINAL SOUND–LYRICSAUDIO2

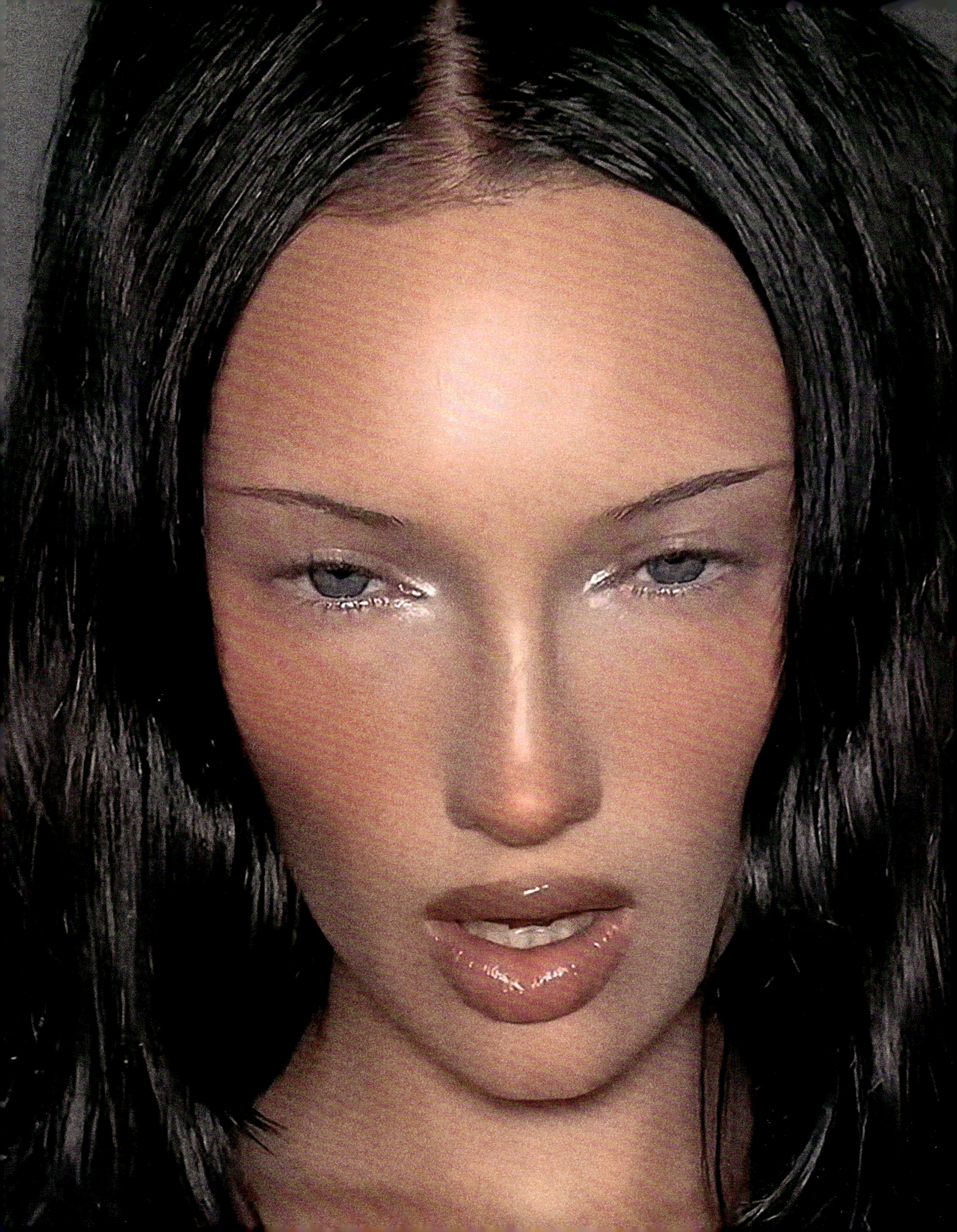

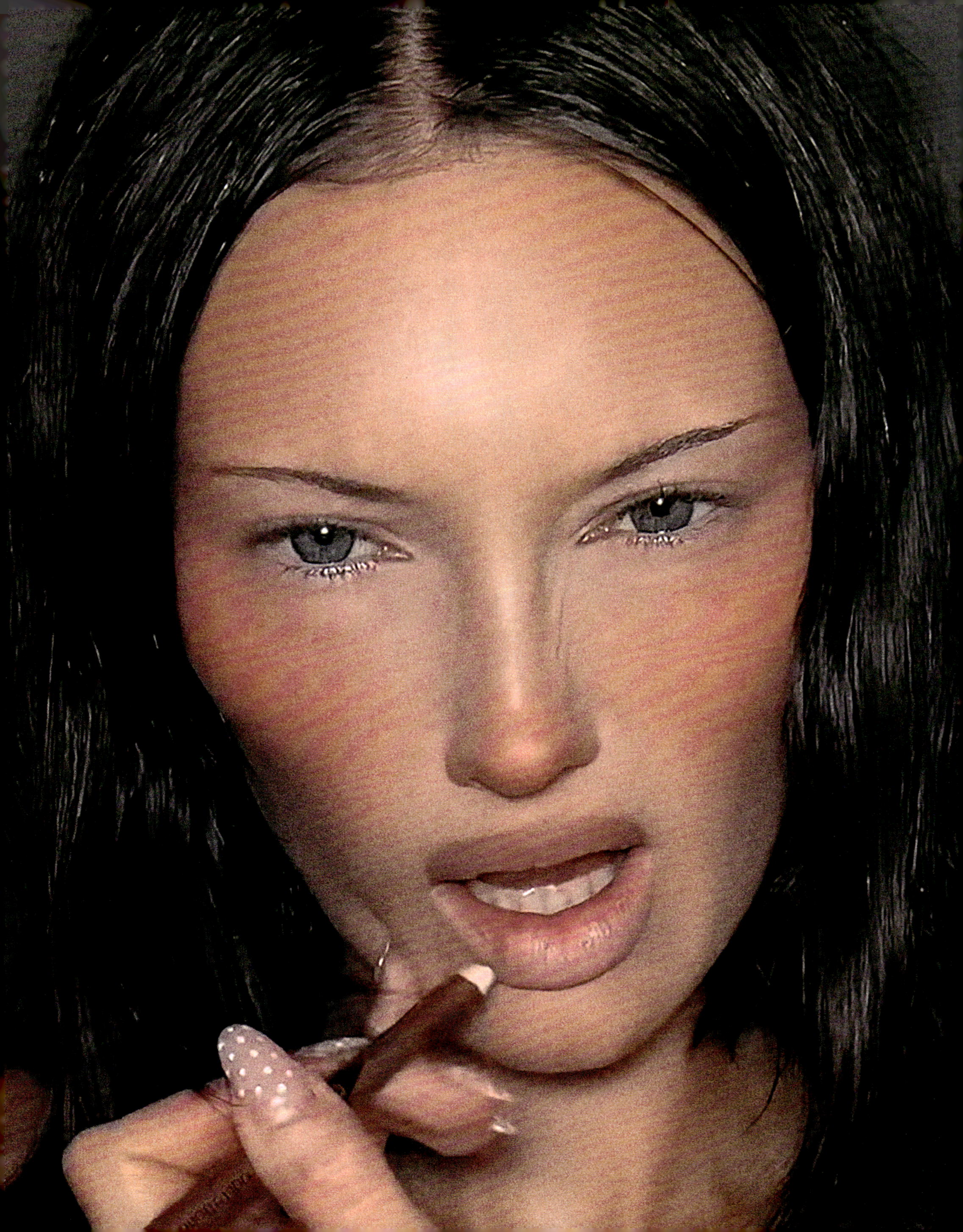

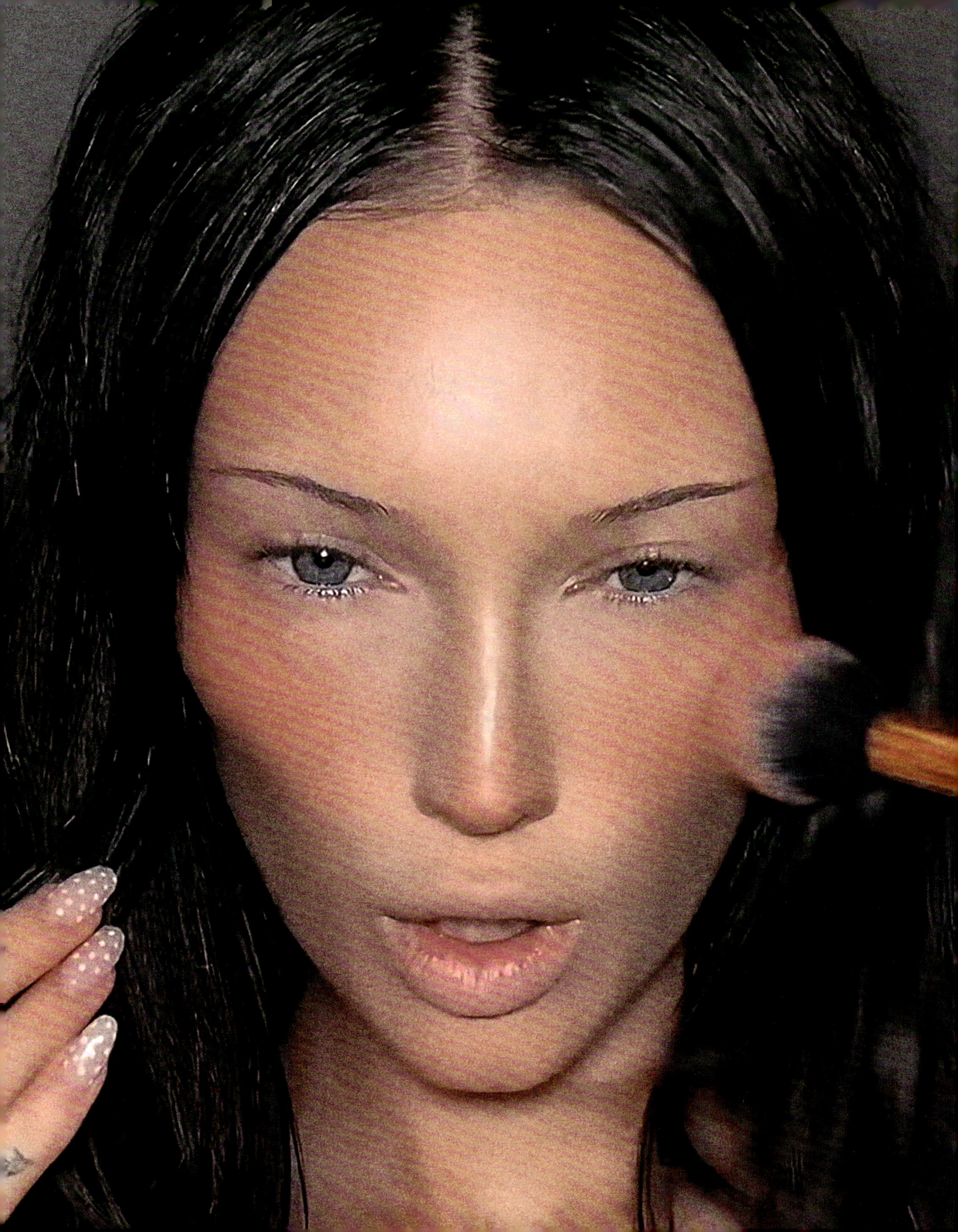

These are stills from a short film that I produced and directed. The quote "Be careful what you feel in silence. Don't allow it to consume you" is very important to me as someone who struggles with ADHD and OCD. I am always moving at such a fast pace. It's easy to become uncomfortable with silence and get stuck in a state of overthinking. I've had to teach myself to use silent, quiet moments as time to reflect and nourish my body and mind. Allowing yourself to be present with your mind is one of the greatest gifts you can give yourself. Don't run from your thoughts. Allow yourself to acknowledge them and work through them.

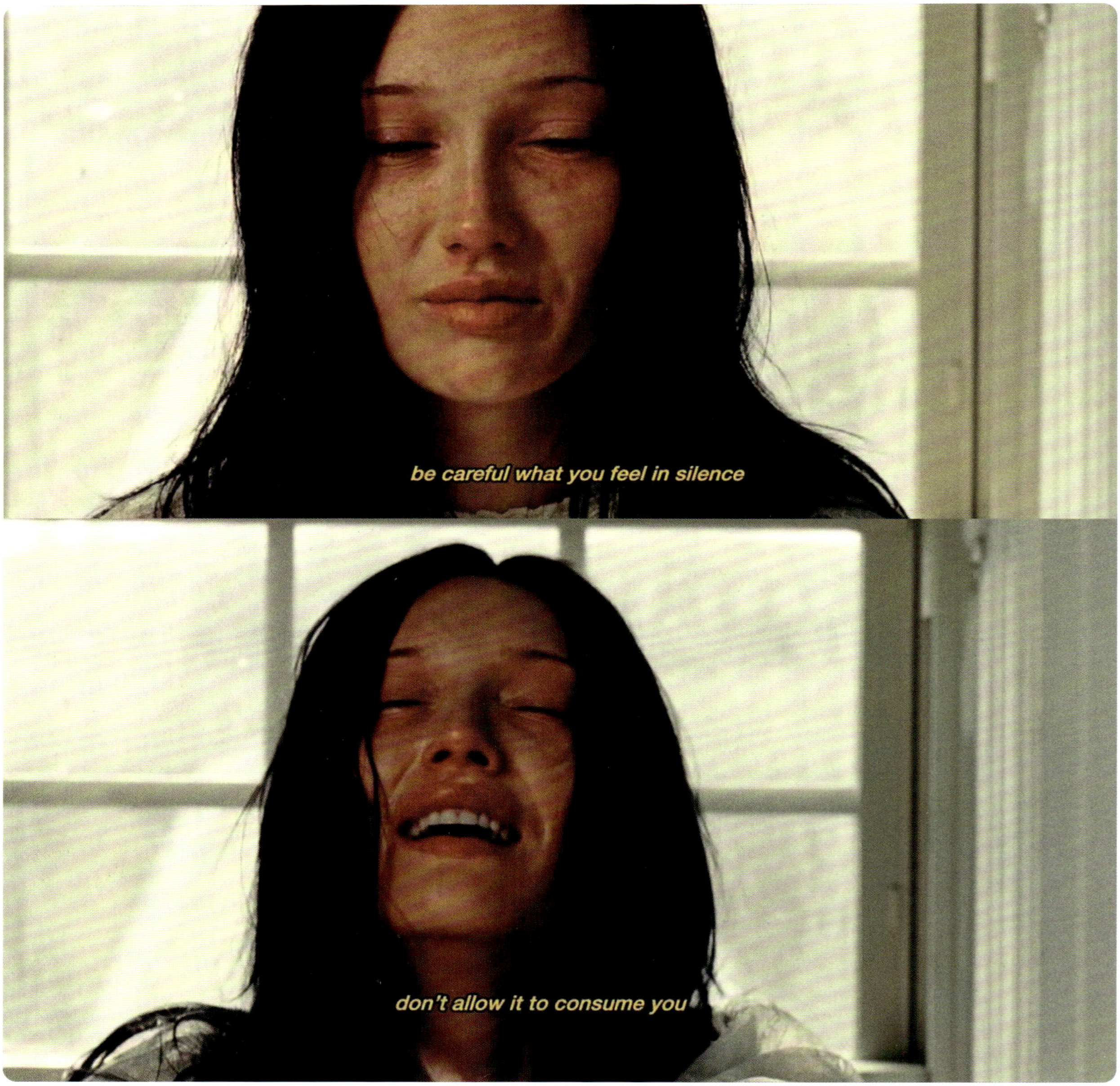

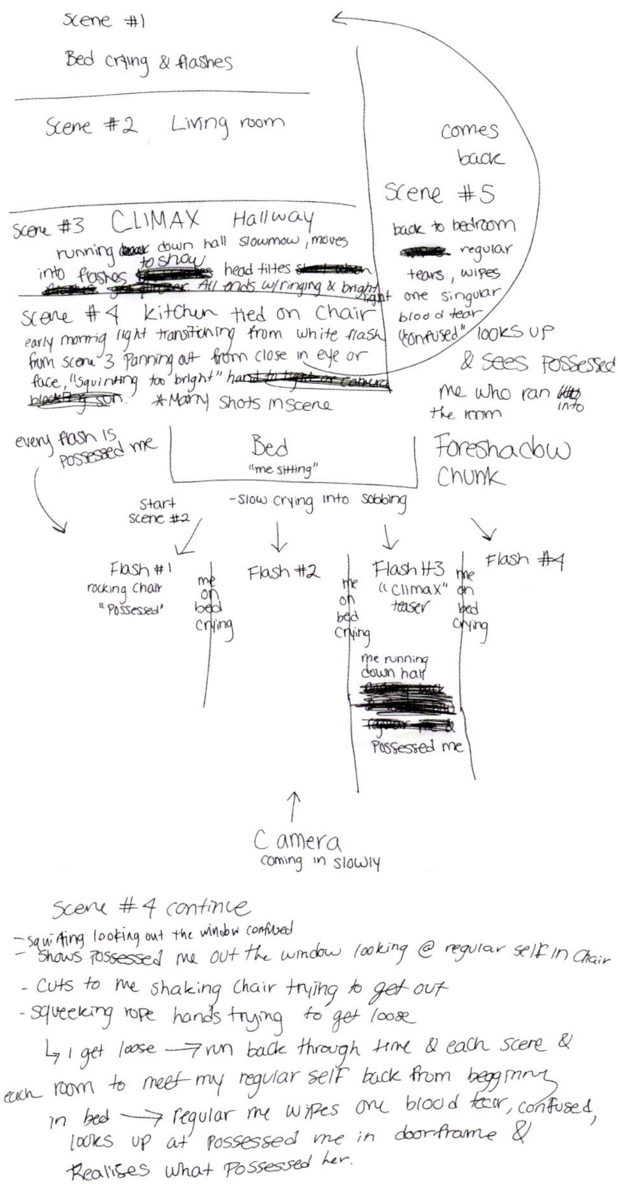

This is a very rough draft script from when I was workshopping my short film. I think it perfectly depicts how my brain works with being all over the place, but, to me, it all made so much sense when jotting it down on paper. Not everything has to be perfect. Let yourself be messy and just let your mind create and flow.

Q When do you feel the safest?

A I feel at night when there are no eyes on me. It feels good to feel enough. I like it when I can just fully be in my natural state.

Q When the world stops watching, what expectation do you find you can finally let go?

A My body image.

Q What surprises you about yourself when you step out of your online persona?

A Sometimes I forget I can be more shy and introverted. A lot of my work is putting myself out there for the world to see, and I've become so comfortable with it that I sometimes forget I still have that quiet side to me.

Q Do you worry that you might run out of creativity?

A There are times when I definitely get into content ruts and feel like I'm running low on creativity, but there are always new ways to feel inspired. It's just about finding them in the right places. A lot of the time, I look to my passions and find inspiration from things I'm passionate about that I haven't fully indulged in yet. For example, I really have a passion for creating short films, so when I was in one of my content ruts, this was something I worked on that gave me the creativity I felt I was missing at the time.

Q Do you ever get emotional while you are washing the day off?

A Of course, that's when I feel like I'm finally able to fully decompress. My therapist says when you go through a process of decompressing, oftentimes you just cry. It's your body's response to release and let out the stress hormone, cortisol.

Q When you wipe off the day, what are you hoping to leave behind?

A I'm hoping to leave behind any pressures I've put on myself throughout the day—resetting and leaving that behind to wake up the next day with a fresh mindset. It's really

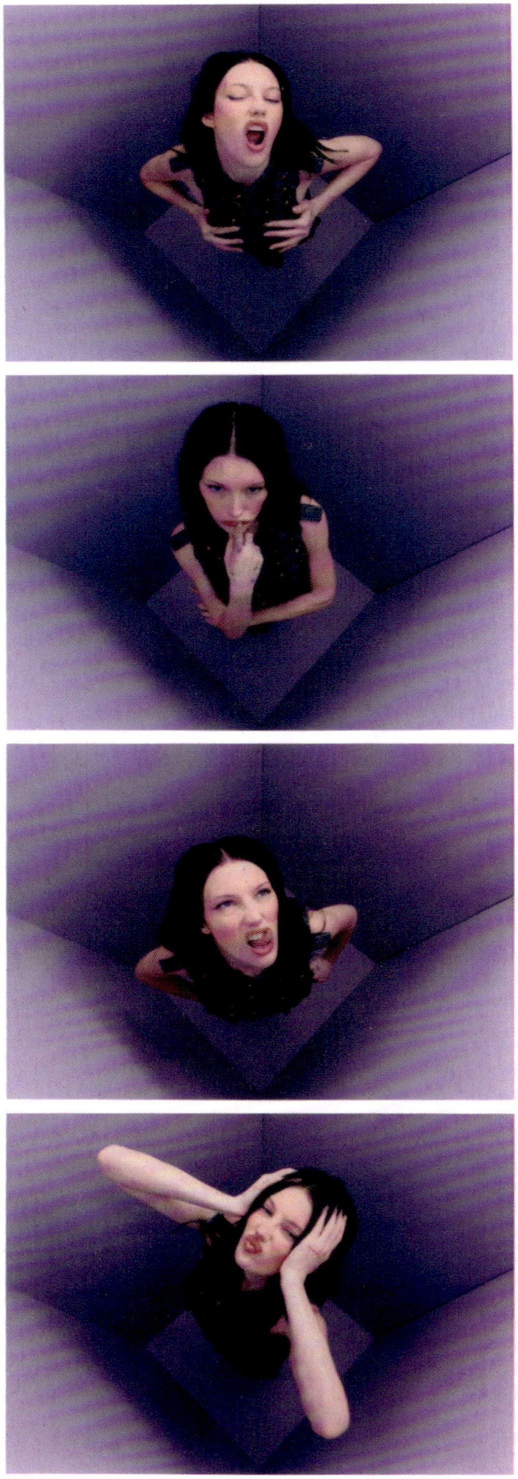

Remember who you are at the end of the day. Find time to be silly with yourself. Life doesn't always have to be taken so seriously.

important because it's not healthy to carry such weight with you day in and day out.

Q What do you do to forgive yourself for expectations that you are unable to meet? What do you do to allow yourself to move on?

A What I like to do to help forgive myself is go through my achievements and my accomplishments to appreciate what I have accomplished so far, whether that's scrolling back down to when I first started on TikTok or going through my camera roll and looking at really special moments. Those visuals remind me that I'm doing my best and what I've always dreamed of.

I tell myself that I've already accomplished so much and I've done so much that I really should live in the present moment, stop trying to fast-forward to the next thing. It's important to dream big and want more, but keep the appreciation close to your heart.

Q What is one belief about yourself that has softened or changed over time?

A My family would always joke that I'm a bossy boots. I think it was just my instinct that I didn't want anyone telling me what to do or how to think. I have such strong creative ideas, and I knew my strong opinions could make me a strong person.

Q It's that trait that has allowed you to get to where you are.

A In my mind, I've traded "bossy" for just having a really strong drive and work ethic.

Q Tell me about a feeling that you chase at night and one you try to avoid.

A I chase adrenaline and dopamine, which I've noticed a lot of other creators talk about. We are so go, go, go and have such big moments in our lives that, at the end of the day, when we do have these smaller, intimate moments with ourselves, our nervous system feels like it's not regulated, and we crave these rushes of something that will make us feel. It takes a lot of work to retrain your mind to not crave these extreme moments and emotions.

Have fun with self-care! I love putting time into curating my accessories, even something as simple as a scrunchie. When you're more intentional with things, I find you begin to appreciate them more in a world of mass consumption.

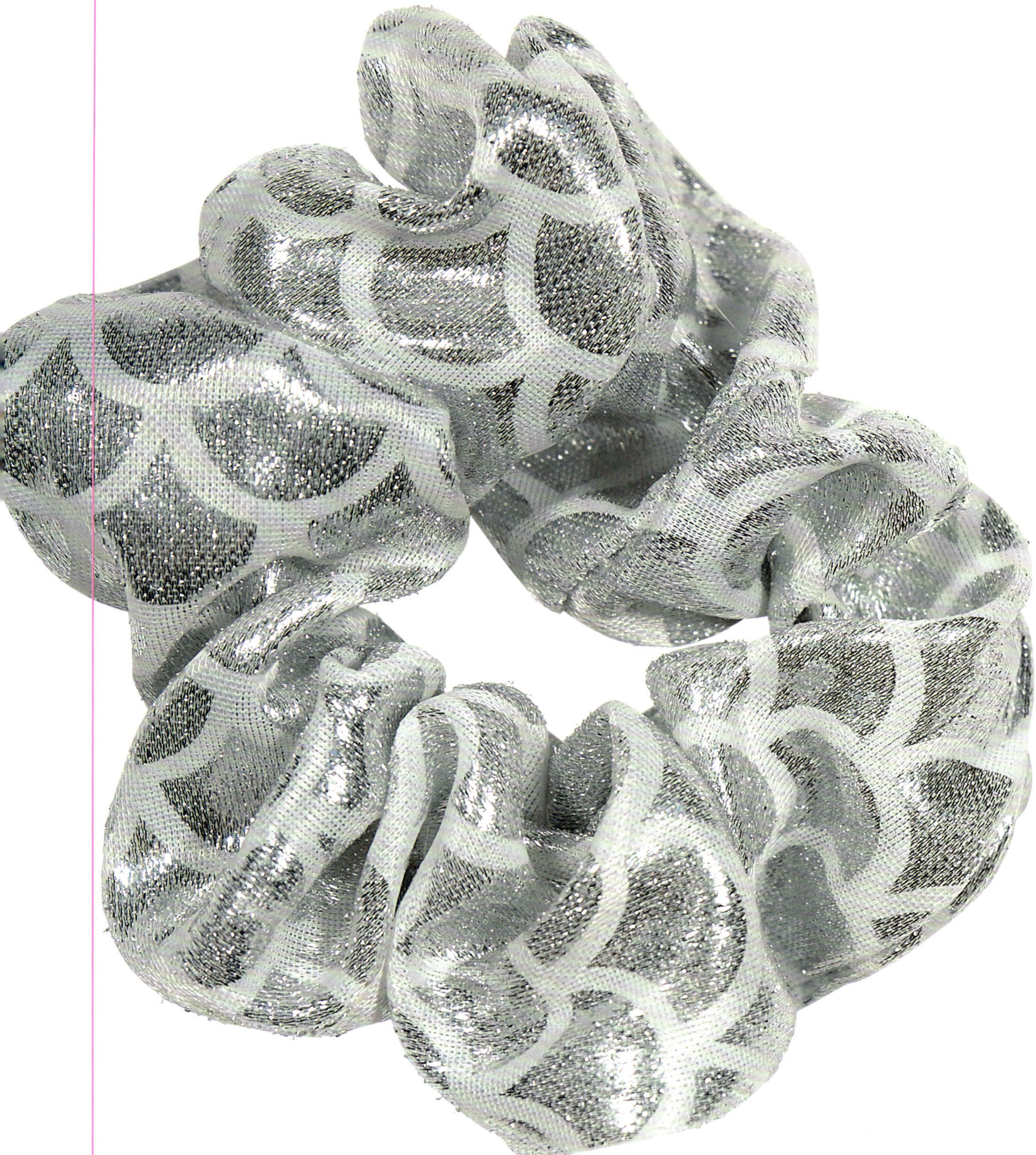

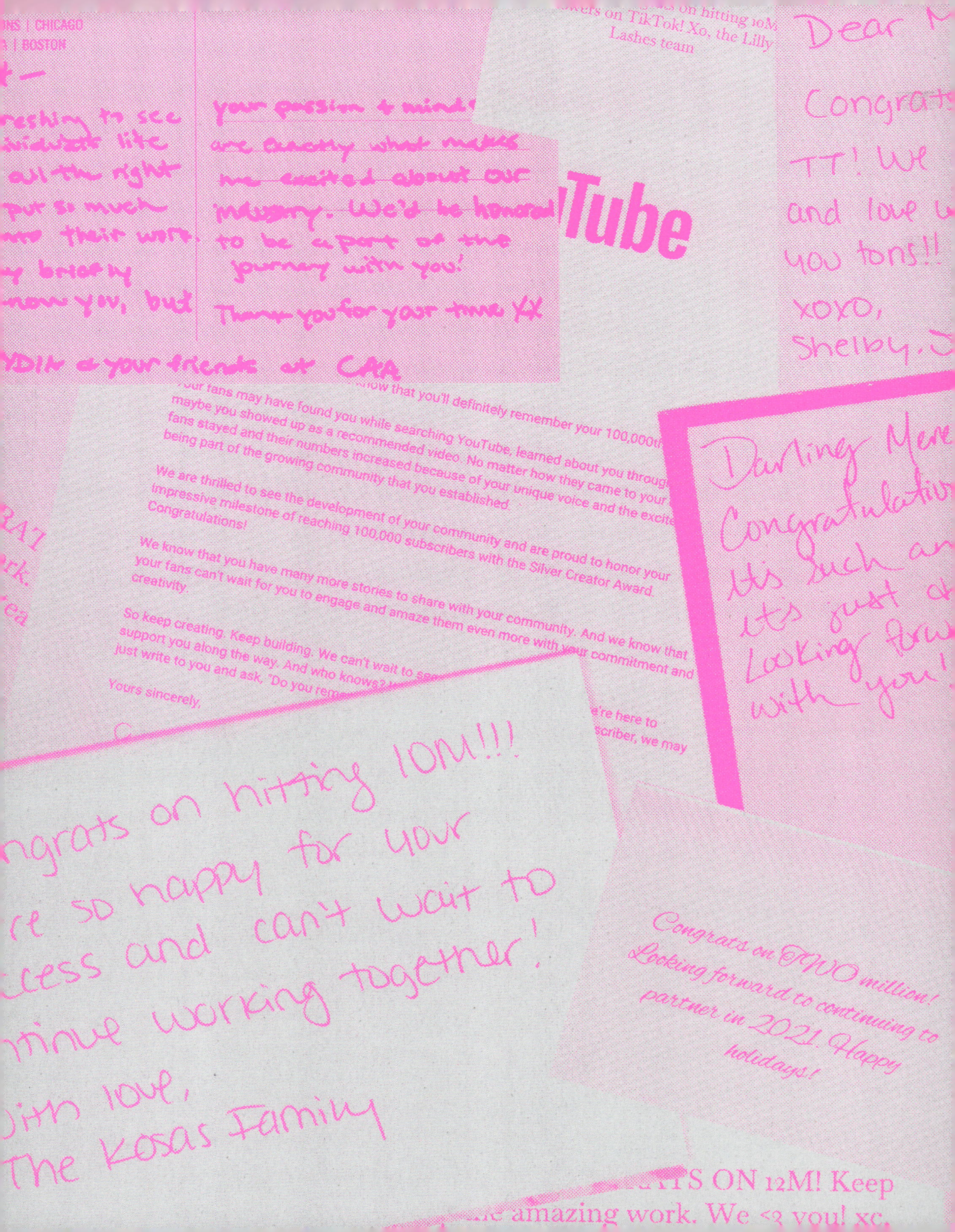

ONS | CHICAGO
A | BOSTON
reshing to see
ndividuals like
all the right
put so much
into their work.
ly briefly
know you, but
your passion & mind-
are exactly what makes
me excited about our
industry. We'd be honored
to be a part of the
journey with you!
Thank you for your time XX
YDIA & your friends at CAA
ers on TikTok! Xo, the Lilly
Lashes team
Tube
Dear M
Congrats
TT! We
and love u
you tons!!
XOXO,
Shelby J
your fans may have found you while searching YouTube, learned about you through
maybe you showed up as a recommended video. No matter how they came to your
fans stayed and their numbers increased because of your unique voice and the excite
being part of the growing community that you established.
We are thrilled to see the development of your community and are proud to honor your
impressive milestone of reaching 100,000 subscribers with the Silver Creator Award.
Congratulations!
We know that you have many more stories to share with your community. And we know that
your fans can't wait for you to engage and amaze them even more with your commitment and
creativity.
So keep creating. Keep building. We can't wait to see
support you along the way. And who knows?
just write to you and ask, "Do you reme
Yours sincerely,
Darling Mere
Congratulatio
Its such an
it's just
Looking forw
with you!
ngrats on hitting 10M!!!
re so happy for your
ccess and can't wait to
ntinue working together!
With love,
The Kosas Family
Congrats on TWO million!
Looking forward to continuing to
partner in 2021. Happy
holidays!
TS ON 12M! Keep
amazing work. We <3 you! xo,

ith–

12 million on
so proud of you
ing you grow! Miss

Benefit

eredith,
Congratulations on making
he Forbes 30 under 30 List!
You are truly one of a kind and
we can't wait to see what 2025 brin
Dare to dream, Darling!
rlotte Tilbury Influencer Tea

n,
on reaching 10M followers!
hievement & I'm sure
beginning!
to sharing the magic

Much Love,
Charlotte xxx

CharlotteTilbury
WWW.CHARLOTTETILBURY.COM
@CTILBURYMAKEUP

Dear Meredith–
Congrats on making Forbes
Creators list!! We are
and proud of you & feel
ful to be a part of
journey. Love you
friends

products and
happy to refill
ur stock! Congrat
aching 13 million
llowers! We ar
thrilled to se
success and
catrice to b

URBANSTEMS

Meredith,
Congratulations on reaching 18M
TikTok!
We are so proud of you, and cannot
wait to see what the future holds.
xx,
Ruhi & the Morph

Don't forget

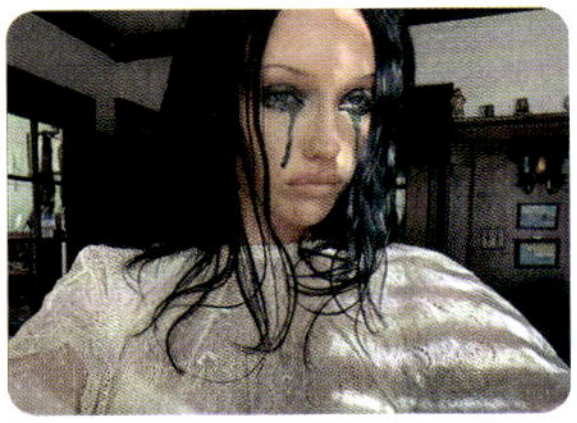

The day we shot the short film was a very emotional day for me. I was acting out all the pain I felt inside and reliving each thought and struggle I was battling. I wanted to prove to myself that I could conquer these thoughts and feelings. I wanted to document the day with behind-the-scenes photos, so I could take myself back to this day and remind myself how strong I am.

Q What does being gentle with yourself look like for you?

A Being gentle with myself is coming to terms with my vulnerabilities, fears, and judgments that I've carried on or absorbed from my surroundings. Recognizing it's normal human instinct to feel that way at times, but also knowing that I am happy with myself and embrace the person that I am.

It's so easy to be hard on ourselves after a full day of expectations and work, as well as judgments, and feeling like we need to fit into a certain box.

Q What advice would you give to someone who hasn't learned how to wind down or to someone who kind of struggles with that? What has helped you?

A I'm still struggling with that, but I will say getting a journal helped me. *The Untethered Souls* by Michael Alan Singer is a really great one because the book prompts you to do different exercises and provides different ways to reframe your thinking, mindset, and your reality. I find it really productive.

Q Do you become more dramatic or more pensive after 11 pm?

A Pensive, for sure. All the emotions hit me at night. It is, unfortunately, the perfect time to think about every conversation and emotion I've ever felt or said in my life.

Q What does morning you thank nighttime you for?

A I would say always washing my face. The worst feeling in the world is waking up, opening your eyes, and feeling crusted makeup everywhere. I can't name a worse feeling. Truly.

Q Do you have a sleep routine, or do you just hope for the best?

A I have a routine. I take melatonin and spray my lavender sleep spray on my sheets. And then I get both my dogs up in my bed and put on my rain sounds on my Hatch alarm clock. I scroll on my phone for a little bit and just detach from reality.

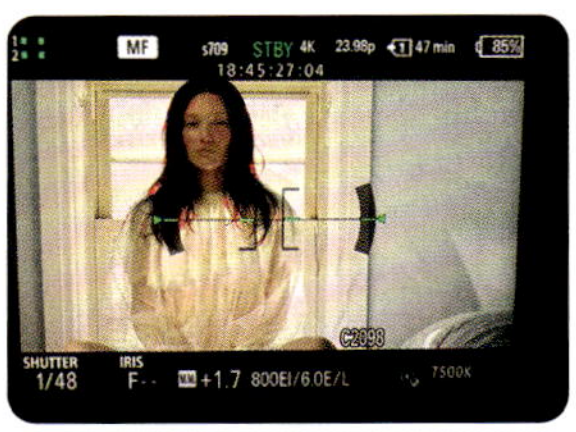

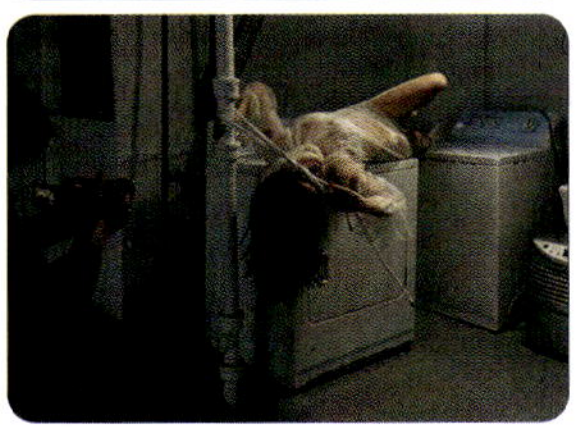

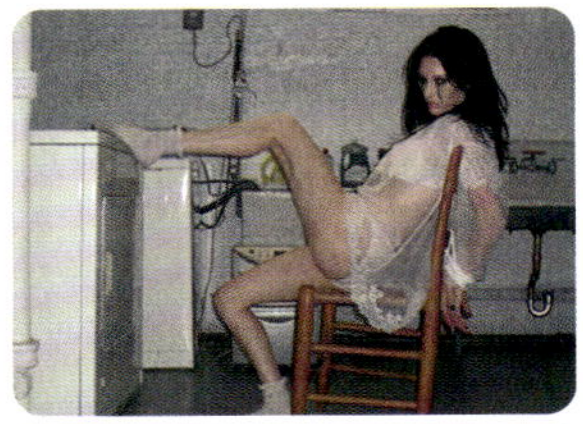

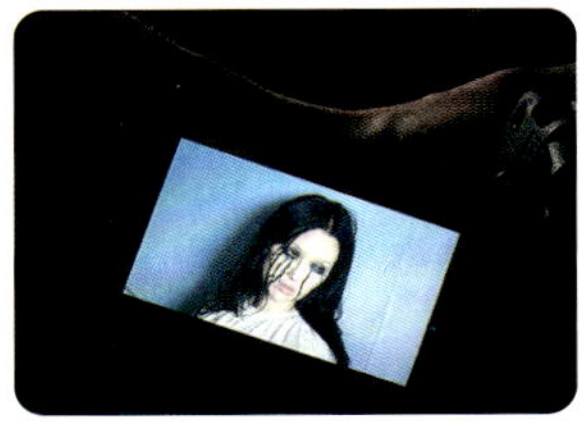

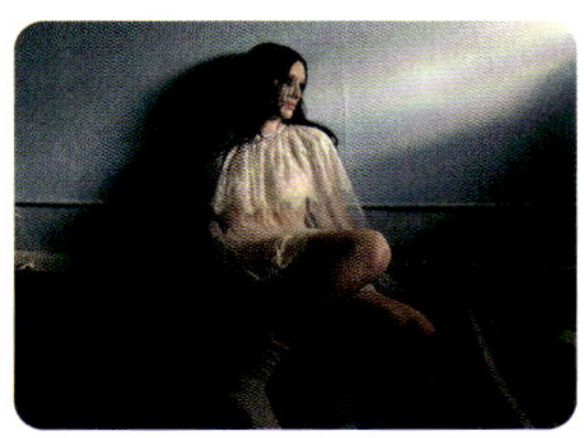

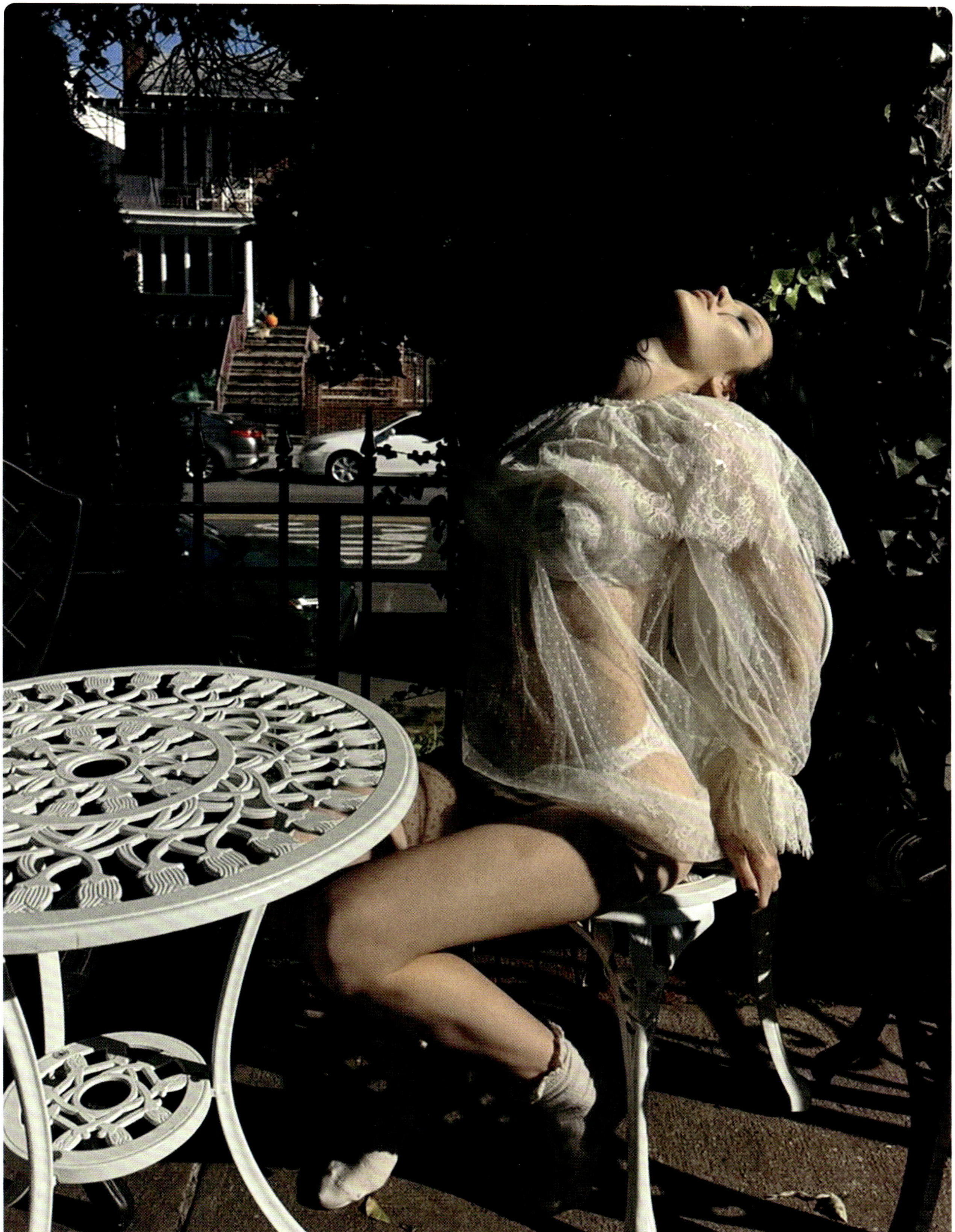

Candles are a way for me to wind down that I like to implement into my routine. I always like to collect matches to remind myself when I go to light my candles of some of my favorite places I've been or brands I've worked with.

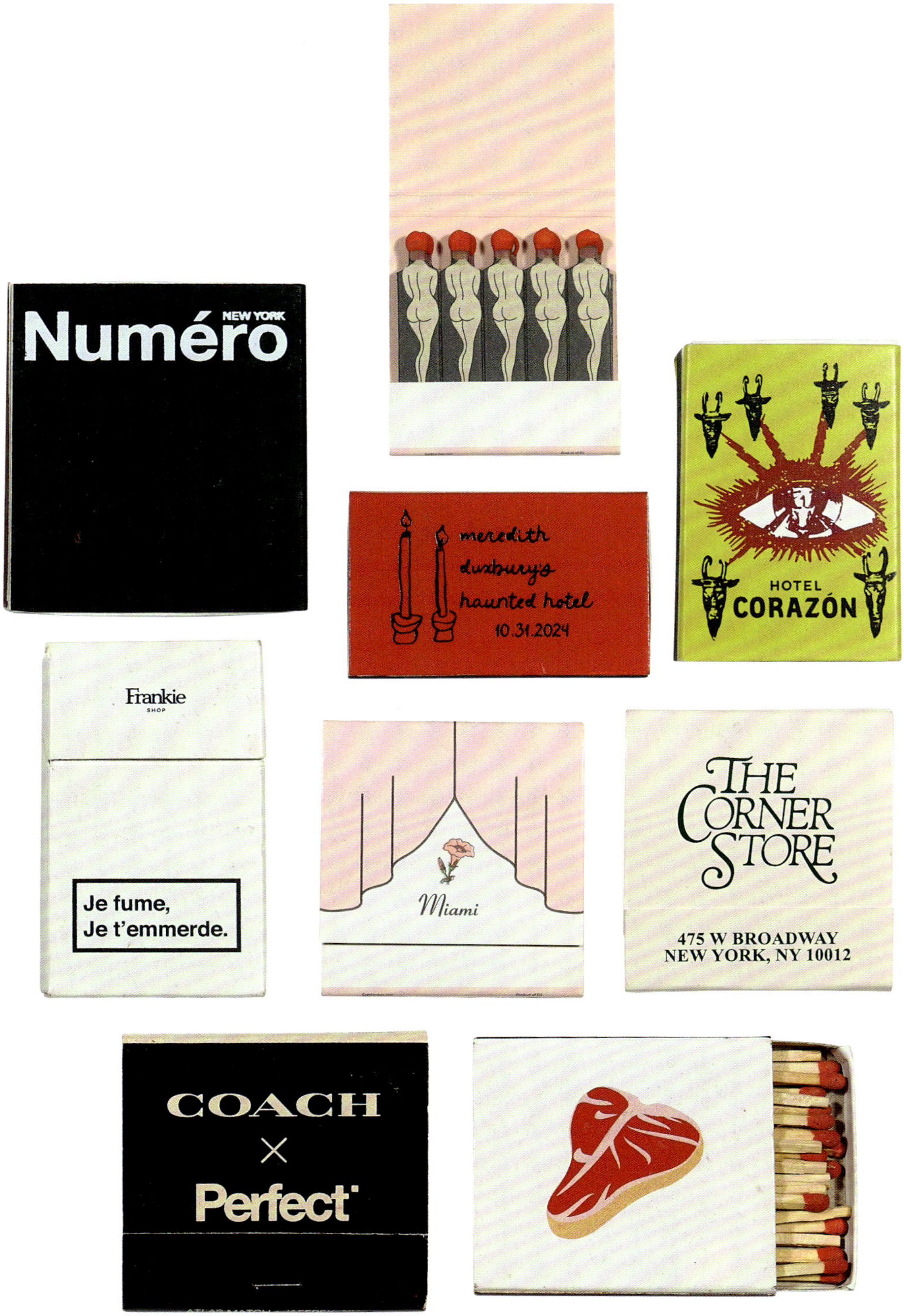

I find art to be a really great way to fill my mind with creative thoughts and feelings. I love collecting pieces that are fun and unique, like this ceramic ashtray, to place around my apartment. When you surround yourself with things that inspire you, you'll find you enjoy being in that space a lot more.

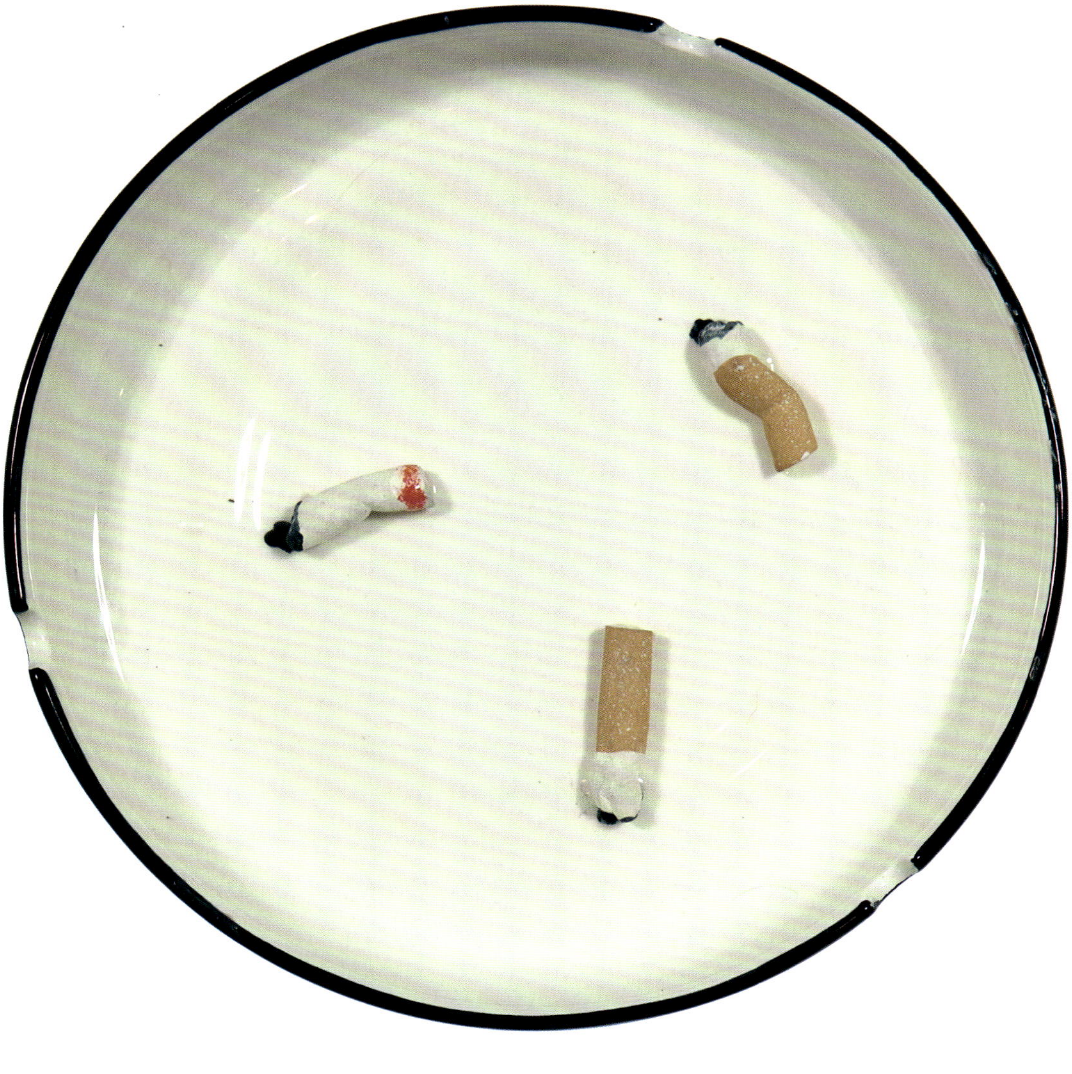

Q What is the last thing you usually think about before you fall asleep? Are you going through your to-do list? What is on your mind?

Be intentional with your nighttime routine. Put your favorite pj's on, and invest in bedding that makes you feel happy when you look at it! Put effort and time into the things you surround yourself with daily. It will add a lot more joy to your life.

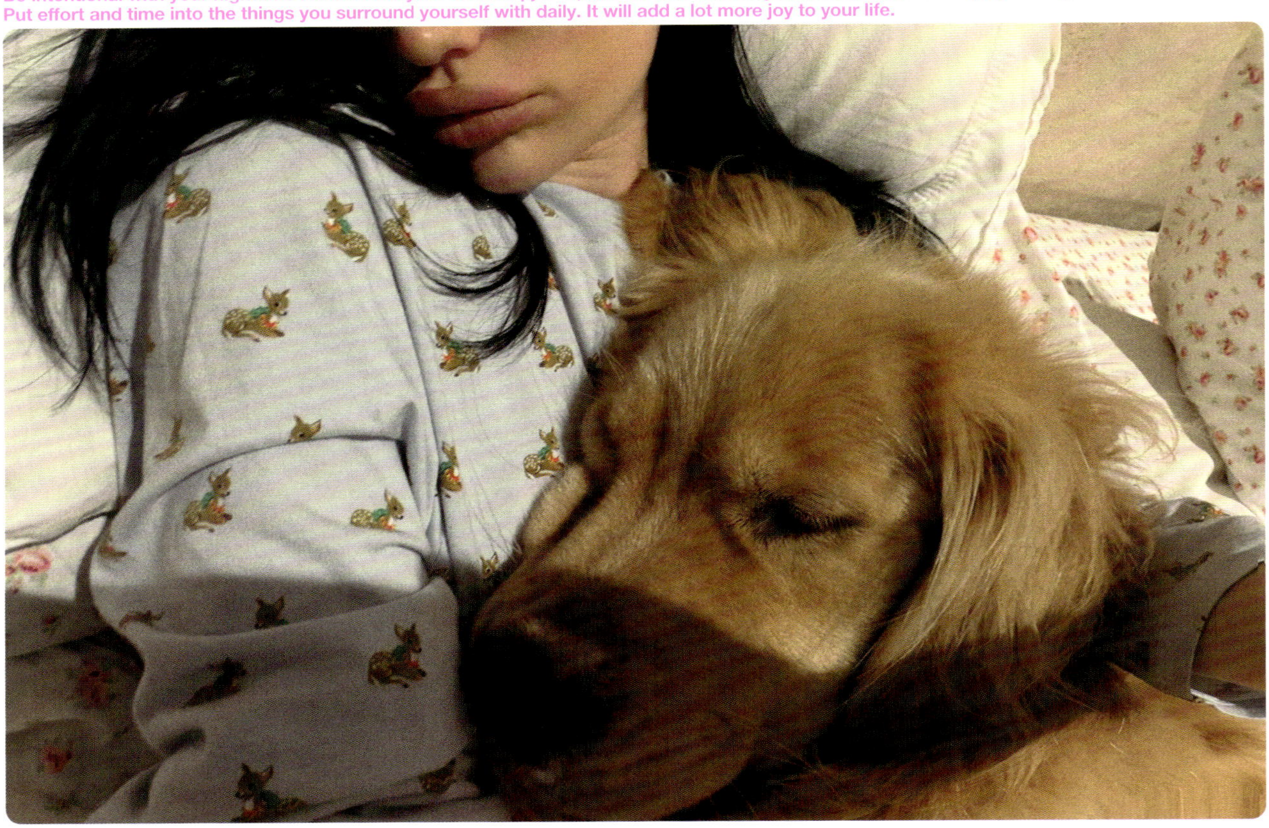

A Like every girl, I reenact in my head every conversation or interaction I've had that day, and worry if I said or did something weird, lol. Not healthy, but it's reality. Or, I make up fake scenarios in my head and then just fall asleep, haha.

Q When you come home, and it is time to take your glam off, what has to come off immediately?

A My foundation, for sure. I don't go straight into rubbing my eyes. For me, it's muscle memory to get the foundation off my face. I always go really in-depth on the skin, and then the eyes come second.

Q What do you use to remove the makeup? Wipes? Micellar water?

A I go in with a melting balm, and then I'll use a cleanser and micellar water.

Q So, you're doing a double cleanse?

A Yes! So important!

Q Okay, be honest. Have you gone to bed in full glam?

A For sure, those 5 am nights will get you, lol.

Q What was your first thought the next morning?

A How long will it take for the pimple to show up, and where is it going to be on my face?

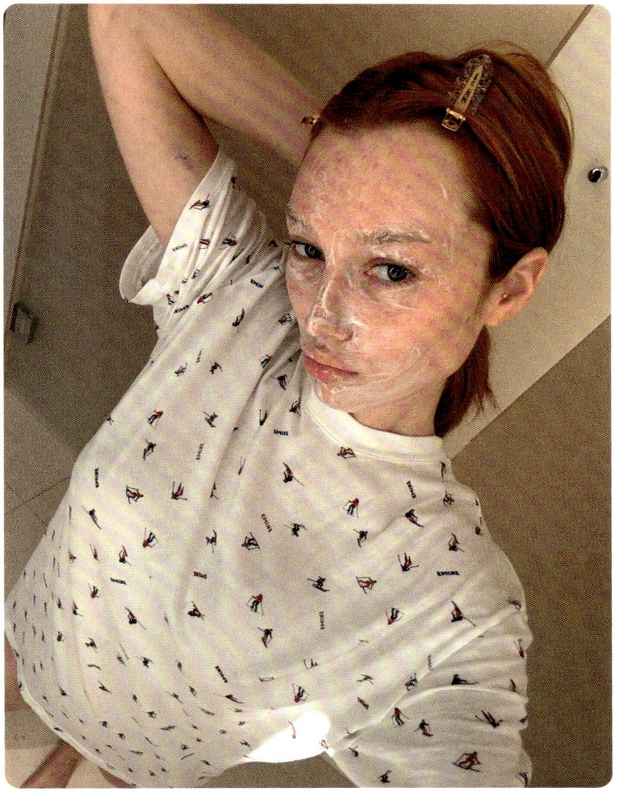

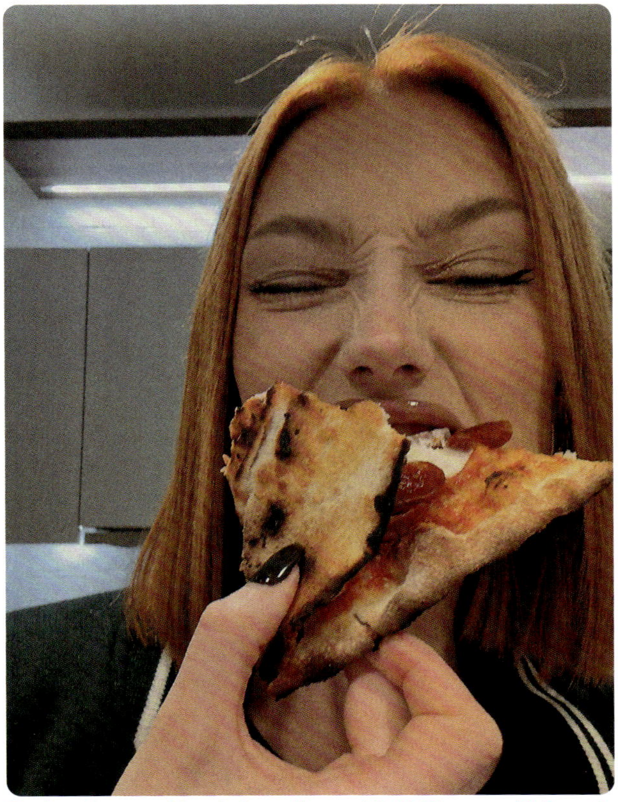

Don't get too caught up in the wellness of it all. Of course, it's important to be healthy, but to me, it's really about having a well-balanced lifestyle. That's being able to enjoy life. It's ok to allow yourself to have pizza or greasy food from time to time!

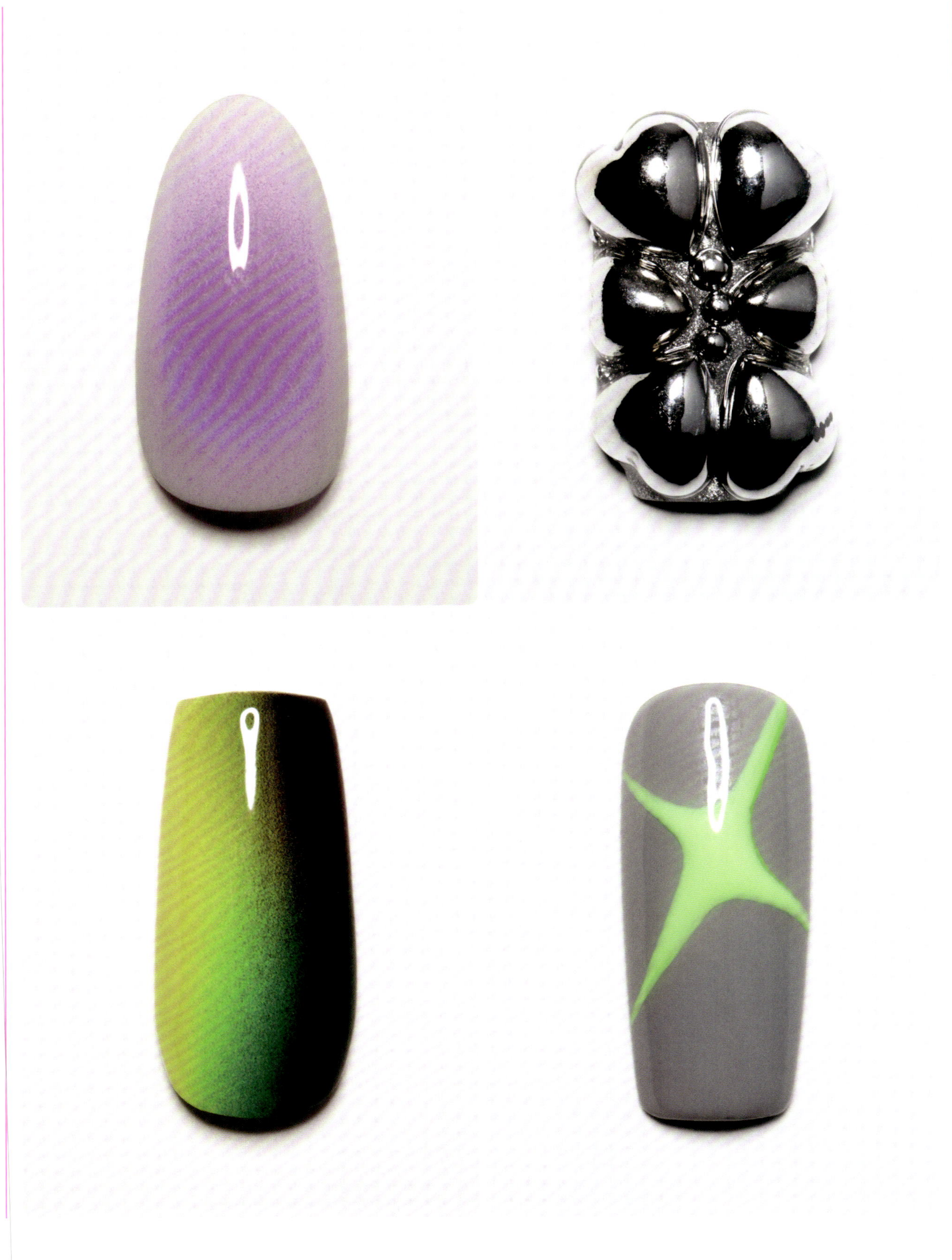

Getting unready isn't just about the process. It's about the thoughts you have throughout the process. Nail care to me is a form of self-care. To me, these press-on nails represent creativity and boldness, which is a great thing to reflect on and make sure you're implementing into your life. I also want to remind everyone it's crucial to take care of yourself and look good for *you*, not just for the outside world.

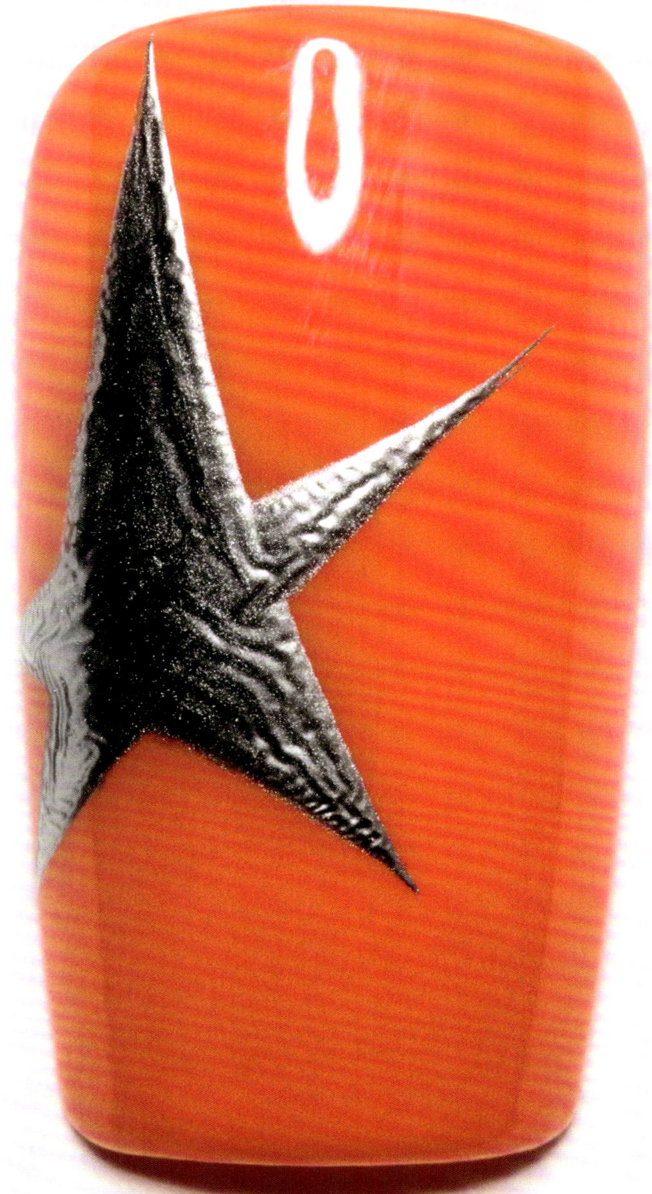

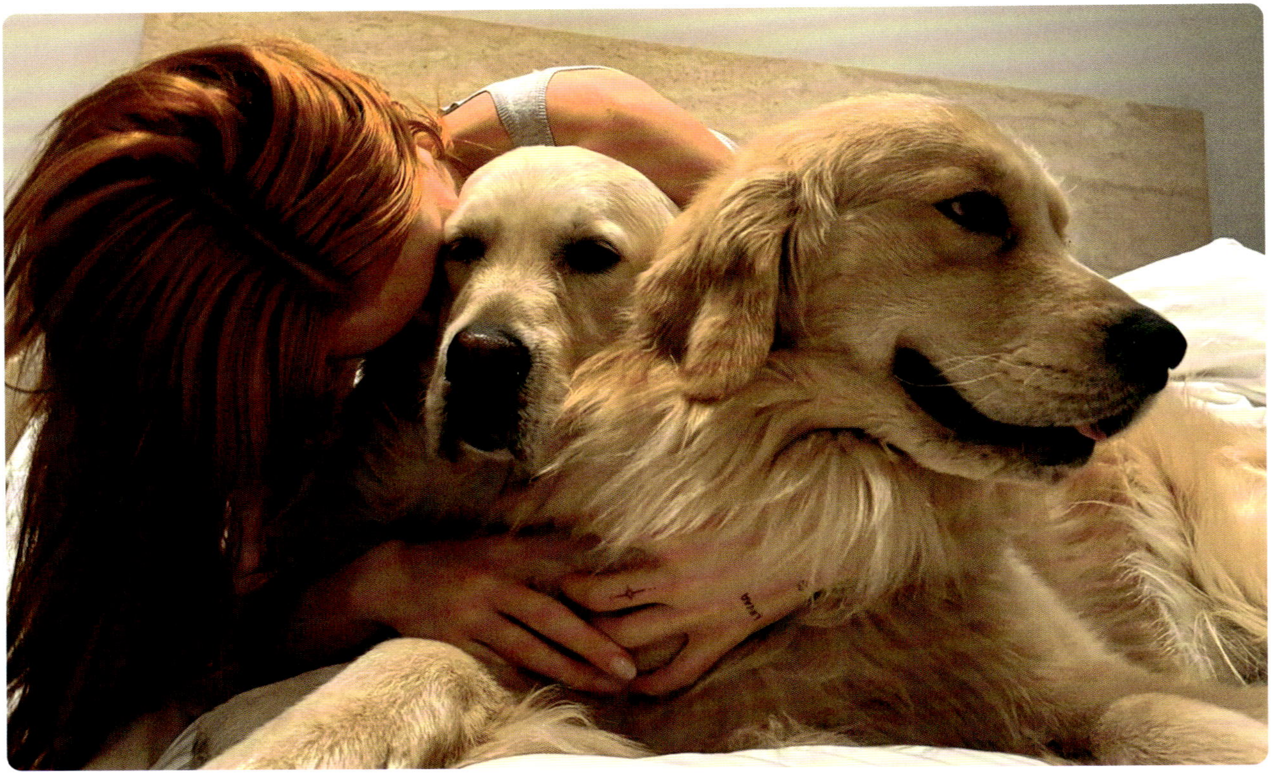

Routine to me is a big part of my life. When I lose that, I feel out of place and get anxious. For my nighttime routine, I love starting with a nice, hot shower with all my favorite products that nourish the body, then taking time to do a face mask, and cuddling with my dogs. After that, I finish off my skincare routine and moisturize my body. Once I'm done with face and body care, I like to make myself a hot tea, put on a favorite pair of pj's, get into cozy, clean sheets, and light a candle on my nightstand. Journaling for ten minutes has always helped me to reflect on my day and think about how I'm feeling mentally. Once I'm ready to head to bed, I put some CBD oil on my temples and on the back of my neck, and spray a lavender sleep spray on my sheets.

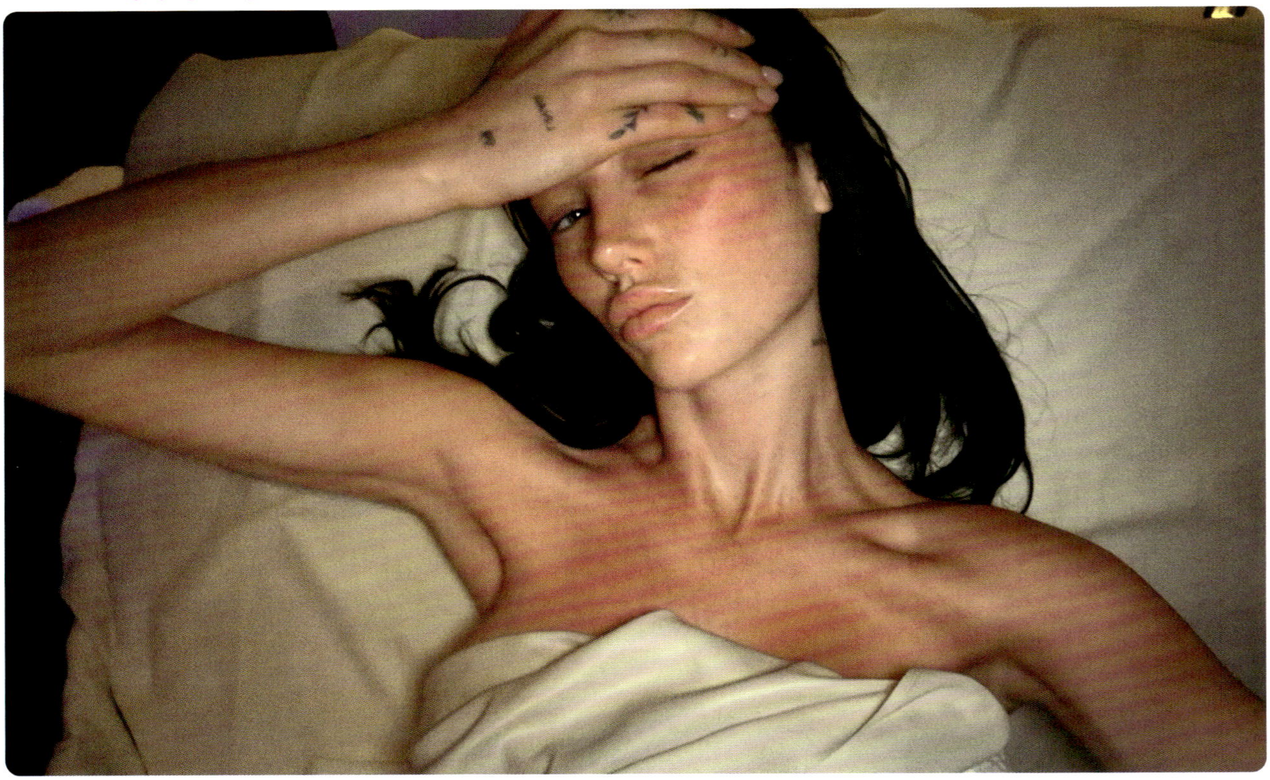

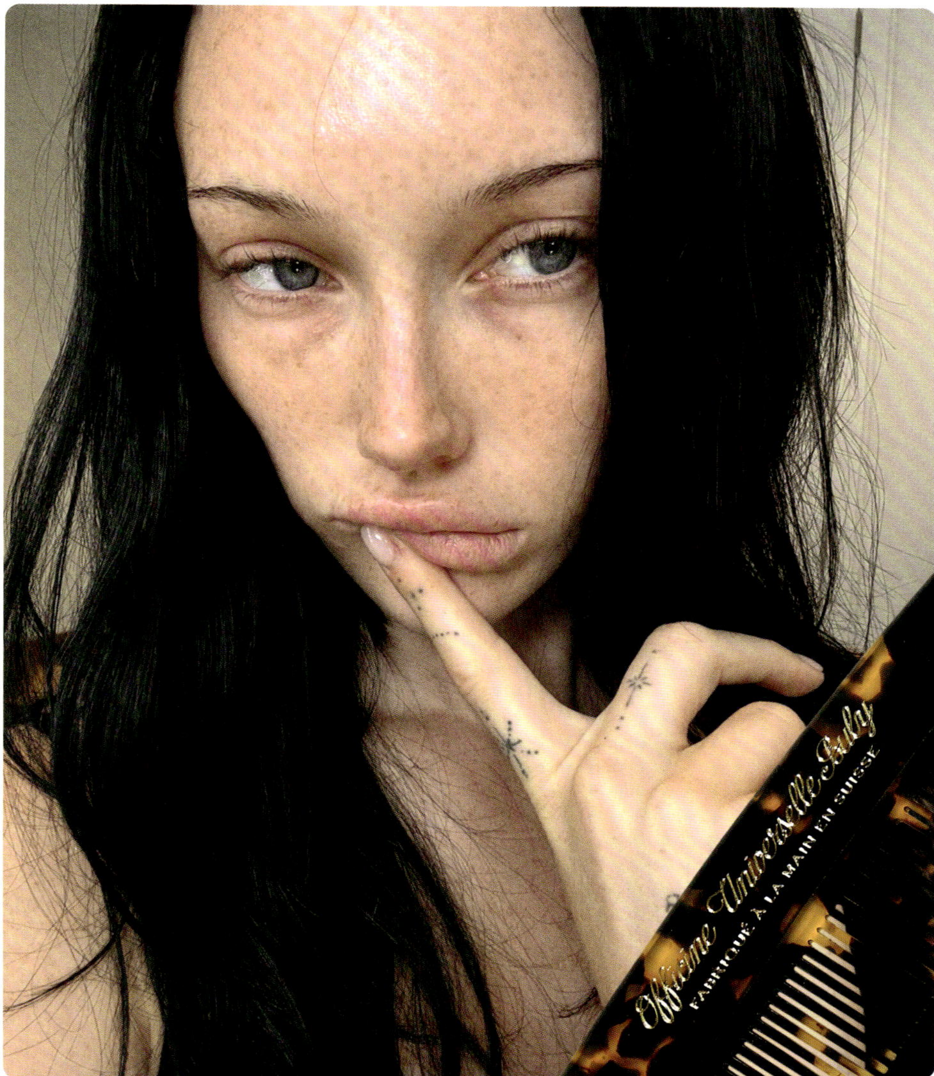

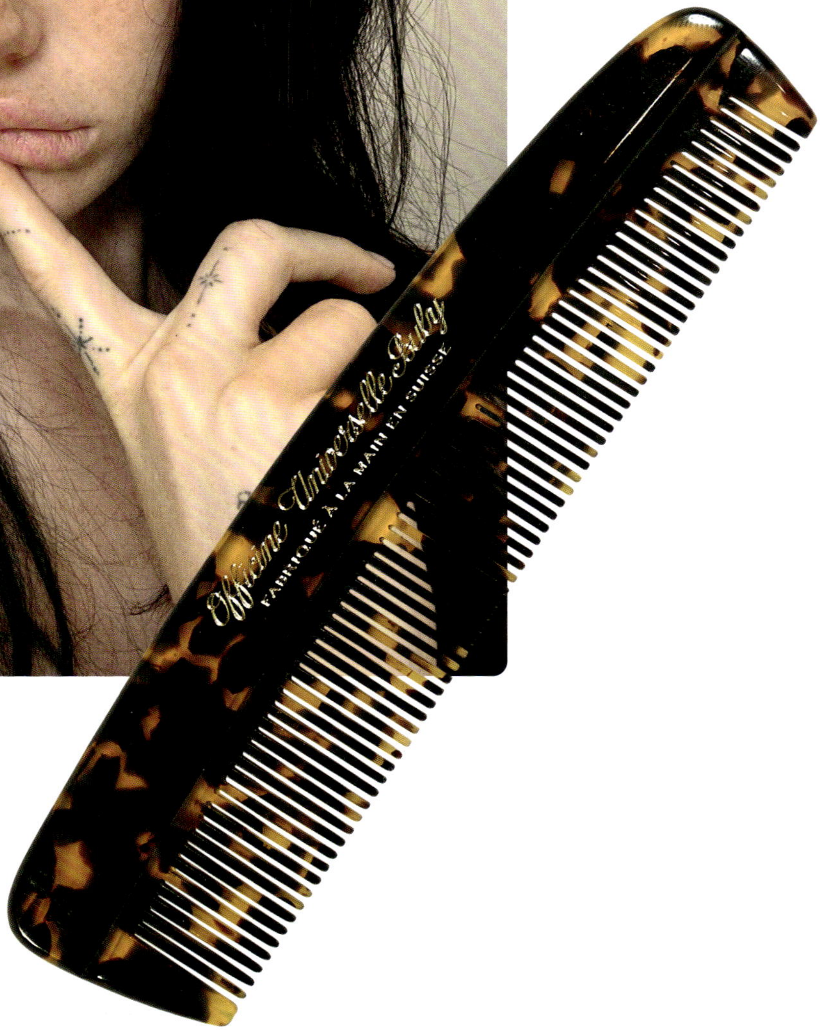

TOP: A moment to let my skin breathe and my freckles shine. CENTER: This was a gift from L'Oréal. It's very special to me because L'Oréal is all about promoting self-worth and encouraging powerful, strong women. Whenever I use this, it reminds me of that message!

CONFESS OR DENY

Q You've used an expired product and hope for the best.
A Oh god no, deny. My skin would hate me.

Q You've ignored the instructions on a mask and rinsed whenever you felt like it.
A Confess. I literally leave hair masks on for three days and face masks overnight. The longer the better, right?

Q You've used body lotion on your face because you ran out of moisturizer.
A Confess, sometimes you don't have an option, lol.

Q You've removed lashes in a car on the way home.
A Confess. I've removed an entire makeup look on the way home from a shoot, I arrive home a brand-new girl, lol.

Q You've secretly loved how dramatic a pimple patch looks.
A Confess. I got these little cute ones from Korea, and they're little emoji hearts and stars. I love using those.

Q You've said to yourself, "I'll wash my makeup brushes tomorrow" more times than you'd like to admit.
A Confess. I have a box of 500 dirty ones waiting to get cleaned.

Q You've done your entire routine in bed.
A Confess. I've made *someone else* do my entire skincare routine, lol.

Q Please elaborate.
A An ex…Oops.

Q You've cried mid-skincare routine at least once.
A Confess. Multiple times.

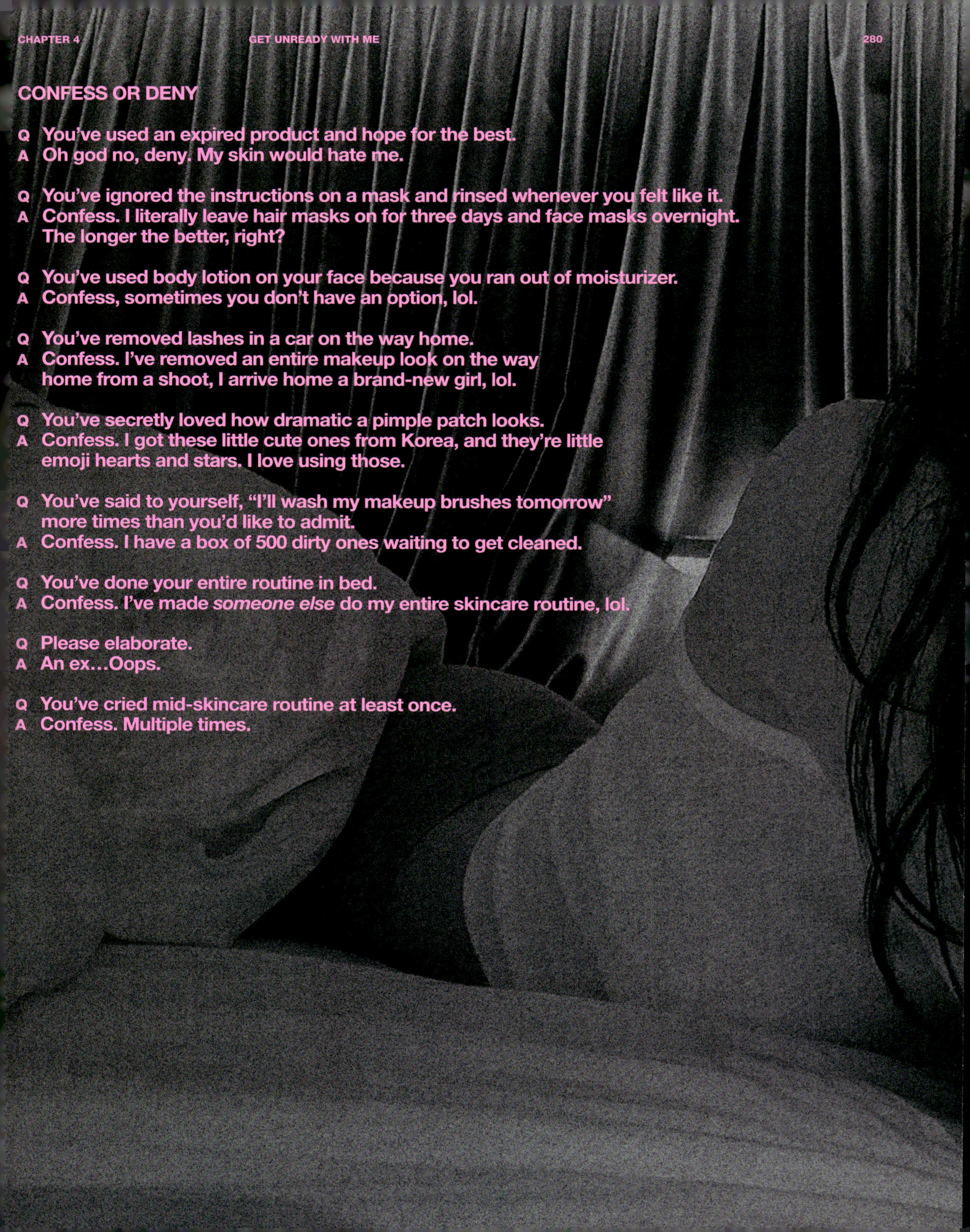

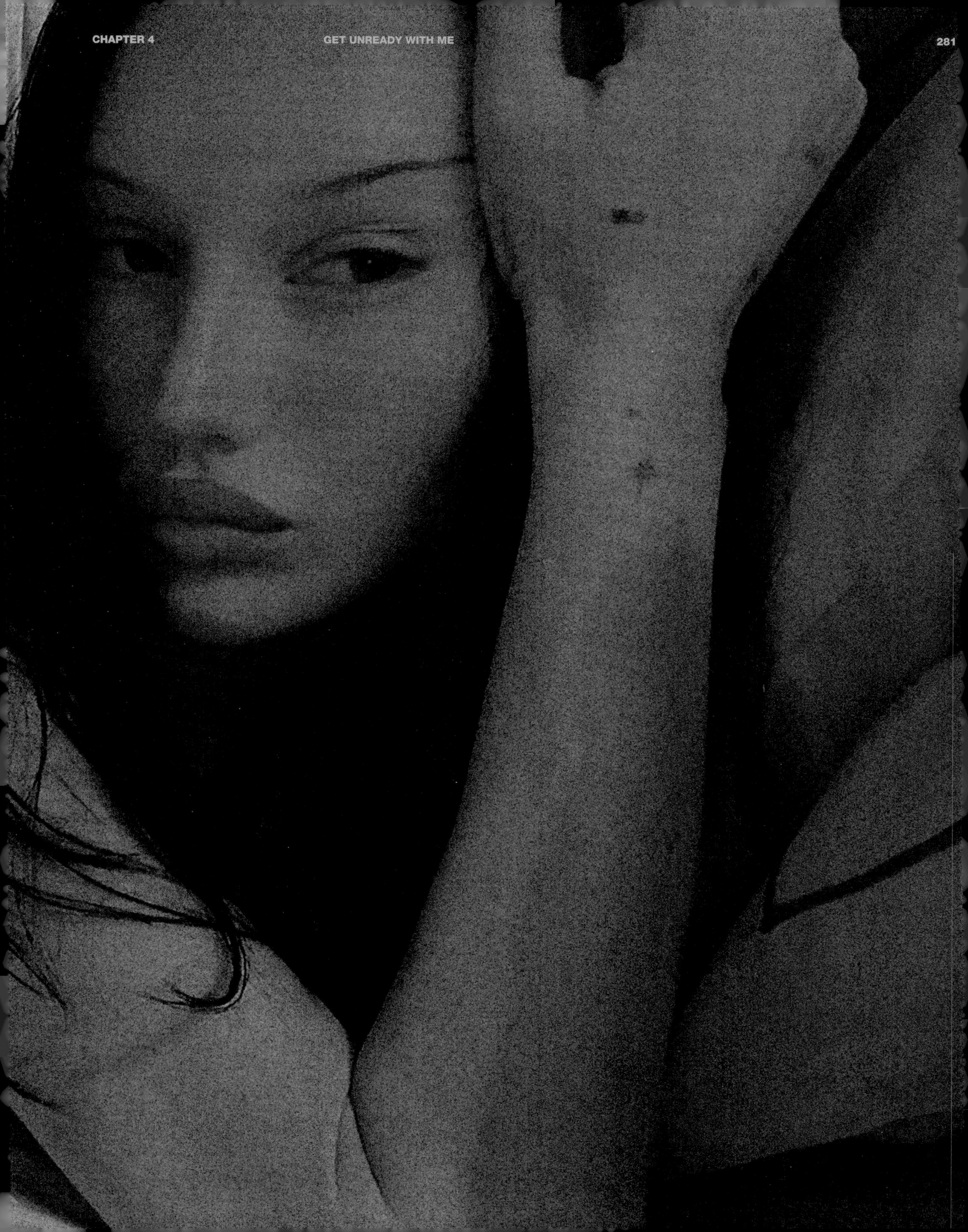

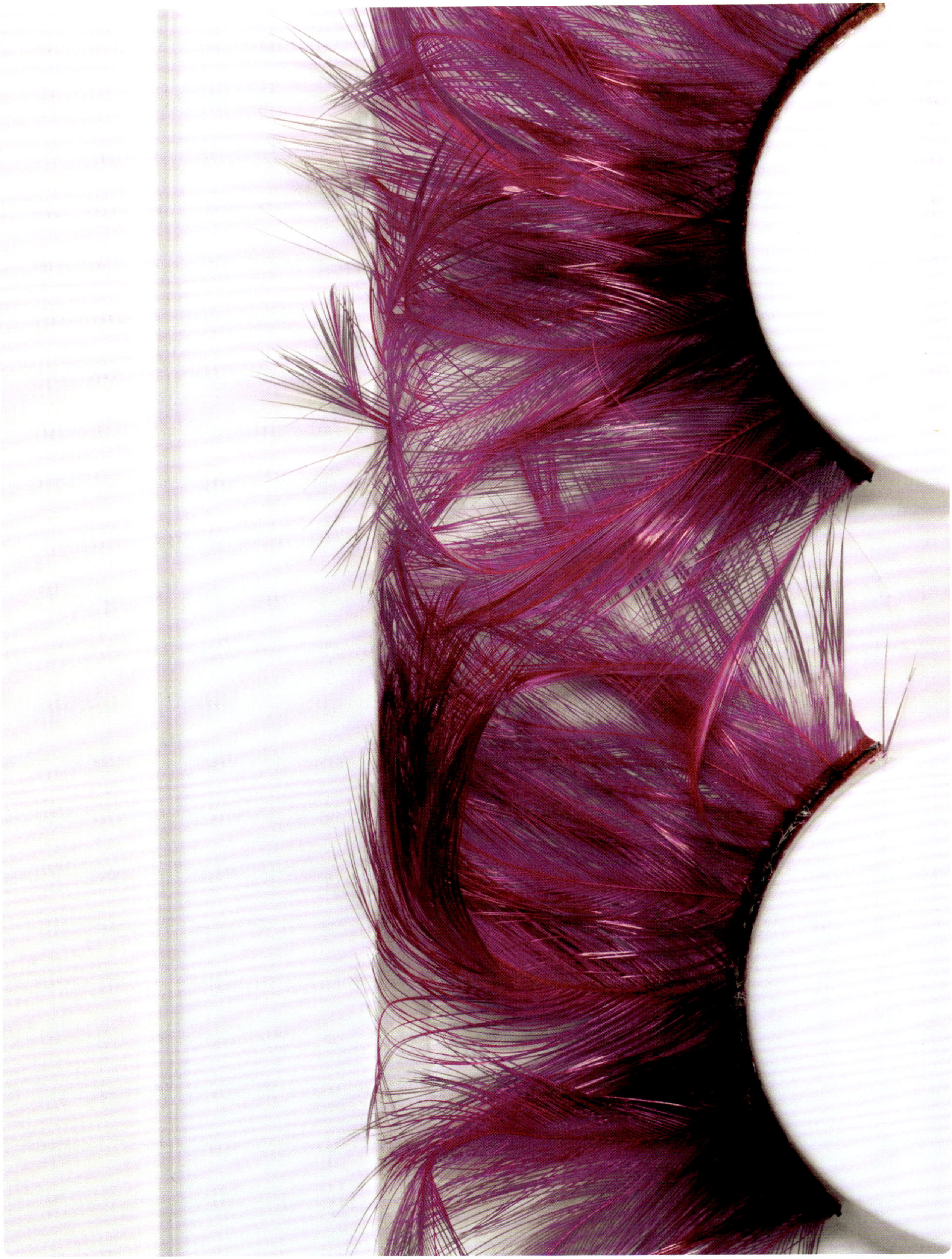

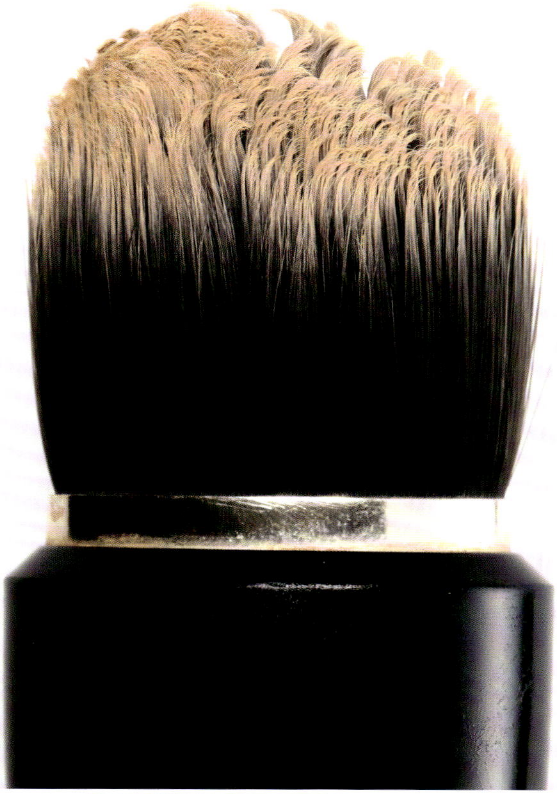

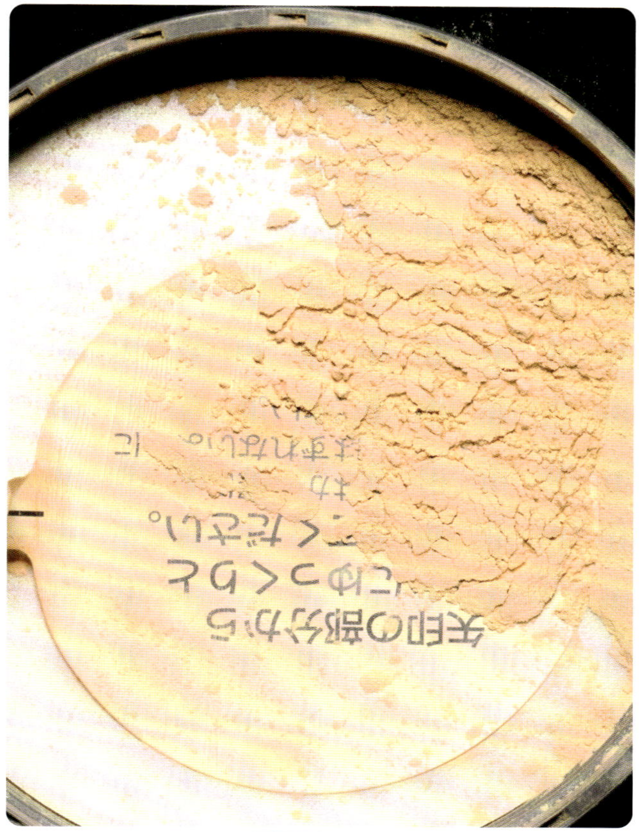
矢印の部分から

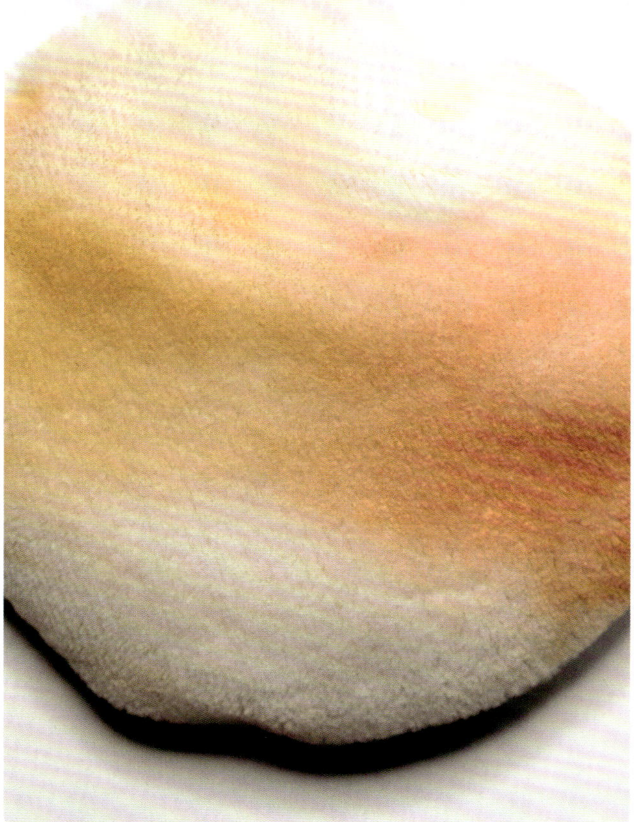

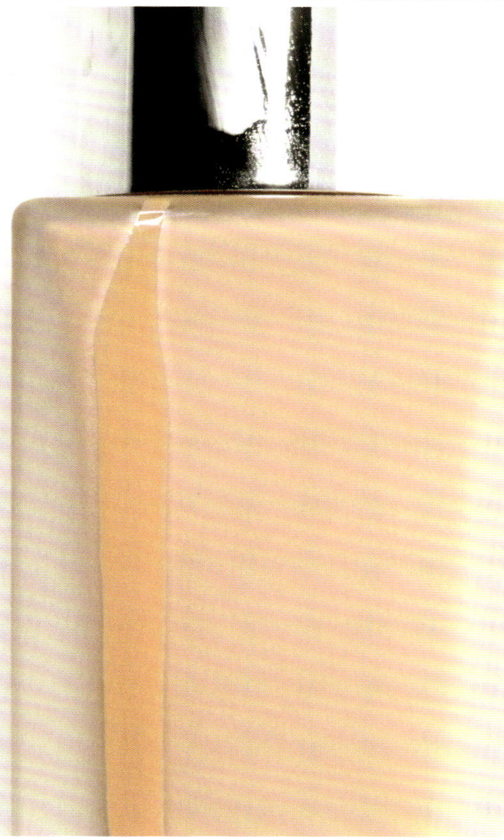

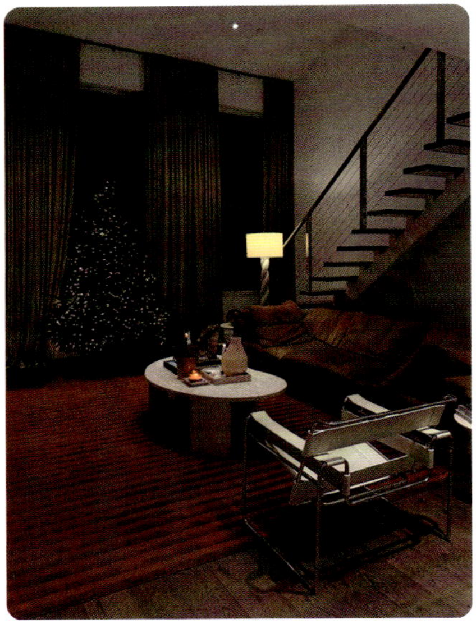

My apartment is my little sanctuary, I designed it all myself! One of my fave side hobbies is interior design.

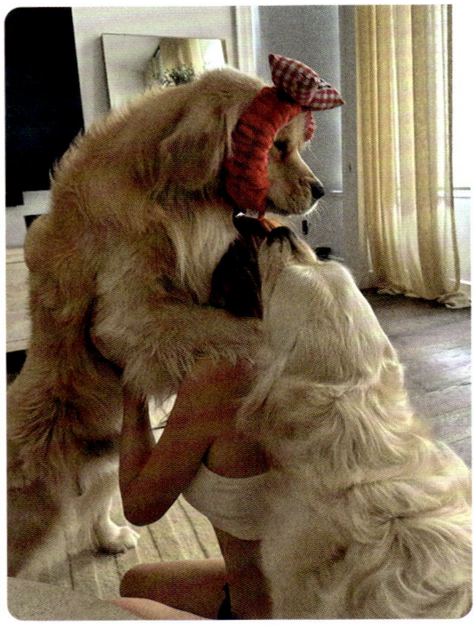

Playing with Crumpet and Pancake is truly the best therapy!

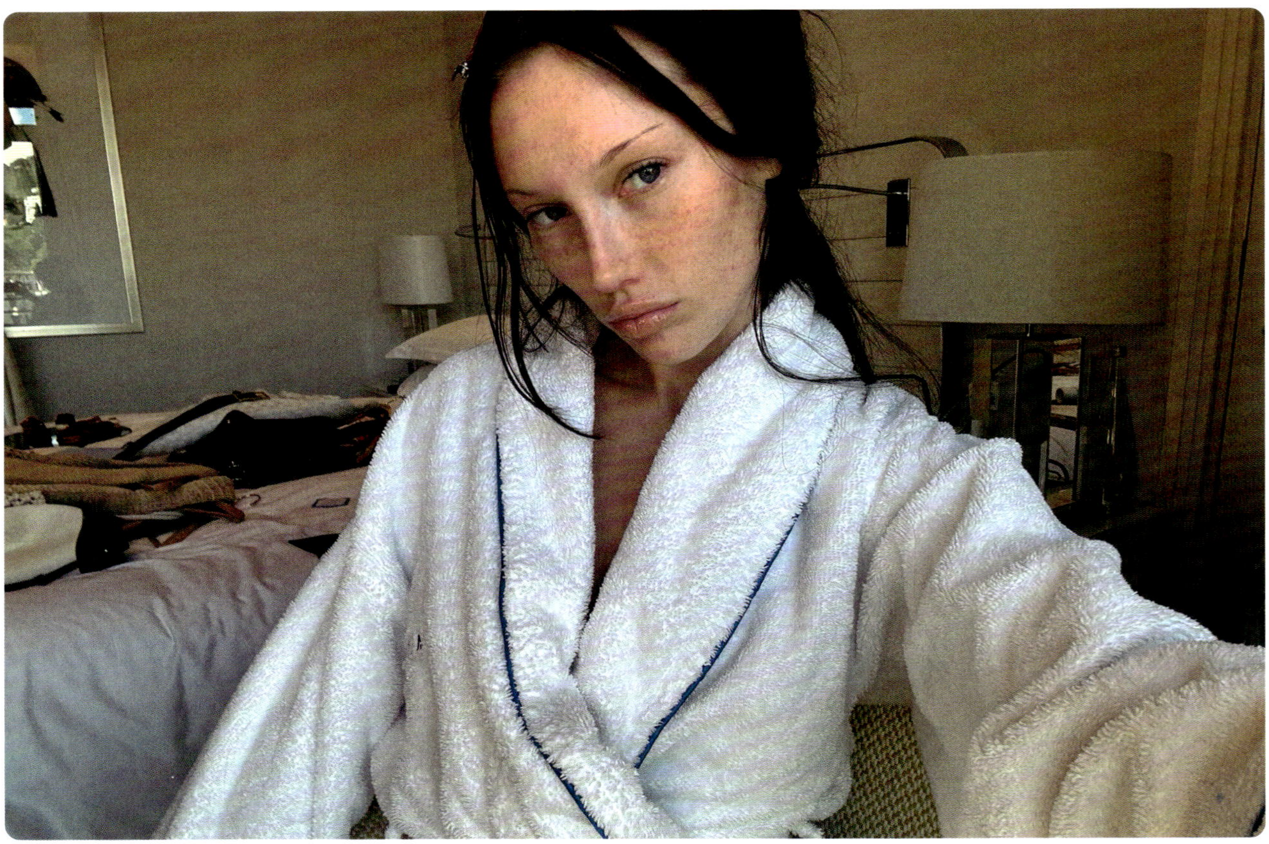

Q What is one thing you do at night that your followers would be shocked to hear? Would they be shocked to find out that you sometimes go to bed with your makeup on?

A I don't think anything is a shock to them anymore. My followers know me so well. I've made videos doing a hungover get unready with me after sleeping in my makeup, lol.

Q What is a nighttime habit that you are low-key embarrassed to admit?

A Honestly, nothing. I'm an open book.

Q Do you ever catch yourself practicing your online voice or shooting your overhead?

A My social media voice definitely doesn't need any more practice, so no—haha. If anything, it needs an off button.

Q What is the strangest thing you've watched on your phone with a face mask on?

A Probably mukbangs and pimple-popping videos.

Q What do you hope tomorrow's version of you remembers from the night before?

A How she was able to overcome the day before, and that every day is a new day. She'll be able to overcome whatever challenges she has the next day as well.

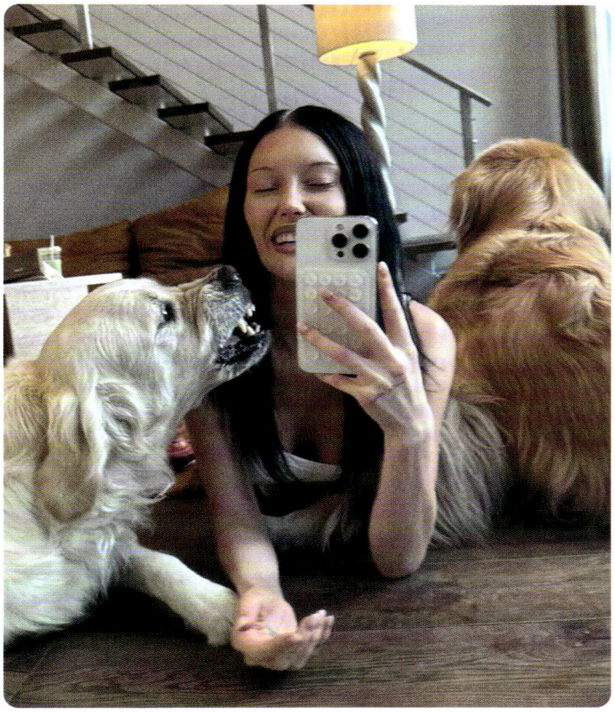

My dogs are my best friends, built-in roommates, and the best company!

OPPOSITE PAGE: Acceptance plays a major role in the way you're going to feel about yourself. Not everything is in your control. Once you learn to let go, you're going to feel a lot lighter. It's so important to feel comfortable in your own skin and, of course, that can be hard when you're struggling with any skin concern like acne or eczema. One thing that has always made me feel at ease is acknowledging that I am not alone. So many people deal with these same issues, and a lot of the time, we exaggerate them to be something they're not. People are not going to remember you for the pimple or blemish you had on your face. They're going to remember you for how you treated them and the person you are on the inside.

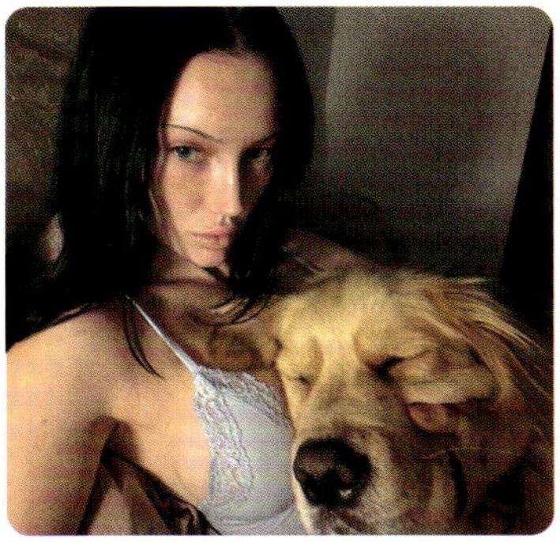

Snuggle time!

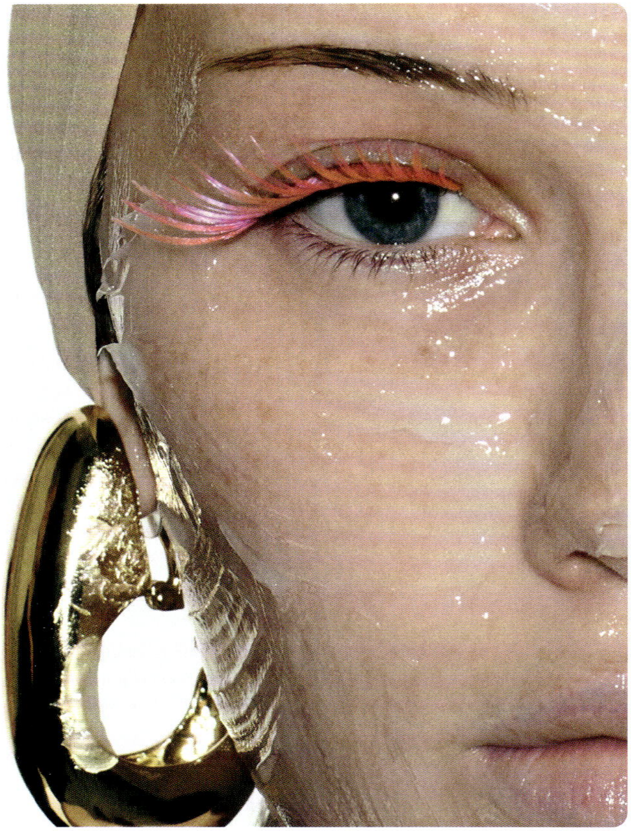

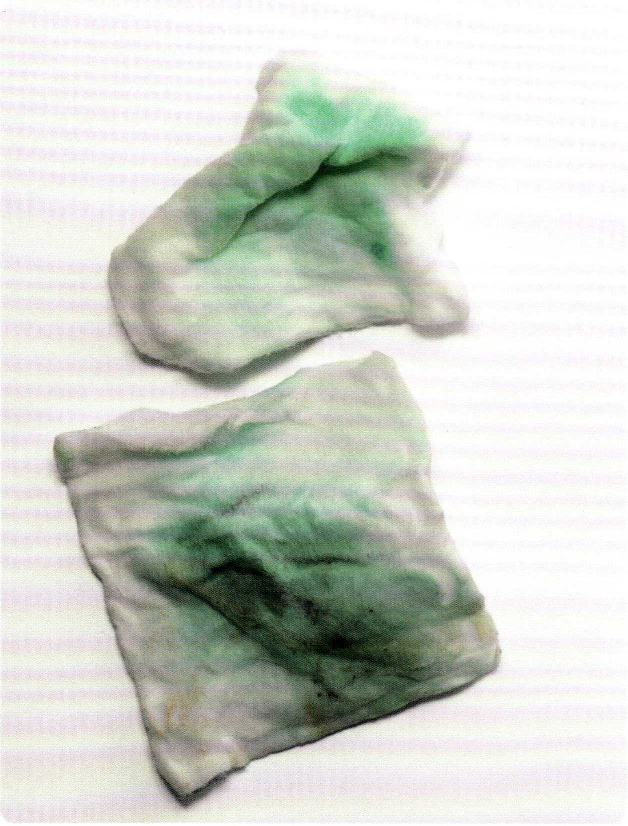

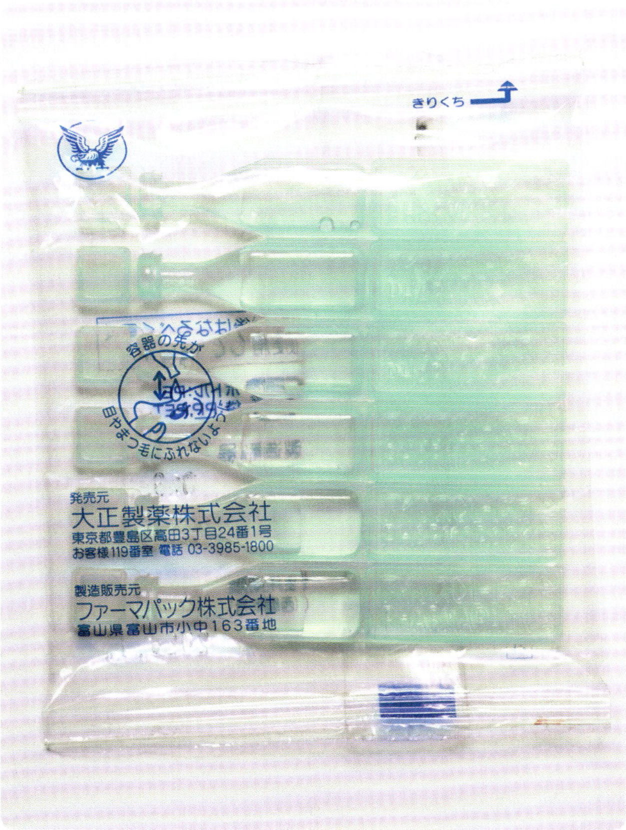
きりくち
発売元
大正製薬株式会社
東京都豊島区高田3丁目24番1号
お客様119番室 電話 03-3985-1800
製造販売元
ファーマパック株式会社
富山県富山市小中163番地

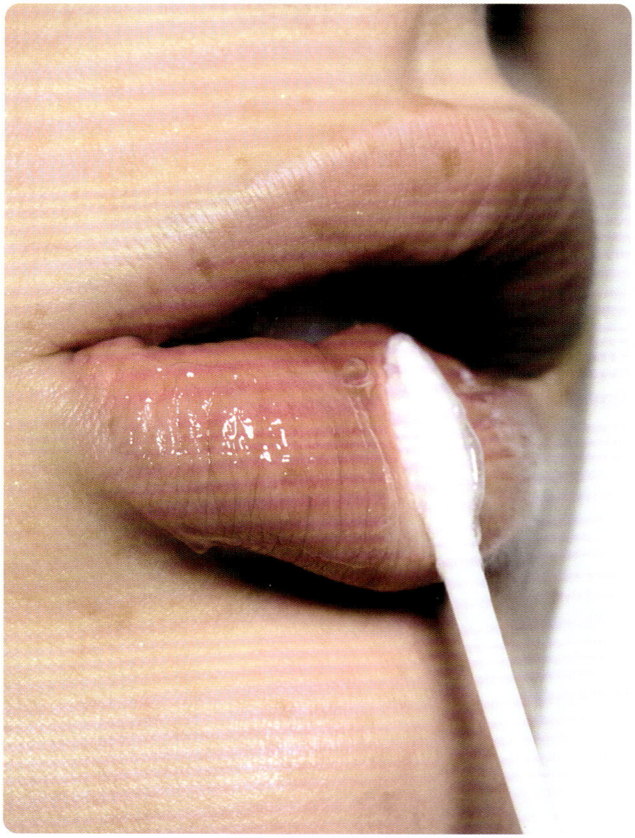

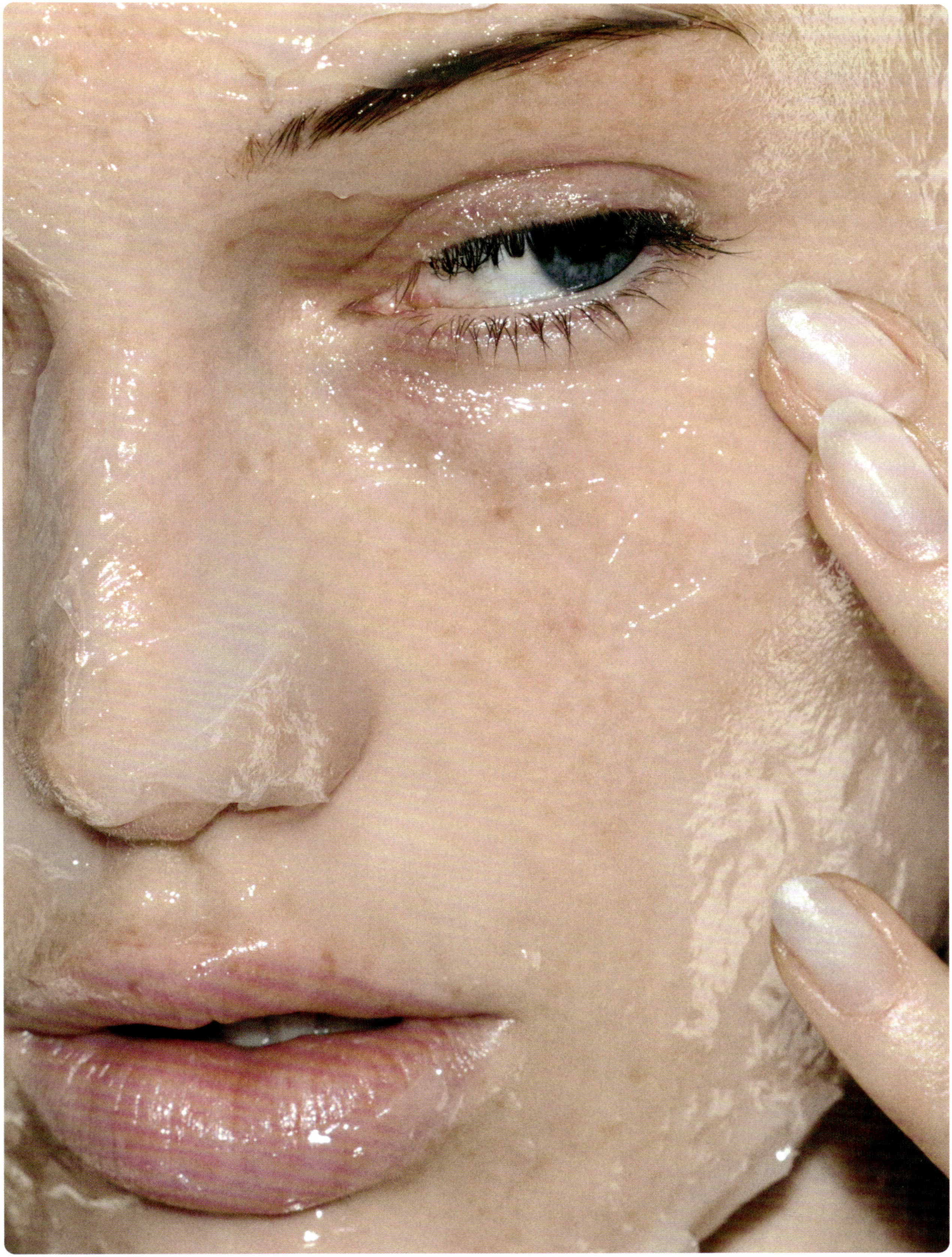

COVER SHOOT

Art Direction:
Graphic Services

Photography:
Kévin Drelon

Production and Studio:
Neighbors

Styling:
Elly McGaw, Frank Reps

Makeup:
Mitch Yoshida, Streeters

Hair:
Edward Lampley, CLM

Manicurist:
Natalie Pavloski, Bridge Artists

Digital Tech:
Max Louis Miller, Neighbors

Makeup Assistant:
Rio Kinoshita

Hair Assistant:
Fallon Seymour

ACKNOWLEDGMENTS

I want to begin by sharing my deepest gratitude to my online community! Thank you for all of your support from the very beginning—from my first video, to my "ten pumps of foundation" and runway moments—and all the way through the making of this book. You believed in me long before I could imagine this moment, and I am here today because of you. I always want to be a safe space of love and support, where people can come to escape and just feel a weight lifted off their shoulders. I will always advocate and stand up for each and every one of you, love you more than my words can describe! Thank you for sticking with me through it all!

To my associate publisher, Anthony Petrillose, and editors, Gisela Aguilar and Julie Schumacher, and the entire team at Rizzoli—thank you for believing in this project. Your support, care, and enthusiasm made this book possible. I am deeply grateful for the trust you placed in my vision and for your support of my creativity every step of the way. I have been a fan of Rizzoli for as long as I can remember. This book would not be what it has come to be without you. Thank you for providing me with such a supportive team to create and express myself.

Thank you to Daise Bedolla for such thoughtful and generous interviews, and for helping shape this book with curiosity and care. Sitting down with you and getting personal was a very special moment I'll always cherish.

I am also incredibly grateful to Sydney Shiffman, my literary agent at CAA, for her guidance, knowledge, and belief in me throughout this process. The countless creative calls and workshopping from a blank space was such a fun process to have your input and involvement in. Thank you for ushering me into a new space and creative challenge that has been so fulfilling.

And to my art directors, Jasmine Holm and Marcus Hollands (Graphic Services), who brought so much talent, imagination, and heart to this project. Thank you for being such a dream to work with and for expanding my creativity in ways I could have never imagined. I have always dreamed of collaborating with a team that sees and aligns with my vision, and you truly have gone above and beyond. Thank you endlessly.

And to Hannah Satzke, my manager: thank you for being a constant source of support, and everything in between. You advocate for me better than anyone I know, and I truly could not have made this book without you. I am beyond grateful for the safe space you provide me to share my thoughts, deepest dreams, and ambitions with you—and not only that, but also for your support in helping me bring them to life.

To Julia McGreevy, my right hand, thank you for the countless hours you've spent with me rummaging through photo archives and mementos, and being a sounding board for my thoughts and ideas throughout this process.

I want to thank the rest of my team, Lydia Fotiadou, Ted Nguyen, Carson Goodwyn, and Julien Clisson, who have helped me to achieve my biggest dreams and the many milestones documented within these pages and beyond! I couldn't have done it without you all. You are a vital part of my team and life, and I wouldn't be where I am without you all by my side.

Finally, to my mom, dad, sister, and brother—thank you for all your love and support over the years, and for nurturing me while growing up, helping me get to where I am today. You have all shaped me into the person I have become, and a part of all of you is in this book. My creativity is what it is because of all of you—you've shown me how important it is to be adventurous, spontaneous, and to have fun. I love you all and am so lucky to have you in my life. Like my dad always says, "Life is not a rehearsal, so dream big and take risks, you only have one life!"

To my angel muffins, Pancake and Crumpet, I love you beyond belief. Even though you cannot read, I must share how grateful I am to have you in my life every day. I've experienced some of my deepest and hardest emotions next to both of you and always feel the biggest comfort just having you in my presence. You've taught me what love is all about without ever saying a word.